WENNER-GREN CENTER
INTERNATIONAL SYMPOSIUM SERIES

VOLUME 39

EXCITOTOXINS

Excitotoxins

Proceedings of an International Symposium held at
The Wenner-Gren Center, Stockholm, August 26–27,
1982

Edited by

Kjell Fuxe
Department of Histology, Karolinska Institutet, Stockholm, Sweden

Peter Roberts
*Department of Physiology and Pharmacology, University of Southampton,
Bassett Crescent East, Southampton, England*

Robert Schwarcz
*Department of Psychiatry, University of Maryland School of Medicine,
Baltimore, Maryland, USA*

Plenum Press · New York and London

QP
363
. E96x
1984

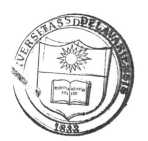

Published 1984 by
PLENUM PRESS, NEW YORK
A Division of Plenum Publishing Corporation
233 Spring Street, New York, N.Y. 10013

ISBN 0–306–41653–0

Printed in Great Britain

CONTENTS

Contents

Contents   vii

LIST OF PARTICIPANTS

Luigi F. Agnati
Depts. of Human Physiology and
Endochronology
University of Modena
Via Campi 287
41100 Modena
Italy

David Bowen
Institute of Neurology
The National Hospital
Queen Square
London WC1N 3BG
England

Joseph Coyle
Dept. of Pharmacology
Johns Hopkins University
School of Medicine
725 North Wolfe Street
Baltimore
Maryland
USA

Ingemar Engberg
Dept. of Physiology
Aarhus University
DK–8000 Aarhus
Denmark

Hans Fibiger
Division of Neurological Sciences
Dept. of Psychiatry
University of British Columbia
Vancouver B. C.
Canada V6T 1W5

Kjell Fuxe
Dept. of Histology
Karolinska Institutet
S–104 01 Stockholm
Sweden

Yehezkel Ben-Ari
Département de Neurophysiologie
Appliquée
Centre National de la Recherche
Scientifique
F–91190 GIF-sur YVETTE
France

J. F. Collins
Dept. of Chemistry
City of London Polytechnic
31 Jewry Street
London EC3N 2EY
England

Michael Cuénod
Institute for Brain Research
University of Zurich
CH–8029 Zurich
Switzerland

Ulf von Euler
Dept. of Physiology
Karolinska Institutet
S–104 01 Stockholm
Sweden

Frode Fonnum
Norwegian Defence Research
Establishment
Division for Toxicology
P. O. Box 25
N–2007 Kjeller
Norway

Christer Köhler
Astra Pharmaceuticals
S-151 85 Södertälje
Sweden

Brian Meldrum
Dept. of Neurology
Institute of Psychiatry
De Crespigny Park
London SE8 AF
England

Victor Nadler
Dept. of Pharmacology
Duke University Medical Center
Durham
North Carolina 27710
USA

William Nicklas
Dept. of Neurology
Rutgers Medical School
University Heights
Piscataway
N. J. 08854
USA

David Ottoson
Dept. of Physiology
Karolinska Institutet
S-104 01 Stockholm
Sweden

Michele Pisa
Dept. of Neurosciences
McMaster University
1200 Main Street West
Hamilton
Ontario
Canada L8N 3Z5

Hugh McLennan
Dept. of Physiology
University of British Columbia
Vancouver B. C.
Canada V6T 1W5

Claude de Montigny
Dept. of Physiology
University of Montreal
CP 6208
Succ A
Quebec H3C 3T8
Canada

Charles Nemeroff
Depts. of Psychiatry a. Medicine
University of North Carolina
School of Medicine
Chapel Hill
North Carolina 27514
USA

John Olney
Depts. of Psychiatry and Neuropathology
Washington University School of Medicine
4940 Audubon Ave.
St Louis
Missouri 63110
USA

Christer Owman
Dept. of Histology
University of Lund
S-223 64 Lund
Sweden

Liane Reif-Lehrer
Eye Research Institute
Harvard Medical School
20 Stainford Street
Boston
Massachusetts 02114
USA

Peter Roberts
Depts. of Physiology and Pharmacology
University of Southampton
Bassett Crescent East
Southampton SO9 3TU
England

Ira Shoulson
Dept. of Neurology
Rochester Medical Center
601 Elmwood Ave.
Rochester
NewYork 14642
USA

Lennart Wetterberg
Dept. of Physiology
St. Görans Hospital
S–112 81 Stockholm
Sweden

Ròbert Schwarcz
Dept. of Psychiatry
University of Maryland School of Medicine
P. O. Box 3235
Maryland 21228
USA

Jeffrey Clifton Watkins
Dept. of Physiology
The Medical School
University Walk
Bristol BS8 1TD
England

William Whetsell
Dept. of Pathology
Division of Neuro-Pathology
858 Madison Ave.
Memphis
Tennessee 38163
USA

PREFACE

This book is the proceedings of an International Wenner-Gren Center Foundation Symposium on "Excitotoxins" held at the Wenner-Gren Center in Stockholm on August 26 and 27, 1982. We are particularly happy that so many of the leading scientists in this field have been able to participate in this symposium. Since the book on "Kainic Acid" appeared in 1978 edited by Dr. McGeers and Dr. John Olney there has been an explosive interest in the research on neuroexcitatory and toxic amino acids. We therefore felt the time was right to bring the leading experts in this field together by organising a symposium on "Excitotoxins". In this way we hoped to have a penetrating and friendly discussion on the mechanisms underlying the neuroexcitatory and neurotoxic properties of excitotoxins and their relationship to the glutamate and aspartate neuron systems of the brain.

In Sweden we have previously had a symposium on "6–hydroxydopamine as a denervation tool in catecholamine research" held in Göteborg, Sweden, July 17–19, 1975 and organized by Drs. Gösta Jonsson, Torbjörn Malmfors and Charlotte Sachs. This symposium illustrated the considerable interest Swedish neuroscientists have had on highly specific neurotoxins, such as 6–hydroxydopamine, 5,6–dihydroxytryptamine and 5,7–dihydroxytryptamine; neurotoxins, which can produce damage to a certain type of transmitter-identified neuron. However, the neurotoxins, kainic acid and ibotenic acid represent another type of an invaluable tool in the experimental studies on brain function.

With the help of these powerful neurotoxins you can analyse the neuronal networks in the brain in a new way, since in a given area it is possible to specifically lesion the postsynaptic components without lesioning the presynaptic component. Thus, axons of passage and afferent inputs into the area, in which the neurotoxins have been injected, are spared, while the nerve cell bodies and the dendrites degenerate. Another important aspect to consider is that the excitotoxins, when injected into the mammallian brain, provide animal models of human pathology, such as Huntington's disease and temporal lobe epilepsy and possibly also presenile and senile dementias. In this way the excitotoxins also give indications as to the possible etiology of neurodegenerative diseases in man. Thus, it seems possible that a deranged metabolism in brain can lead to the formation of endogenous excitotoxins related to glutamate and aspartate.

In order to develop drugs which can prevent nerve cell degeneration in the brain it will become of paramount importance to better understand the molecular mechanism of action of kainic acid and of ibotenic acid and how the binding sites for these excitotoxins relate to the various classes of receptors for excitatory amino acids. Obviously, the development of potent antagonists or modulators of the kainate and ibotenate binding sites could represent a new possible type of treatment of neurodegenerative diseases and of epilepsia. Finally, another aspect to consider is that the research on excitotoxins may lead to new ideas in the field of human surgery. Thus, it may be speculated that some excitotoxins (bound to specific receptor agonists or antagonists) can specifically bind to certain target cells where they may exert their neuroexcitatory and neurotoxic actions.

This year the secretary of the Wenner-Gren Foundation, Professor Y. Zotterman died after working for the Foundation for many years. We will always remember him as a wonderful person and an outstanding sensory physiologist who was in love with the neurosciences. He enthusiastically initiated and supported Wenner-Gren Symposia including the present one. We are very grateful to Mrs. Gun Hultgren at the symposium secretariat for her excellent assistance.

We are very much indepted to the following sponsors, who made this symposium possible:

The Swedish Medical Research Council
American Cyanamid Company, USA
Astra Pharmaceuticals, Sweden
Beecham Pharmaceuticals, England
CIBA-GEIGY Ltd., Switzerland
CIBA-GEIGY AB, Sweden
Committee to Combat Huntington's Disease Inc., USA
Ferring, AB, Sweden
Fidia Research Laboratories, Italy
Hoechst Aktiengesellschaft, West Germany
Hoffman-La Roche Inc., USA
Leo AB, Sweden
AB H. Lundbeck & Co, Sweden
E. Merck, West Germany
Sandoz AB, Sweden
Sandoz Ltd, Switzerland
Shering Corporation, USA
Synthélabo, France

Kjell Fuxe
   Karolinska Institutet, Stockholm, Sweden
Peter Roberts
   University of Southampton, England
Robert Schwarcz
   University of Maryland, USA

EXCITOTOXIC AMINO ACIDS: LOCALIZATION, CHEMISTRY, PHYSIOLOGY, PHARMACOLOGY AND BIOCHEMISTRY

Chairman: U. S. von Euler

IDENTIFICATION OF EXCITATORY AMINO ACID PATHWAYS IN THE MAMMALIAN NERVOUS SYSTEM

F. FONNUM, V. M. FOSSE, and C. N. ALLEN

Norwegian Defence Research Establishment, Division of Toxicology,
P. O. Box 25, N–2007 Kjeller, Norway.

INTRODUCTION

Although the short-lasting excitatory action of glutamate on neurons was demonstrated more than 20 years ago (Curtis and Watkins, 1960), it has proved difficult to confirm its role as a neurotransmitter in the mammalian CNS. Unlike other putative neurotransmitters, glutamate fullfills a multitude of tasks in the brain. It is involved in energy metabolism and fatty acid synthesis, incorporated into proteins and peptides and is even a precursor for the inhibitory neurotransmitter GABA. In addition its action as a neuroexcitant has been regarded as universal and non-specific.

In the last 5 years, however, several new methods (Table 1) have been applied to define and characterize specific glutamate pathways in the mammalian brain (for discussion: Fonnum and Malthe-Sørenssen, 1981). One should not forget, however, that evidence for glutamate as a transmitter at the neuromuscular junction of invertebrates, e.g. the locust, started to accumulate 15 years ago (Usherwood, et al, 1968).

Table 1.

BIOCHEMICAL METHODS FOR IDENTIFICATION OF GLUTAMERGIC TERMINALS:

1. HA UPTAKE STUDIES (AUTORADIOGRAPHY & BIOCHEMISTRY)
2. AMINO ACID LEVEL
3. ANTEROGRADE OR RETROGRADE AXONAL TRANSPORT
4. ELECTRICAL OR K^+ STIMULATED RELEASE
5. IMMUNOHISTOCHEMISTRY
6. GLUTAMATE ENZYMES

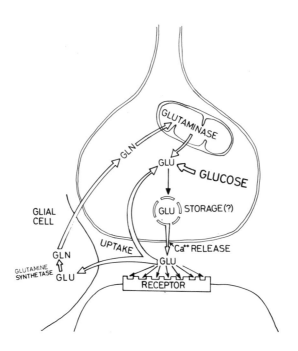

Fig. 1.   Schematic drawing of a glutamergic synapse.

The most commonly used method to identify a glutamergic pathway is
the high affinity uptake of L-glutamate or D-aspartate, measured
either in a sucrose homogenate or autoradiographically in a brain
slice (Table 1).   The uptake system does not distinguish between
D- and L-Asp or L-Glu, whereas D-Glu is a good inhibitor (Balcar
and Johnston, 1972, 1973; Davies and Johnston, 1976).   This allows
us to use the metabolically stable D-Asp as a false transmitter.

THE VISUAL SYSTEM

The pyramidal cells in layer 6 of visual cortex projects ipsilater-
ally to the lateral geniculate body (Gilbert and Kelly, 1975).
Ablation of visual cortex was accompanied by a severe reduction in
high affinity uptake of both D-Asp and L-Glu in the ipsilateral
lateral geniculate body (Table 2).   Similarly there was a substantial reduction in L-Glu levels, but not in that of other amino acids
including Asp, demonstrating that a large glutamate pool was lost
when the corticogeniculate terminals degenerate (Table 2).   Further,
injection of the false transmitter [3]H D-Asp into the lateral geniculate body leads to labelling of cells in layer 6 of visual cortex
(Baughman and Gilbert, 1980).   This is an example of retrograde

transport of the transmitter from the terminal region to the cell bodies (Cuenod, et al, 1981). Also release experiments confirmed that glutamate was the excitatory transmitter of the cortico-geniculate pathway. Depolarization of geniculate slices with K^+ lead to a Ca^{++} dependent release of both endogenous glutamate and exogenously added ^{3}H D-Asp. The release of both compounds were reduced after lesion of the cortical input (Table 2, Fig. 2). Therefore, the corticogeniculate pathway fullfills the 4 most commonly used criteria to demonstrate that Glu is a transmitter.

Table 2

THE EFFECT OF VISUAL CORTEX ABLATION ON TRANSMITTER PARAMETERS IN LATERAL GENICULATE BODY.

PARAMETER			% OF NORMAL
HA $[^3H]^{.}$ D-Asp	uptake		30
HA $[^3H]^{.}$ L-Glu	uptake		40
HA $[^3H]^{.}$ GABA	uptake		95
Glu	level		72
Asp	level		95
Gln	level		108
GABA	level		100
K^+-evoked release of $[^3H]$-D-Asp			51
K^+-evoked release of L-Glu			62

Pyramidal cells in the visual cortex also project to several other areas in brain such as superior colliculus and pulvinar (Carpenter, 1976; Lund, 1978).Visual cortex ablation was accompanied by a 40-50% decrease in uptake of D-Asp and L-Glu, and a significant reduction in the Glu level in superior colliculus (Lund Karlsen and Fonnum, 1978). In this case, however, there was no retrograde transport to visual cortex after injection of D-Asp in superior colliculus (Baughman and Gilbert, 1980). After visual cortex ablation the reduction in uptake in superior colliculus is only 10% of that in lateral geniculate body. The possible glutamergic pathway could therefore be too diffuse to allow detection by this method. This is a discrepancy which warrants further investigation. Recently we have obtained evidence based on reduction in HA-uptake and release of endogenous Glu (Figure 2) that also the cortico-pulvinar pathway uses Glu as its transmitter (Fosse and Fonnum, to be published). Complete transection of the total cortical input to the pontine nuclei reduced the uptake of D-Asp and L-Glu by more than

60%, showing that Glu/Asp are strong candidates also in this case
(Storm-Mathisen, pers. communication. A major part of this input
is probably derived from the visual cortex (Carpenter, 1976).

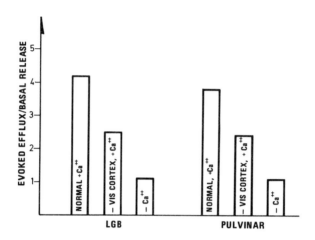

Fig. 2.   The effect of visual cortex ablation on K[+]-evoked release
           of endogenous L-glutamate from LGB and pulvinar.

Although Glu is considered as a major transmitter in the pigeon
optic nerve (Cuenod, et al, 1981), the evidence is not as strong
for the retinotectal projection of mammalian species. Applications
of the techniques outlined in Table 1 have shown that at the most
only 5-15% of the retinal ganglion cells use Glu or Asp as their
transmitter in the rat.

There is good electrophysiological evidence that Glu is the transmitter of the photoreceptor cells and bipolar cells in the retina
(Redburn, 1981). The most compelling (histochemical) evidence has
been obtained by autoradiogrphy after uptake into the goldfish
retina. From these studies Glu may be considered as the transmitter of the rods whereas Glu and Asp may function as the transmitter of the red and green sensitive cones (Marc and Lam, 1982). The
immunohistochemical localization of aspartate transaminase in the
cone cells and terminals of the guinea pig retina has been taken as
evidence for Asp/Glu as a transmitter of these cells (Altschuler,
et al, 1982). As will be discussed below, there is not a close
correlation between the level of aspartate transaminase and the
density of Glu/Asp terminals.

GLUTAMERGIC FIBRES FROM VISUAL CORTEX

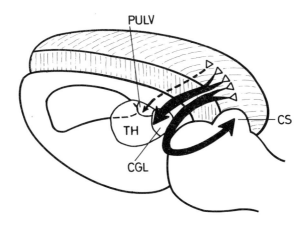

Fig. 3.   Distribution of Glu-fibres from visual cortex, in the rat.
CS, superior colliculus; TH, thalamus; Pulv, pulvinar;
CGL, lateral geniculate body.

BASAL GANGLIA INCLUDING NUCLEUS ACCUMBENS

Neostriatum exhibits a high level of Glu uptake and low glutamate
decarboxylase activity compared to globus pallidus and substantia
nigra.   The ablation of the entire hemicortex was followed by a 70%
reduction in HA Glu-uptake, 20-40% reduction in endogenous Glu, 70%
reduction in the release of ^{3}H Glu formed from ^{3}H Gln and 40% reduction in release of endogenous Glu in neostriatum (Fonnum, et al,
1981; Walaas, 1980; Reubi and Cuenod, 1979; Rowlands and Roberts,
1980).

Removal of cortical afferents to the striatum results in a parallel
decrease in glutamate binding and HA Glu uptake.   The sodium dependent glutamate binding is reduced by 40% after intrastriatal injection of kainic acid, while HA Glu uptake is unaffected (Vincent
and McGeer, 1980).   In addition labelled D-Asp is retrogradely
transported from neostriatum to neocortex (Cuenod, et al, 1981).
Several independent investigations therefore support the concept
that Glu is the transmitter of the corticostriatal pathway (Divac,
et al, 1977; Fonnum, et al, 1981; McGeer and McGeer, 1979; Kim,
et al, 1977).   The glutamergic corticostriatal neurons may modulate
    the release of dopamine from nigrostriatal terminals (Roberts

GLUTAMERGIC FIBRES FROM CORTEX TO CAUDATOPUTAMEN AND NUCLEUS ACCUMBENS

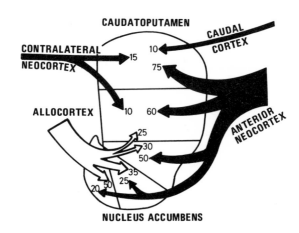

Fig. 4. The origin and distribution of putative Glu fibres in the caudatoputamen and nucleus accumbens, in the rat. Numbers indicate % reduction in HA Glu-uptake after cortical ablation.

and Sharif, 1978), while serotonin may modulate the synthesis of dopamine (de Belleroche and Bradford, 1980). There are also indications that glutamate release from striatal terminals are regulated by dopamine (Roberts and Rowlands, 1980).

Anatomical and neurochemical evidence indicate that <u>nucleus accumbens</u> may be regarded as part of ventral neostriatum (Walaas and Fonnum, 1979; Heimer, 1978; Goldman and Nauta, 1977). Transection of fimbria/fornix was accompanied by a 50% decrease and frontal cortex ablation by an additional 25% decrease in Glu uptake in nucleus accumbens (Walaas and Fonnum, 1979, 1980; Walaas, 1981). In agreement with anatomical studies there is a distinct quantitative difference between the distribution of cortical and fornix fibres to the different parts of neostriatum/nucleus accumbens as summarized in Fig. 4 (Fonnum, <u>et al</u>, 1981; Walaas, 1981).

The existence of cortical input to globus pallidus and substantia nigra has long been disputed. However, ablation of frontal cortex was accompanied by a 20-50% loss of Glu uptake in <u>substantia nigra</u> which indicated the presence of a glutamergic cortico-nigral projection. Retrograde transport of ^{3}H D-Asp from substantia nigra to

frontal cortex (Cuenod, et al, 1982), and electropharmacological
studies support this concept (Collingridge and Davies, 1979), see
Fig. 5.

GLUTAMERGIC FIBRES FROM FRONTAL NEOCORTEX

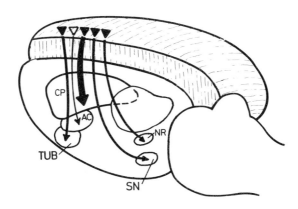

Fig. 5.   The distribution of glutamergic fibres from frontal neocortex, in the rat. CP, caudatoputamen; Ac, nucleus accumbens; Tub, olfactory tubercle; SN, substantia nigra;
nr, nucleus ruber.

It has previously been suggested that phosphate activated glutaminase was associated with GABAergic terminals to a greater extent than
with glutamergic terminals (McGeer and McGeer, 1979). We have recently found that a small but significant part of glutaminase (20%) in
neostriatum was lost after cortical ablation. Similar findings have
been made independently by Nicklas (1979) and Bradford (1982). In
addition, the level of glutaminase was more closely correlated to
HA Glu uptake than to GAD activity (Table 3) in regions of basal
ganglia.

**GLUTAMERGIC FIBRES FROM NEOCORTEX
INCLUDING PARIETAL CORTEX**

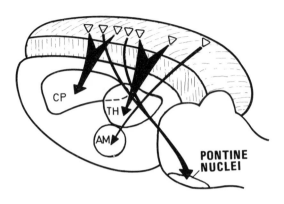

Fig. 6. The distribution of glutamergic fibres from neocortex, including parietal cortex, in the rat. CP, caudatoputamen;
TH, thalamus; Am, nucleus amygdala.

Table 3.

LOCALIZATION OF HA UPTAKE OF GLUTAMATE, GAD AND GLUTAMINASE IN
BASAL GANGLIA

	HA Glu	GAD	GLNase	Sol ASP-T
STRIATUM	6.05	14.4	73	1.3
GLOBUS PALLIDUS	0.86	42.3	32.5	1.2
SUB NIGRA	0.61	55.1	33.1	-

Arbitrary units.

Aspartate transaminase is localized in brain as two isoenzymes, one
localized in cytoplasma and the other in mitochondria (Fonnum,
1968). There was no difference in the level of the cytoplasmic iso-
enzyme (Table 3) between regions in basal ganglia with high and low
Glu uptake activity. In a separate experiment we have compared the
level of the two isoenzymes to HA Glu uptake in 6 regions of brain
without finding any striking correlation. Neither can the distribution of the enzyme explain local exesses in the concentrations of
glutamate and aspartate in areas of the cat spinal cord (Graham and

Aprison, 1969). Kainic acid injection into the striatum (Nicklas, et al, 1979) and interruption of the habenula-interpeduncular tract (Sterri and Fonnum, 1980), which will both affect non-glutamergic fibres, leads to significant loss of aspartate transaminase in the terminal regions. We therefore suggest that the positive immuno-histochemical localization of aspartate transaminase in putative glutamergic terminals in retina (Altschuler, et al, 1982) and bio-chemically in the cochlear nucleus (Wenthold, 1981) may not be gene-rally valid. The patterns of enzyme activity may only reflect the general metabolic compartments in the tissue (Graham and Aprison, 1969).

Table 4

AMINO ACID CONCENTRATIONS IN NORMAL AND DECORTICATED RAT NEOSTRIATUM DURING SEVERE HYPOGLYCEMIA

| | NORMAL | | OPERATED | |
| | NOR | GLY | NOR | GLY |
		μmoles/gm protein		
GLU	97±11	48±10	71±11	75±11
ASP	15± 3	54±10	13± 2	29± 5
GLN	43± 7	6± 2	56±10	41±16
GABA	17± 3	14± 3	16± 3	18± 4
TAU	69±11	88±16	67±13	88±15

NOR = NORMAL
GLY = HYPOGLYCEMIC

The normal and decorticated sides of rat neostriatum represent two similar regions with high and low density of glutamergic terminals. Induction of hypoglycemia by injection of insulin showed a much faster conversion of glutamine to Glu and Asp in neostriatum rich in glutamergic terminals. This is the first indication in the literature that the turnover of transmitter Glu is much faster than that of metabolic Glu (Table 4).

OTHER CORTICAL PROJECTIONS

Thalamus is among the regions in brain with the highest Glu uptake. Autoradiography of thalamic slices after ^{3}H D-Asp uptake showed a variable uptake in the different thalamic nuclei (Fonnum, et al, 1981). Hemidecortication was accompanied by a large reduction (70%) in D-Asp uptake and loss in both glutamate (40%) and aspartate (15%) on the ipsilateral side of the lesion (Fonnum, Storm-Mathisen and Divac, 1981).

Removal of specific cortical regions such as the sensorimotor region in rat and cat was accompanied by a large reduction in both Glu up-take and Glu level in the ventro-lateral thalamic nuclei (Young, et al, 1981; Bromberg, et al,1980).

Cortical ablations, particularly those involving the mediofrontal part, was accompanied by a substantial loss (60%) in D-Asp uptake in the olfactory tubercle. The cortical projections (Figure 5)

therefore probably contain Asp/Glu as a transmitter.

Lesions in the pyriform cortex, which also involved fibres from the enthorinalis cortex, reduced Glu uptake in the amygdala by more than 50%. Amygdala (Figure 6) also received fibres from the medio-frontal cortex in addition to the other regions (Heimer, 1978), but they must be quantitatively less important.

Ablation of the sensorimotor cortex in cat was accompanied by a significant loss in high affinity glutamate uptake in the nucleus ruber (44% loss), and cervical and lumbar region of the spinal cord (37 and 24% loss). In none of these regions were there a fall in the levels of Glu of Asp (Young, et al, 1981). Electrophysiological studies have indicated that Glu is a major candidate as the pyramidal tract neurotransmitter (Stone, 1976 a,b) and endogenous Glu is also released from rostral spinal cord after electrical stimulation (Fagg, et al, 1978).

ALLOCORTICAL PROJECTIONS

The pyramidal cells in CA-3 hippocampus project bilaterally through fimbria-fornix to the lateral but not medial part of septum (Lorente de Nó, 1934; Swanson and Cowan, 1977). When the fimbria-fornix was transected there was a fall in the Glu uptake and Glu level in lateral septum, but not the medial septum. The fall in these parameters, in accordance with the anatomical finding, were more pronounced when the fimbria-fornix was bilaterally transected (Fonnum and Walaas, 1980; Storm-Mathisen and Woxen Opsahl, 1978). By electrical stimulation of the fimbrial-septal slice we were able to demonstrate an evoked release of ^{3}H D-Asp from the septal terminals (Malthe-Sørenssen, Skrede and Fonnum, 1980). The release was Ca^{++} dependent and did not occur with leucine or GABA under the same conditions. The hippocampal-septal projections (Figure 7) is a pathway with strong evidence favouring Glu as its transmitter.

The pyramidal cells, particularly in the subiculum, project through fornix to several brain regions (Swanson and Cowan, 1977; Meibach and Siegel, 1977). Interruption of fornix was accompanied by 40-70% reduction in Glu uptake and between 15-35% reduction in the Glu level in nucleus of the diagonal band, bed nucleus of striae terminalis, nucleus accumbens, mediobasal hypothalamus and corpus mammillare. In some cases there were also a small reduction in the level of aspartate. From these observations it is clear that the hippocampal pyramidal cells, particular those in subiculum, constitutes an important center for glutamergic fibres which distribute widely into the brain.

HIPPOCAMPAL PATHWAYS

The hippocampal formation contains several excitatory systems which are well characterized and organized in distinct laminae (Figure 8). The main input to the region arises from the enthorinal cortex via perforant path which terminate on the dendrites of the granular cells in area dentatae and to the molecular layer of hippocampus. Surgical lesion of this pathway had lead to a reduction in Glu uptake demonstrated both biochemically (Storm-Mathisen, 1977a; Nadler, et al, 1976) and autoradiographically (Storm-Mathisen, 1977a). Further there was a reduction in release of endogenous Glu, but no change in the level of Glu or Asp after the lesion (Nadler, et al, 1976).

GLUTAMERGIC FIBRES FROM HIPPOCAMPUS-SUBICULUM

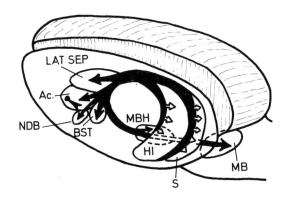

Fig.7. The distribution of glutamergic fibres in the fimbria/fornix, in the rat. LAT.SEP., lateral septum; Ac, nucleus accumbens; NDB, nucleus of the diagonal band; BST, bed nucleus of stria terminalis; MBH, mediobasal hypothalamus; MB, mammillary body; S, subiculum; HI, hippocampus.

DISTRIBUTION OF GLUTAMERGIC FIBRES IN HIPPOCAMPUS

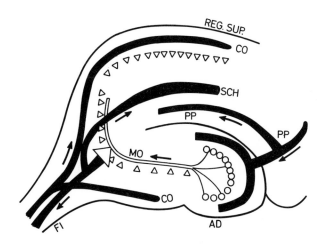

Fig.8.   The distribution of glutamergic fibres in the hippocampus. REG.SUP., regio superior; CO, commissural fibres; SCH, Schaffer collaterals; PP, perforant path; MO, mossy fibres; FI, fimbria; AD, area dentata.

There is, however, some disagreement whether the <u>commissural hippo-campal fibres</u> employ Glu or Asp, or both. Transection of these fibres was accompanied by a preferential reduced release of Asp from hippocampal slices (Nadler, <u>et al</u>, 1976), whereas the same lesion reduced the endogenous level of Glu in stratum oriens in hippocampus (Nitsch, <u>et al</u>, 1979).

The collaterals of the hippocampo-septal fibres, the so-called <u>Schaffer collaterals</u>, terminate mainly in the stratum radiatum of hippocampus CA1. Surgical interruption of the CA3-CA1 projection was accompanied by a reduced autoradiographically and biochemical-ly uptake of D-Asp particularly in stratum radiatum CA1 (Storm-Mathisen, 1977 a,b). Electrical stimulation of the Schaffer col-lateral fibres in the transverse hippocampal slice evoked a Ca^{++} dependent release of ^{3}H D-Asp (Malthe-Sørenssen, <u>et al</u>,1979) and L- ^{3}H Glu (Wieraszko and Lynch, 1979). These findings together with the work on the hippocampo-septal fibres make a strong case for Glu as transmitter in the Schaffer collaterals.

The axons of the granule cells, the so-called <u>mossy fibres</u>, exhibit a small uptake of D-Asp which is retained after treatment of the hippocampus with kainic acid (Heggli, <u>et al</u>, 1981). This may indi-cate that a few of these fibres contain Glu/Asp as their transmit-ter.

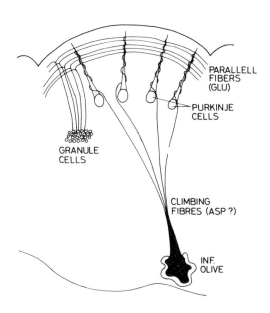

Fig. 9. The distribution of glutamergic/aspartergic fibres in the cerebellum.

CEREBELLUM

Selective destruction of <u>granule cells</u> (Figure 9) in the cerebellum
of hamsters by a viral infection decreases the HA Glu/Asp uptake and
the level of endogenous Glu (Young, <u>et al</u>, 1974). Subsequent investigations including X-ray induced granule cell degeneration
(Sandoval and Cotman, 1978) and studies with mutant mice (McBride,
<u>et al</u>,1976) have substantiated this observation. Furthermore, the
postnatal accumulation of high affinity binding sites for L-glutamate
(Foster and Roberts, 1978) coincides with the major phase of granule
cell formation (de Barry, <u>et al</u>, 1980). The notion that the cerebellar granule cells are glutamergic is therefore well founded.

The <u>climbing fibres</u> (Figure 9) may employ either Asp or Glu as
transmitter. This has been inferred from experiments in which the
inferior olive was destroyed by an injection of 3-acetylpyridine
(Nadi, <u>et al</u>,1977), after which a decrease in endogenous Asp is observed.

AUDITORY NERVE

Destruction of the cochlea in guinea pigs decreases the endogenous
levels of Glu and Asp in the <u>nucleus cochlearis</u>, and the release
of endogenous Glu (Wenthold and Gulley, 1978; Wenthold, 1979). A
decrease in glutaminase and aspartate aminotransferase is observed
after destruction of the auditory nerve (Wenthold, 1980). In addition pharmacological evidence from studies with the cat support
the notion that the auditory nerve contains glutamergic fibres
(Martin and Adams, 1979).

VAGUS NERVE

Primary <u>afferent fibers of arterial baroreceptors</u> terminate in the
medulla oblongata within the middle third of the nucleus tractus
solitarii, NTS (Heymans and Neil, 1958). Injection of L-Glu into
the intermediate NTS elicits hypotension, bradycardia and apnea
simulating baroreceptor reflexes. Ablation of the nodose ganglion
results in selective reduction in high affinity L-Glu uptake in the
NTS (Talman, <u>et al</u>, 1980). Acute hypertension is observed after
local injection of the rigid Glu analogue kainic acid into NTS
(Talman, Perrone and Reis, 1981). Finally, glutamate diethyl ester
(GDEE) antagonises the effect of L-Glu, as well as blocking the
naturally occurring baroreflex (Talman,<u>et al</u>, 1981). All these
observations are consistent with the proposed role of L-Glu as
neurotransmitter of baroreflex afferents.

REFERENCES

Altschuler, R.A., Mosinger, J.L., Harnison, G.G., Parakhal, M.H. , and Wenthold, R.J (1982). Nature, 298, 657-659.
Balcar, V.J., and Johnston, G.A.R (1972). J. Neurochem., 19, 2657-2666.
Balcar, V.J., and Johnston, G.A.R (1973). J. Neurochem., 20, 529-539.
Baughman, R.W., and Gilbert, C.D (1980). Nature, 287, 848-850.
Bradford, H.F (1982) In press.
Bromberg, M.B., Penney, J.B. Jr., Young, A.B., and Stephenson, B (1980). Neurology, 30, 396.
Carpenter, M.B (1976). Human Neuroanatomy. 7th Ed. Williams & Williams Co., Baltimore.
Collingridge, G., and Davies, J (1979). Neuropharmacology, 18, 193-199.
Cuénod, M., Beaudet, A., Canzek, V., Streit, P., and Reubi, J.C (1981). In Glutamate as a Neurotransmitter (Eds. G Di Chiara and G.L. Gessa) pp. 57-78, Raven Press, N.Y.
Cuénod, M., Bagnoli, P., Beaudet, A., Rustioni, A., Wiklund, L., and Streit, P (1982). In Cytochemical Methods in Neuroanatomy (Eds. S.L. Palay and V. Chan-Palay) Alan R.Liss, N.Y. In press.
Curtis, D.R., and Watkins, J.C (1960). J. Neurochem., 6, 117-141.
Davies, L.P., and Johnston, G.A.R (1976). J. Neurochem., 26, 1007-1014.
de Barry, J., Vincendon, G., and Gombos, G (1980). FEBS Lett., 109, 175-179.
De Belleroche and Bradford, H.F (1980). J. Neurochem., 35, 1227-1234.
Divac, I., Fonnum, F., and Storm-Mathisen, J (1977). Nature, 266, 377-378.
Fagg, G.E., Jordan, C.C., and Webster, R.A (1978). Brain Res., 158, 159-170.
Fonnum, F (1968). Biochem. J., 106, 401-412.
Fonnum, F., and Malthe-Sørenssen, D (1981). In Glutamate: Transmitter in the Central Nervous System (P.J. Roberts, J. Storm-Mathisen and G.A.R. Johnston, Eds.), pp. 205-222, J. Wiley & Sons, New York.
Fonnum, F., and Walaas, I (1978). J. Neurochem., 31, 1173-1181.
Fonnum, F., Storm-Mathisen, J., and Divac, I (1981). Neuroscience, 6, 863-873.
Fonnum, F., Søreide, A., Kvale, I., Walker, J., and Walaas, I (1981). In Glutamate as a Neurotransmitter. (Eds. G. Di Chiara and G.L. Gessa) Raven Press, N.Y., pp. 29-41.
Foster, A.C., and Roberts, P.J (1978). J. Neurochem., 31,1467-1477.
Gilbert, C.D, and Kelly, J.P (1975). J. Comp. Neurol., 163,81-105.
Goldman, P.S., and Nauta, H.J.H (1977). J. Comp. Neurol., 171,369-385.
Graham, L.T. Jr., and Aprison, M.H (1969). J. Neurochem., 16, 559-566.
Heggli, D., Aamodt, A., and Malthe-Sørenssen, D (1981). Brain Res., 230, 253-262.
Heimer, L (1978). In Limbic Mechanisms. (Eds. K.E. Livingston and O. Hornykiewicz), Plenum Press, N.Y., pp. 95-187.
Heimer, L., and Wilson, R.D (1975). In Perspectives in Neurobiology. (Ed. M.Santini), pp. 177-193, Raven Press, N.Y.
Heymans, C., and Neil, E (1958). Reflexogenic Area of the Cardiovascular System. Churchill, London.

Kim, J.S., Hassler, R., Haug, P., and Paik, K.S (1977). Brain Res., 132, 370-374.
Lorente de Nó, R (1934). J. Psychol. Neurol.(Leipzig) 46,113-177.
Lund, R.D (1978). Development and Plasticity of the Brain. An Introduction. Oxford University Press, N.Y.
Lund-Karlsen, R., and Fonnum, F (1978). Brain Res., 151, 457-467.
McBride, W.J., Aprison, M.H., and Kusano, K (1976). J. Neurochem., 26, 867-870.
McGeer, E.G., and McGeer, P.L (1979). J. Neurochem., 32, 1071-1075.
Malthe-Sørenssen, D., Skrede, K.K., and Fonnum, F (1979). Neuroscience, 4, 1255-1263.
Malthe-Sørenssen, D., Skrede, K.K., and Fonnum, F (1980). Neuroscience, 5, 127-133.
Marc, R.E., and Lam, D.M.L (1981). Proc. Natl. Acad. Sci. USA, 78, 7185-7189.
Martin, M.R., and Adams, J.C (1979). Neuroscience, 4, 1097-1105.
Meibach, R.C., and Siegel, A (1977). Brain Res., 124, 197-224.
Nadi, N.S., Kanter, D., McBride, W.J., and Aprison, M.H (1977). J. Neurochem., 28, 661-662.
Nadler, J.V., Vaca, K.W., White, W.F., Lynch, G.S., and Cotman, C.W (1976). Nature, 260, 538-540.
Nicklas, W.J., Nunez, R., Berl, S., and Duvoisin, R (1979). J. Neurochem., 33, 839-844.
Nitsch, C., Kim, J-K., and Shimada, Y (1979). In Progr. in Brain Res., 51, 193-201. Elsevier/North-Holland.
Redburn, D (1981). In Glutamate as a neurotransmitter (G. Di Chiara and G.L. Gessa, Eds.). Raven Press, New York, pp. 79-89.
Reubi, J.C., and Cuénod, M (1979). Brain Res., 176, 185-188.
Roberts, P.J., and Sharif, N.A (1978). Brain Res., 157, 391-395.
Roberts, P.J., and Rowlands, G.J (1980). Proc. of the Br. Physiol. Soc., 137P-138P.
Rowlands, G.J., and Roberts, P.J (1980). Exptl. Brain Res., 39, 239-240.
Sandoval, M.E., and Cotman, C.W (1978). Neuroscience, 3, 199-206.
Sterri, S., and Fonnum, F (1980). J. Neurochem, 35, 249-254.
Stone, T.W (1976a). Expermentia, 32, 581-583.
Stone, T.W (1976b). J. Physiol., (London) 257, 187-198.
Storm-Mathisen, J (1977a). Brain Res., 120, 379-386.
Storm-Mathisen, J (1977b). Progr. in Neurobiology, Vol. 8,119-181.
Storm-Mathisen, J., and Woxen Opsahl, M (1978). Neurosci. Lett., 9, 65-70.
Swanson, L.W., and Cowan, W.S.M (1977). J. Comp. Neurol., 172, 49-84.
Talman, W.T., Perrone, M.H., and Reis, D.J (1980). Science, 209, 813-815.
Talman, W.T., Perrone, M.H., and Reis, D.J (1981). Circulat. Res., 48, 292-298.
Talman, W.T., Perrone, M.H., Scher, P., Kwo, S., and Reis, D.J (1981). Brain Res., 217, 186-191.
Usherwood, P.N.R., Machele, P., and Leaf, G (1968). Nature, 219, 1169-1172.
Vincent, S.R., and McGeer, E.G (1980). Brain Res., 184, 99-108.
Walaas, I (1980). In États Déficitaires Cérébraux Liés a l'Âge, Symposium Bel-Air VI. (Ed. R. Tissot). Georg. Libraire de l'université, Geneve, pp. 47-82.
Walaas, I (1981). Neuroscience, 6, 399-405.
Walaas, I., and Fonnum, F (1979). Brain Res., 177, 325-336.
Walaas, I., and Fonnum, F (1980). Neuroscience, 5, 1691-1698.

Wenthold, R.J (1979). Brain Res., 162, 338-343.
Wenthold, R.J (1980). Brain Res., 190, 293-297.
Wenthold, R.J (1981). In Glutamate as a Neurotransmitter (Eds:
  G. Di Chiara and G.L. Gessa) Raven Press, N.Y., pp. 69-78.
Wenthold, R.J., and Gulley, R.L (1978). Brain Res., 158, 295-302.
Wieraszko, A., and Lynch, G (1979). Brain Res., 160, 372-376.
Wilkin, G.P., Garthwaite, J., and Balázs, R (1982). Brain Res.,
  244, 69-80.
Young, A.B., Oster-Granite, M.L., Herndon, R.M., and Snyder, S. H
  (1974). Brain Res., 73, 1-13.
Young, A.B., Bromberg, M.B., and Penney, J.B. Jr (1981).
  J. Neurosci., 1, 241-249.

ELECTROPHYSIOLOGICAL ACTIONS OF KAINATE AND OTHER EXCITATORY AMINO ACIDS, AND THE STRUCTURE OF THEIR RECEPTORS

H. McLENNAN, G. L. COLLINGRIDGE and S. J. KEHL

Department of Physiology, University of British Columbia, Vancouver, B. C., Canada V6T 1W5

RECEPTORS FOR THE EXCITATORY AMINO ACIDS

It is more than 20 years since Curtis and his colleagues demonstrated that the naturally occurring acidic amino acids L-glutamate and L-aspartate depolarize and excite neurones of the mammalian spinal cord (Curtis, et al., 1959; 1960), and that similar excitatory effects could be elicited by a variety of other compounds chemically related to the natural substances (Curtis and Watkins, 1960; 1963). Curtis and Watkins (1960) set forth the criteria which seemed to be optimal for excitatory effect - "The optimum distance between the amino group and one of the acidic groups of the excitatory amino acids is 2 or 3 carbon atoms. The other acidic group is optimally situated α with respect to the amino group" - and since all active compounds possessed these three polar groups, one cationic and two anionic, it was concluded that reaction with a single population of three-point attachment sites took place. It should however be noted that more recent evidence has been obtained indicating that the reaction of more than one molecule of an amino acid is required for functional activation to occur (McLennan and Wheal, 1976a). It was further noted that the "receptor" was not stereoselective, although for many of the more potent substances the "non-natural" D- configuration appeared to confer a greater excitatory activity.

Since those days the situation has, predictably, become much more complex. It is now well-known that, for example, there are high-affinity uptake processes which accept some of the excitatory amino acids including the naturally-occurring ones (Logan and Snyder, 1972), but not the more potent non-endogenous compounds (Balcar and Johnston, 1972). Processes of this type can be expected to have a profound effect upon the apparent potency of any substance exogenously administered to the vicinity of a neurone in vitro and as well upon the time course of its action (Cox et al., 1977). It is also known that the lengths of time for which different agonists can activate receptors to permit ionic fluxes across neuronal membranes vary ("channel open times") (Gration et al., 1981), and this factor too will contribute to apparent potencies. Finally, as will be considered below in greater detail, it is now clear that several classes of recognition site exist for the amino acids, more than one of which may accept a given agonist, and all of these receptor types apparently coexist upon many or all central neurones.

There is now a reasonable concurrence of evidence derived mainly from studies in the spinal cord that at least three different amino acid receptors can be identified. Engberg and his colleagues have measured the electrophysiological sequelae of the extracellular administration of the compounds to motoneurones, and on the basis of the patterns of depolarization and altered conductances produced have concluded that the substances which they tested could be allocated to one of three groups (Engberg, et al., 1979; Lambert, et al., 1981). In the first group were placed L-glutamate and L-aspartate, L-homocysteate and quisqualate; in the second ibotenate, D-homocysteate and N-methyl-D-aspartate (NMDA); and in the third, kainate only. Similar results have been obtained by MacDonald and Wojtowicz (1982) on cultured spinal neurones.

These data agree very well with the results of pharmacological studies of the actions of antagonists of the excitatory effects of the amino acids. The first antagonist to be described was L-glutamate diethylester (GDEE), which Haldeman, et al., (1972) and Haldeman and McLennan (1972) showed to have a selective action against glutamate-induced excitations but little against those produced by aspartate or DL-homocysteate. Although subsequent work indicated that GDEE could have some effect against aspartate also (McLennan and Wheal, 1976b), it is now accepted that there are a number of excitants whose actions are almost or entirely unaffected by it and others such as quisqualate whose actions are selectively blocked (McLennan and Lodge, 1979; McLennan and Liu, 1982).

In 1977 the first of a number of other compounds with a quite different spectrum of antagonistic action was described (Hall, et al., 1977; Biscoe, et al., 1977). α-Aminoadipate had little effect against glutamate-induced excitations and more powerfully reduced those produced by aspartate, but its most striking effects were against NMDA whose actions had proven to be entirely untouched by GDEE (Biscoe, et al., 1978; McLennan and Hall, 1978; Lodge, et al., 1978). The antagonistic activity resided with the D(-) isomer (DαAA), and subsequent work has shown a similar behaviour for other longer chain analogues of glutamate (Davies and Watkins, 1979).

The actions of various amino acid excitants can indeed be classified by their sensitivity to blockade by GDEE and DαAA, and if the agonists are listed in order of susceptibility the two ranks are virtual converses one of the other; that is, those substances whose effects are most reduced by GDEE are almost unaffected by DαAA and vice versa (Hicks, et al., 1978; McLennan and Lodge, 1979; McLennan, 1981). Only one substance, kainate, gives rise to excitations which are relatively resistant to both antagonists, and on this basis it has been concluded once more that three distinct receptor sites exist (McLennan, 1981; Watkins, et al., 1981). One is activated by L-glutamate and quisqualate and blocked by GDEE (the "quisqualate receptor"), a second is stimulated by NMDA, ibotenate and a number of other compounds and antagonized by DαAA (the "NMDA receptor") while the third is activated by kainate but no specific antagonist to it has yet been described. Certain excitants, among them L-aspartate, presumably can interact to some degree with both of the first two classes of receptor albeit with different affinities, since their actions are affected both by GDEE and DαAA although not necessarily to the same degree.

Other and more potent compounds have been developed as NMDA receptor antagonists, of which the most powerful is the Ω-phosphonate analogue of aminoadipate, 2-amino-5-phosphonovalerate (Davies, et al., 1981a). This compound has an identical pattern of effect against various agonists as does DαAA (McLennan and Liu, 1982) and apparently reacts little if at all with quisqualate or kainate receptors. Once more the blocking effect is attributable entirely to the D(-) isomer (Stone, et al., 1981; Davies and Watkins, 1982; McLennan, 1982a).

No selective antagonist is known, other than GDEE, for quisqualate receptors; and although there are compounds which are able to block kainate-induced excitations (Davies, et al., 1981b; Davies and Watkins, 1981), these compounds are also NMDA antagonists (McLennan and Liu, 1982) and one of them, 2,3-piperidine dicarboxy-late, can show quite marked excitatory effects of its own which limits its usefulness as a pharmacological tool (Collingridge, et al., 1982a).

Certain additional pieces of information are known respecting the chemical and physical nature of these various receptors. Evidence derived from the use of both agonists and antagonists which are molecularly constrained suggests that the NMDA receptor accepts its ligands in a relatively extended conformation, while the quisqualate receptor has a greater affinity for "folded" molecules (McLennan, et al., 1982). Kainate has certain structural similarities to an extended form of glutamate (Johnston, et al., 1974) but as noted above does not react with the NMDA receptor. The fact that hydrogenation of the isopropylene side chain of the kainate molecule abolishes its excitatory potency (Johnston, et al., 1974) indicates that this portion of the molecule must in some way be involved in addition to the usual three charged groups in order for receptor activation to occur, which emphasizes once again the uniqueness of the kainate receptor.

EFFECTS OF KAINIC ACID ON NEURONAL ELECTRICAL ACTIVITY

Shinozaki and Konishi (1970) were the first to demonstrate the powerful excitatory action of kainate administered electrophoretically to single cortical neurones, an effect which has been confirmed by many other investigators and for cells in many other parts of the nervous system. Unlike other amino acid excitants it has a rather slow time course of action when tested in electrophoretic experiments (see, for example, Fig. 3 in Hutchinson, et al., 1978), in part probably due to the lack of an uptake mechanism which would contribute to the termination of its effect (Cox, et al., 1977; Johnston, et al., 1979). There is evidence that kainate is bound to some regions in the hippocampus where certain synapses believed to be amino acid-mediated are known to terminate (Foster, et al., 1981), although other kainate receptors are certainly extrasynaptic (Davies, et al., 1979). Finally systemic (Olney, et al., 1974) or intracerebral (Schwarcz and Coyle, 1977) inject-ion of kainate in low doses is powerfully cytotoxic, with an action preferentially against dendrites and neuronal somata, although with prolonged exposures and/or higher doses axons and terminals may be affected as well (Nadler, et al., 1978; Wuerthele, et al., 1978; Tissari and Onali, 1982). These so-called local actions of kainate are observable also after injections of other of the excitatory amino acids with a degree of effectiveness roughly in line with their activities as neuronal excitants (Schwarcz, et al., 1978; Nadler, et al., 1982); however there is no indication of a specificity for any one of the classes of excitatory receptor in this connection, that is to say NMDA agonists (NMDA, ibotenate) and quisqualate agonists (quisqualate, glutamate) as well as kainate itself can elicit effects. This prompted Evans (1981) to write "It is possible therefore that the excitotoxic actions may be produced by any treatment that results in prolonged increase of neuronal membrane conductance". The report by Sloviter and Damiano (1981a) that long continued electrical stimulation can reproduce some of the toxic effects of kainate in the hippocampus might be interpreted as supporting this point of view.

There are however some special features to the actions of kainate when contrasted with other excitatory amino acids. Its administration produces not only local cytotoxicity but also distant brain damage, particularly to limbic structures. This action appears to be related to a kainate-induced status epilepticus, for Ben-Ari, et al., (1980a) have correlated the extent of distant damage with the development and spread of convulsive activity and have further shown that treat-ment with diazepam, which reduces the spread of convulsions, also attenuates the cytotoxic consequences (Ben-Ari, et al., 1979; 1980b). The convulsant (Hommes and Obbens, 1973) and distant toxic actions of kainate are duplicated by folate (pteroyl-L-glutamate) (Olney, et al., 1981a) although this substance is without any "local" toxic action. Folate has been reported as having a weak excitatory action on cortical cells (Davies and Watkins, 1973) but is without such effect in the spinal cord or trigeminal nucleus (McLennan, 1982b; Evans, et al., 1982).

Recently there has been much study of the actions of kainate upon cells in the hippocampus. The pyramidal cells of this structure, and particularly those of the CA3 region, are exquisitely sensitive both to the cytotoxic (Nadler, et al., 1980) and excitatory (de Montigny and Tardif, 1981; Robinson and Deadwyler, 1981) effects of kainate. This region of the brain is of much interest also in that it demonstrates the electrophysiological phenomenon known as long-term potentiation, which was first described by Bliss and Lømo (1973) and Bliss and Gardner-Medwin (1973) in the area dentata but which is now recognized as occurring throughout the hippocampus. Long-term potentiation which is produced by brief high frequency activation of an afferent pathway (Andersen, et al., 1980), is manifested as a marked enhancement in the number of cells synchronously firing and contributing to a "population spike" (Andersen, et al., 1971). It is associated with an increased EPSP (Andersen, et al., 1980); at dentate granule cells with an enhanced release of glutamate (Dolphin, et al., 1982) which is believed to be the transmitter of the afferent fibres in the perforant path (Hicks and McLennan, 1979; Wheal and Miller, 1980); and with enhanced D-aspartate release from the CA1 region (Skrede and Malthe-Sørenssen, 1981).

Brief electrophoretic administration of kainate to the stratum pyramidale in the CA1 region of a hippocampal slice causes a short period of over-depolarization of the cells during which the population spike evoked by stimulation of the Schaffer collateral pathway (stratum radiatum) is blocked, but this is succeeded by a period during which the population spike is increased for a considerable time (Collingridge and McLennan, 1981). Smaller electrophoretic doses give potentiations which are neither as great nor last as long but are usually not preceded by the initial depression seen with higher amounts. Identical effects are observed if the site of application of kainate is to the dendritic regions of the cells, which suggests that interaction at synaptic receptors is involved. A similar sequence of events can be seen with brief (ca. 1 min.) superfusions of the slice with kainate save that with a concentration of 10^{-4}M (i.e. with the administration in toto of 0.1 µmole) there is a brief enhancement of the response which is succeeded by depression and only thereafter by a second prolonged phase of potentiation. With concentrations of 10^{-5}M kainate or less, the phase of depression does not appear (Fig. 1); and when other excitatory amino acids were tested, none could reproduce the whole spectrum of kainate effect. Glutamate and aspartate showed only the brief initial enhancement (as also does acetylcholine (Collingridge and McLennan, 1981)),while NMDA and ibotenate (up to 10^{-4}M) intensely depolarized the cells but following which there was no potentiation. Effects obtained with quisqualate normally resembled those with glutamate, but occasionally weak and short-lived kainate-like actions were observed. Similar sequences of events have been found at CA3 pyramidal cells with mossy fibre stimulation and in the dentate gyrus with stimulation of the medial or lateral (Fig. 2) perforant path.

The prolonged potentiating action of kainate appears to be largely a postsynaptic phenomenon for several reasons. There is ordinarily no alteration in the amplitude of the fibre volley which can be recorded in stratum radiatum; however the extracellular field EPSP is characteristically reduced (Fig. 1) presumably due to the induced depolarization in the dendrites of the cells. Preliminary results indicate that the potentiating action of kainate is unchanged in the presence of low calcium and high magnesium ion concentrations in the perfusing fluid. The release of labelled D-aspartate evoked by stimulation of afferent inputs to pyramidal cells (Malthe-Sørenssen, et al., 1979) is presumably from activated presynaptic terminals; and neither spontaneous release nor that evoked by high potassium is increased by kainate (C. Tong, unpublished observations in the authors' laboratory). Finally, that the effect is not simply due to a generalized increase in neuronal excitability is indicated by the lack of effect of kainate upon antidromic responses elicited by stimulation of the alveus (Fig. 1). Kainate's effects thus are probably confined to the postsynaptic target cells of the afferent inputs and involve mechanisms at synaptic sites where the binding of kainate has been shown to occur (Foster, et al., 1981).

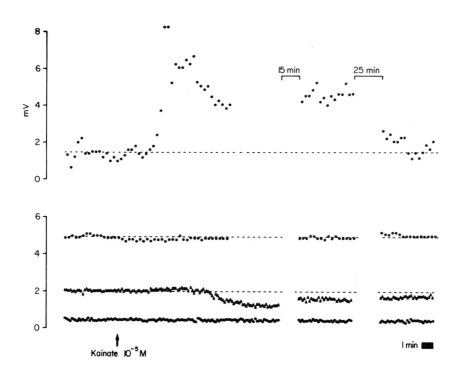

Fig. 1.   The action of kainate (10^{-5}M) superfused for 1 min. over a
           hippocampal slice. Recordings were made in the CA1 region, and
           the graphs, from above downwards, plot the peak amplitudes of
           the population spike and the antidromic spike evoked by stimula-
           tion of the alveus (both recorded from stratum pyramidale), the
           extracellular EPSP and presynaptic fibre volley (from stratum
           radiatum). Kainate has caused potentiation of the population
           spike and a later depression of the EPSP but no change in the
           antidromic or fibre volley responses.

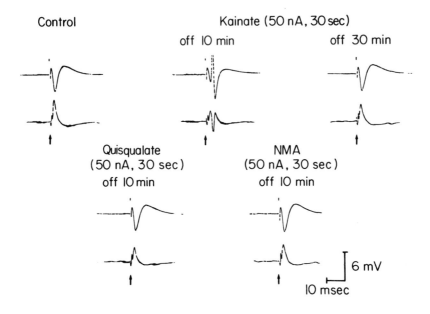

Fig. 2.   The effects of amino acids administered electrophoretically on
the excitation of dentate granule cells by stimulation of the
lateral perforant path. The upper record of each pair was from
the cell body region and the lower from the dendritic zone. Ten
min. after the end of administration kainate had potentiated the
population spike and depressed the EPSP: quisqualate and N-
methyl-aspartate were without effect. Negativity upwards.

There is however also the possibility that another process is involved. Douglas,
et al., (1982) have demonstrated, again at dentate granule cells with stimulation
of the perforant path, that long-term potentiation was prevented by stimulation
of the contralateral hippocampus which activated inhibitory interneurones
impinging upon the granule cells. The effect was postsynaptic and bicuculline-
sensitive. The possibility that long-term potentiation may be due, at least in
part, to reduced tonic inhibition therefore merits consideration.

Fig. 3 shows that in the CA1 region a stimulus delivered to the alveus preceding
the stratum radiatum volley by 30 msec caused a substantial inhibition of the
population spike. However administration of kainate augmented the population
spike to the same absolute amplitude whether or not the inhibitory input was

stimulated, i.e. at the peak of the potentiation the inhibition was abolished, and recovery was slow. This is the converse of the effect reported by Douglas, et al., (1982), and suggests the possibility that kainate-induced potentiations and those evoked by stimulation have a common origin, i.e. to a diminution in the degree of tonic inhibitory influence impinging upon the pyramidal cells, and Sloviter and Damiano (1981b) have made similar observations at dentate granule cells.

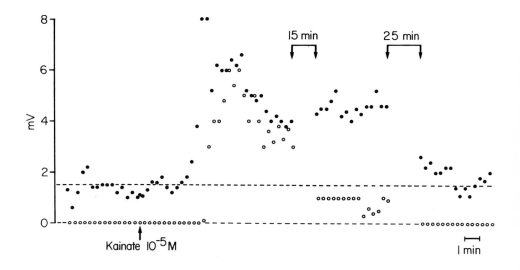

Fig. 3.   The action of kainate (10^{-5}M, 1 min.) upon the amplitude of the CA1 population spike in the absence (filled dots) and presence (open circles) of a preceding inhibitory stimulus. The uninhibited control response is identical to that shown in Fig. 1.

However in the authors' experience (unpublished observations) a loss of inhibition has not been marked during electrically-induced long-term potentiation.

Although none of the other excitatory amino acids can mimic these effects of kainate as noted above, folic acid perfused over a slice can do so (Fig. 4), although ca. 100-fold higher concentrations are needed. Most of the electro-physiological features of kainate administration are reproduced by folate and on the few occasions when it was tested apparently also by its metabolite N^5-methyl-5,6,7,8-tetrahydrofolate (MTHF), and it may be recalled that folate and MTHF elicit distant brain damage as does kainate but are without the latter's excitatory actions or local toxic effects. MTHF reacts with kainate binding sites (Ruck, et al., 1981); however Roberts, et al., (1981) have claimed that its toxic reaction is not due to activation of kainate receptors, and Auker, et al., (1982) have claimed that the folates do not mimic the action of kainate in the olfactory cortex. In this last case however the concentrations of the folates used in the experiments illustrated (10^{-4}M) may have been too low since we have found this to be a threshold dose in hippocampus and the responses which Auker, et al., show for kainate are themselves quite small. The situation is thus complex; however so far as the electrophysiological phenomena in hippocampus are concerned only folate and MTHF among the amino acids have been found able to mimic the effects of kainate in CA1 (Collingridge, et al., 1982b).

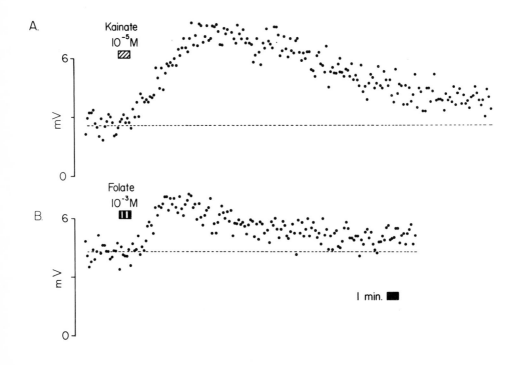

Fig. 4.   A comparison in the same slice of the effects of brief super-fusions of (A) 10^{-5}M kainate and (B) 10^{-3}M folate, upon the amplitude of CA1 population spikes.

EPILEPTIFORM ACTIVITY EVOKED BY KAINATE AND FOLATE IN THE CA3
REGION OF THE HIPPOCAMPUS

In addition to its local toxic effect on the hippocampus which is most notable
in the CA3 region (Olney, et al., 1979; Nadler, et al., 1981; and many others),
the local or systemic injection of kainate has a marked epileptogenic effect
again most noticeable in CA3 (Ben-Ari, 1981). It was noted earlier that
the administration of kainate mimics the effect of a tetanus in causing long-term
potentiation in hippocampal pathways, and it can also elicit epileptiform bursting activity in the CA3 region of the slice (Lothman, et al., 1981).

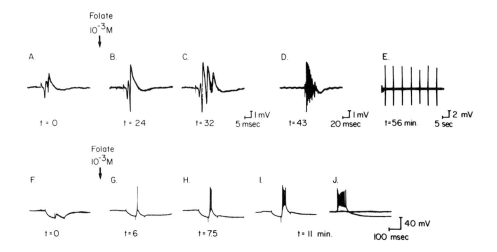

Fig. 5.   The effects of 10 min. superfusions of folate, beginning at t=0,
          upon the amplitude and number of population spikes recorded in
          pyramidal cells. The traces were taken at the times indicated
          under each record. A-E: extracellular recording in CA3.
          Spontaneous bursts (E) were observed some 40 min. after folate
          perfusion was started. F-J: intracellular records from a CA3
          neurone, illustrating the gradually increasing amplitude of the
          mossy fibre-evoked depolarization produced by folate, associated
          with the appearance of a single (G) and later multiple (H,I)
          action potentials. The response is superimposed on an hyper-
          polarizing pulse in F-I. J: a spontaneous burst superimposed
          on a baseline to show the prolonged hyperpolarization which
          follows the burst. Negativity downwards.

When either kainate (10^{-7}M) or folate (5.10^{-4}-10^{-3}M) are perfused over a slice
there is an initial potentiation of the extracellularly recorded population spike
(Fig. 5B), following which a second and eventually multiple population spikes
develop (Fig. 5C,D). With intracellular recording during folate administration
it can be observed that this progression is due to the increasing firing of
bursts of action potentials by individual cells associated with a larger underlying depolarization (Fig. 5F-I). The bursts appear to be terminated by the
sudden development of a profound and lengthy hyperpolarization (Fig. 5J). At
this stage also the bursts will occur "spontaneously" (Fig. 5E), i.e. without
afferent stimulation, but in all other respects the spontaneous bursts greatly
resemble those which follow activation of the afferent input. The interval

between spontaneous bursts is <u>ca</u>. 4-5 sec., and is presumably determined by the
duration of the hyperpolarizing phases. Return to a resting condition requires
one to several hours.

Once more it appears that an inhibitory mechanism, or lack of it, may be involved
in the genesis of these epileptiform manifestations. Figure 6A illustrates the
inhibition of the second response in CA3 when paired pulses were delivered, in
this case to the fimbria, with an interval of 25 msec.

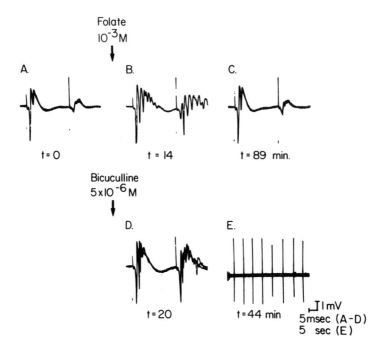

Fig. 6.   The loss of paired pulse inhibition induced by 10 min. perfusions
           with folate or bicuculline methochloride. CA3: fimbrial stimu-
           lation evoked an antidromic spike followed by a small orthodromic
           response. A: control; B: partial loss of inhibition associated
           with a larger initial and appearance of multiple population
           spikes; C: recovery 60 min. after cessation of folate perfusion.
           D: 20 min. after bicuculline perfusion was started; E: spon-
           taneous bursting after 44 min. of bicuculline perfusion. A-C, E:
           single sweeps, D: 3 superimposed traces. Negativity downwards.

Fourteen minutes after starting perfusion with folate (10^{-3}M) the inhibition was
much reduced and potentiation of the response with an evoked bursting pattern was
evident (Fig. 6B). Spontaneous bursts were also occurring. One hour after
cessation of the folate perfusion recovery had occurred (Fig. 6C); however a
seemingly identical sequence of changes to give the epileptiform pattern associated with loss of paired pulse inhibition and the development of spontaneous bursting was elicited by perfusion with the GABA antagonist bicuculline methochloride
(Fig. 6D,E), and hippocampal inhibitions are known to be GABA mediated (Curtis,
et al., 1970; Skrede and Malthe-Sørenssen, 1981b). Therefore a loss of inhibition
induced by folate (and kainate) may be postulated to contribute to the potentiation of responses in CA3 and to the development of the quasi-status epilepticus.

A similar process has been implicated in the production of penicillin-induced epilepsy (Dingledine and Gjerstad, 1979), and in cerebral cortex a morphologically demonstrable loss of inhibitory synapses is associated with the development of epileptic activity (Ribak and Reiffenstein, 1982). Any mechanism which causes reduction of the inhibitory input to CA3 pyramidal cells apparently is sufficient for these effects to occur; thus Krnjević, et al., (1981) and Haas (1982) have described a cholinergically-mediated disinhibition in hippocampal slices and we have found that brief perfusion of slices with 5×10^{-6}M carbachol can also induce both multiple evoked population spikes and spontaneous bursts, from which recovery is again slow.

DISCUSSION

The actions of kainic acid in the nervous system are clearly multiple and complex. It is powerful neuronal excitant which structurally resembles a somewhat extended form of glutamate but does not react with the "extended" NMDA receptor since its effects are not blocked by the potent and specific NMDA antagonists. Similarly its excitatory actions are resistant to GDEE, an antagonist of the quisqualate/glutamate receptors. On these grounds the existence of a special kainate receptor has been suggested, a proposition strengthened by the fact that saturation of the side chain in the kainate molecule abolishes its excitatory activity thus indicating the involvement of the isopropylene function in the kainate receptor. Only the chemically related domoate (Biscoe, et al., 1976) and possibly the neurolathyrogen β-N-oxalyl-L-α,β-diaminopropionate (Pearson and Nunn, 1981) have been suggested as reacting with the excitatory kainate receptor, and no special endogenous agonist for it has been recognized. Binding studies have been interpreted to indicate that kainate receptors may indeed be a subset of glutamate receptors, and in support of this view Riveros and Orrego (1982) could identify glutamate as the only ligand present in extracts of synaptosomes which reacted with kainate binding sites.

Kainate shares with many other excitatory amino acids the ability to cause local cellular damage when injected into brain tissue. That there is some parallelism between apparent excitatory potency and ability to induce neuronal destruction (Nadler, et al., 1981; but see Seil, et al., 1978) prompted the coining of the term " excitotoxins" for this group of compounds (Olney, 1978). Nevertheless differences between kainate and other members of the group are evident. It now is apparent that, as originally reported by Biziere and Coyle (1978) and McGeer, et al., (1978) for the neostriatum, destruction of a major excitatory input protects the cells against the effects of a subsequent kainate injection, and similar observations have been made in other areas including the dentate gyrus and at the pyramidal cells of the hippocampus (Köhler, et al., 1978; Nadler and Cuthbertson, 1980). The protective effect of deafferentation is not confined to inputs which are likely to be amino acid-mediated but is peculiarly specific for the toxic actions of kainate since other amino acid excitants continue to be destructive (Schwarcz and Köhler, 1980). Finally, deafferentation does not change the sensitivity of neurones to excitation by kainate (McLennan, 1980), so that whereas the term "excitotoxin" may be applicable to the other excitatory amino acids, kainate seems unique in this respect also and owes even its local destructive properties to a process different from that applying to the others, i.e. in all probability to a special receptor which may not be the same as that giving rise to excitation.

The ability of kainate to evoke distant brain damage and to produce epileptiform activity in certain limbic structures, most notably the hippocampus, seems dependent on yet another quite different mechanism and one which also is at least not directly related to excitation. The distant toxic actions and the epileptogenic effects of kainate are mimicked by folate and some of its metabolites (Olney, et al., 1981a,b), and Collingridge, et al., (1982b) have suggested that these actions could be related to the property exhibited by both kainate and folate to induce long-term changes in the synaptic responsiveness of hippocampal cells. Although kainate is a powerful excitatory agent in hippocampus and elsewhere, the doses used to elicit potentiation caused only a small and sometimes undetectable depolarization and increase in conductance recorded in the soma of pyramidal cells. Similarly small changes were observed with folate, and thus alterations in the passive properties of somal membranes do not seem to be directly involved with the enhancement of synaptically evoked responses; however that depolarization occurring in the dendrites contributes to the effect must be considered. In other situations also neither folate itself nor the metabolites which have been tested are appreciably excitatory, indeed one of the latter, MTHF, is a weak antagonist of NMDA and kainate excitations (McLennan, 1982b) and of glutamate uptake (Roberts, et al., 1981). The evidence suggests that the actions of kainate and folate to potentiate effects in the hippocampus are in part at least due to disinhibition of a GABA-mediated process since bicuculline induces a similar set of electrophysiological events (Fig. 6).

Thus at least three distinct actions of kainate can be described in the nervous system, one giving rise to its excitatory effects on neurones, a second producing local cytotoxic actions which is different from the first since toxicity disappears with deafferentation while excitation is unaltered, and a third responsible for the epileptogenic and probably secondarily the distant damaging effects in the brain. This third effect seems likely also to be the one implicated in the long-term pharmacological actions of kainate which can be demonstrated in the hippocampus. The number of distinct receptor types mediating these three actions of kainate is a matter of continuing debate amongst the authors.

ACKNOWLEDGEMENTS

The authors' work described in this paper is supported by a grant to HMcL from the Medical Research Council of Canada. GLC is a Fellow of the Killam Foundation and SJK holds an MRC Studentship.

REFERENCES

Andersen, P., T.V.P. Bliss and K.K. Skrede (1971). Exp. Brain Res. 13, 208–221.
Andersen, P., S.H. Sundberg, O. Sveen, J.W. Swan and H. Wigström (1980). J. Physiol. (London) 302, 463–482.
Auker, C.R., D.J. Braitman and S.L. Rubinstein (1982). Nature, 297, 583–584.
Balcar, V.J. and G.A.R. Johnston (1972). J. Neurochem. 19, 2657–2666.
Ben-Ari, Y. (1981). Glutamate as a Neurotransmitter, pp. 385–394, Raven Press, New York.
Ben-Ari, Y., E. Tremblay, O.P. Ottersen and R. Naquet (1979). Brain Res. 165, 362–365.
Ben-Ari, Y., E. Tremblay and O.P. Ottersen (1980a). Neuroscience, 5, 515–528.
Ben-Ari, Y., E. Tremblay, O.P. Ottersen and B.S. Meldrum (1980b). Brain Res. 191, 79–97.
Biscoe, T.J., R.H. Evans, P.M. Headley, M.R. Martin and J.C. Watkins (1976). Br. J. Pharmac. 58, 373–382.
Biscoe, T.J., R.H. Evans, A.A. Francis, M.R. Martin, J.C. Watkins, J. Davies and A. Dray (1977). Nature, 270, 743–745.
Biscoe, T.J., J. Davies, A. Dray, R.H. Evans, M.R. Martin and J.C. Watkins (1978). Brain Res. 148, 543–548.
Biziere, K., and J.T. Coyle (1978). Neurosci. Letts. 8, 303–310.
Bliss, T.V.P., and A.R. Gardner-Medwin (1973). J. Physiol. (London) 232, 357–374.
Bliss, T.V.P., and T. Lømo (1973). J. Physiol. (London) 232, 331–356.

Collingridge, G.L., S.J. Kehl and H. McLennan (1982a). J. Physiol. (London) in press.
Collingridge, G.L., S.J. Kehl and H. McLennan (1982b). Exp. Brain Res. submitted for publication.
Collingridge, G.L., and H. McLennan (1981). Neurosci. Letts. 27, 31–36.
Cox, D.W.G., M.H. Headley and J.C. Watkins (1977). J. Neurochem. 29, 579–588.
Curtis, D.R., J.W. Phillis and J.C. Watkins (1959). Nature, 183, 611.
Curtis, D.R., J.W. Phillis and J.C. Watkins (1960). J. Physiol. (London) 150, 656–682.
Curtis, D.R., D. Felix and H. McLennan (1970). Br. J. Pharmac. 40, 881–883.
Curtis, D.R., and J.C. Watkins. (1960). J. Neurochem. 6, 117–141.
Curtis, D.R., and J.C. Watkins (1963). J. Physiol. (London) 166, 1–14.
Davies, J., R.H. Evans, A.A. Francis and J.C. Watkins (1979). J. Physiol. (Paris) 75, 641–645.
Davies, J., A.A. Francis, A.W. Jones and J.C. Watkins (1981a). Neurosci. Letts. 21, 77–81.
Davies, J., R.H. Evans, A.A. Francis, A.W. Jones and J.C. Watkins (1981b). J. Neurochem. 36, 1305–1307.
Davies, J., and J.C. Watkins (1973). Biochem. Pharmacol. 22, 1667–1668.
Davies, J., and J.C. Watkins (1979). J. Physiol. (London) 297, 621–635.
Davies, J., and J.C. Watkins (1981). Brain Res. 206, 172–177.
Davies, J., and J.C. Watkins (1982). Brain Res. 235, 378–386.
de Montigny, C., and D. Tardif (1981). Life Sci. 29, 2103–2111.
Dingledine, R., and L. Gjerstad (1979). Brain Res. 168, 205–209.
Dolphin, A.C., M.L. Errington and T.V.P. Bliss (1982). Nature, 297, 496–498.
Douglas, R.M., G.V. Goddard and M. Riives (1982). Brain Res. 240, 259–272.
Engberg, I., J.A. Flatman and J.D.C. Lambert (1979). J. Physiol. (London) 288, 227–261.
Evans, R.H. (1981). Neurosci. Res. Prog. Bull. 19, 347–354.
Evans, R.H., R.G. Hill, T.S. Salt and D.A.S. Smith (1982). J. Pharm. Pharmacol. 34, 191–192.
Foster, A.C., E.E. Mena, M.T. Monaghan and C.W. Cotman (1981). Nature, 289, 73–75.
Gration, K.A.F., J.L. Lambert, R.L. Ramsey, R.P. Rand and P.N.R. Usherwood (1981). Brain Res. 230, 400–405.
Haas, H.L. (1982). Brain Res. 233, 200–204.
Haldeman, S., R.D. Huffman, K.C. Marshall and H. McLennan (1972). Brain Res. 39, 419–425.
Haldeman, S., and H. McLennan (1972). Brain Res. 45, 393–400.
Hall, J.G., H. McLennan and H.V. Wheal (1977). J. Physiol. (London) 272, 52–53P.
Hicks, T.P., J.G. Hall and H. McLennan (1978). Can. J. Physiol. Pharmacol. 56, 901–907.
Hicks, T.P., and H. McLennan (1979). Can. J. Physiol. Pharmacol. 57, 973–978.
Hommes, O.R., and E.A.M.T. Obbens (1972). J. Neurol. Sci. 16, 271–281.
Hutchinson, G.B., H. McLennan and H.V. Wheal (1978). Brain Res. 141, 129–136.
Johnston, G.A.R., D.R. Curtis, J. Davies and R.M. McCulloch (1974). Nature, 248, 804–805.
Johnston, G.A.R., S.M.E. Kennedy and B. Twitchin (1979). J. Neurochem. 32, 121–127.
Köhler, C., R. Schwarcz and K. Fuxe (1978). Neurosci. Letts. 10, 241–246.
Krnjević, K., R.J. Reiffenstein and N. Ropert (1981). Neuroscience, 6, 2465–2474.
Lambert, J.D.C., J.A. Flatman and I. Engberg (1981). Glutamate as a Neurotransmitter, pp. 205–216, Raven Press, New York.
Lodge, D., P.M. Headley and D.R. Curtis (1978). Brain Res. 152, 603–608.
Logan, W.J., and S.H. Snyder (1972). Brain Res. 42, 413–431.
Lothman, E.W., R.C. Collins and J.A. Ferrendelli (1981). Neurology, 31, 806–812.

MacDonald, J.F., and J.M. Wojtowicz (1982). Can. J. Physiol. Pharmacol. 60, 282-296.

Malthe-Sørenssen, D., K.K. Skrede and F. Fonnum (1979). Neuroscience, 4, 1255-1263.

McGeer, E.G., P.L. McGeer and K. Singh (1978). Brain Res. 139, 381-383.

McLennan, H. (1980). Neurosci. Letts. 18, 313-316.

McLennan, H. (1981). Glutamate as a Neurotransmitter, pp. 253-262, Raven Press, New York.

McLennan, H. (1982a). Eur. J. Pharmacol. 79, 135-137.

McLennan, H. (1982b). Eur. J. Pharmacol. 79, 307-310.

McLennan, H., and J.G. Hall (1978). Brain Res. 149, 541-545.

McLennan, H., T.P. Hicks and J.R. Liu (1982). Neuropharmacology, 21, 549-554.

McLennan, H., and J.R. Liu (1982). Exp. Brain Res. 45, 151-156.

McLennan, H., and D. Lodge (1979). Brain Res. 169, 83-90.

McLennan, H., and H.V. Wheal (1976a). Can. J. Physiol. Pharmacol. 54, 70-72.

McLennan, H., and H.V. Wheal (1976b). Neuropharmacology, 15, 709-712.

Nadler, J.V., and G.J. Cuthbertson (1980). Brain Res. 195, 47-56.

Nadler, J.V., B.W. Perry and C.W. Cotman (1978). Nature, 271, 676-677.

Nadler, J.V., B.W. Perry, C.Gentry and C.W. Cotman (1980). J. comp. Neurol 192, 333-359.

Nadler, J.V., D.A. Evenson and G.J. Cuthbertson (1981). Neuroscience, 6, 2505-2517.

Olney, J.W. (1978). Kainic Acid as a Tool in Neurobiology, pp. 95-121, Raven Press, New York.

Olney, J.W., V. Rhee and O.L. Ho (1974). Brain Res. 77, 507-512.

Olney, J.W., T. Fuller and T. de Gubareff (1979). Brain Res. 176, 91-100.

Olney, J.W., T.A. Fuller and T. de Gubareff (1981a). Nature, 292, 165-167.

Olney, J.W., T.A. Fuller, T. de Gubareff and J. Labruyere (1981b). Neurosci. Letts. 25, 185-191.

Pearson, S., and P.B. Nunn (1981). Brain Res. 206, 178-182.

Ribak, C.E., and R.J. Reiffenstein (1982). Can. J. Physiol. Pharmacol. 60, 864-870.

Riveros, N., and F. Orrego (1982). Brain Res. 236, 492-496.

Roberts, P.J., G.A. Foster and E.M. Thomas (1981). Nature, 293, 654-655.

Robinson, J.H., and S.A. Deadwyler (1981). Brain Res. 221, 117-127.

Ruck, A., S. Kramer, J. Metz and M.J.W. Brennan (1981). Nature, 287, 852-853.

Schwarcz, R., and J.T. Coyle (1977). Brain Res. 127, 235-249.

Schwarcz, R., and C. Köhler (1980). Neurosci. Letts. 19, 243-249.

Schwarcz, R., D. Scholz and J.T. Coyle (1978). Neuropharmacology, 17, 141-151.

Seil, F.J., W.R. Woodward, N.K. Blank and A.L. Leiman (1978). Brain Res. 159, 431-435.

Shinozaki, H., and S. Konishi (1970). Brain Res. 24, 368-371.

Skrede, K.K., and D. Malthe-Sørenssen (1981a). Brain Res. 208, 436-441.

Skrede, K.K., and D. Malthe-Sørenssen (1981b). Neurosci. Letts. 21, 71-76.

Sloviter, R.S., and B.P. Damiano (1981a). Neurosci. Letts. 24, 279-284.

Sloviter, R.S., and B.P. Damiano (1981b). Neuropharmacology, 20, 1003-1011.

Stone, T.W., M.N. Perkins, J.F. Collins and K. Curry (1981). Neuroscience, 6, 2249-2252.

Tissari, A.H., and P.L. Onali (1982). Pharmacol. Res. Comm. 14, 83-89.

Watkins, J.C., J. Davies, R.H. Evans, A.A. Francis and A.W. Jones (1981). Glutamate as a Neurotransmitter, pp. 263-273, Raven Press, New York.

Wheal, H.V., and J.J. Miller (1980). Brain Res. 182, 145-155.

Wuerthele, S.M., K.L. Lovell, M.Z. Jones and K.E. Moore (1978). Brain Res. 149, 489-497.

TWO TYPES OF EXCITATORY AMINO ACID RESPONSES IN THE CAT CAUDATE NUCLEUS

P. L. HERRLING

Wander Research Institute (a Sandoz Research Unit), Wander Ltd., P. O. Box 2747, CH–3001 Berne, Switzerland

ABSTRACT

Caudate neurons were recorded with intracellular microelectrodes in halothane anaesthetized cats. Excitatory amino acids and some of their antagonists were applied by microiontophoresis. The agonists exhibited two types of responses, both of which consisted of gradual membrane depolarizations; however, in type 1 this was associated with repetitive, relatively regular firing, whereas in type 2 action potentials generally occurred on additional abrupt depolarizations reaching amplitudes of more than 20 mV and which lasted up to 500 ms.

Glutamic and quisqualic acid elicited type 1 excitations exclusively. N-methyl-D,L-aspartic, N-methyl-D-aspartic and the endogenous compound quinolinic acid caused type 1 excitations in about one third of the caudate neurons and type 2 excitations in the rest. When quinolinic and N-methyl-D,L-aspartic acid were applied to the same neurons they always displayed the same effects. Aspartic acid showed mixed effects but type 1 always seemed to predominate.

At low doses, the antagonist D-alpha-aminoadipic acid inhibited only type 2 effects, whereas higher doses also reduced type 1 responses. On the same cells, however, antagonism of type 2 effects was always predominant. 2,3-Cis-piperidine dicarboxylic acid also selectively inhibited the effects of N-methyl-D,L-aspartic acid, but at high doses it potentiated aspartic and glutamic acid-induced excitations.

Cortically evoked EPSPs were unaffected even by high doses of DAA. High frequency stimulations of the cortico-caudate pathway never resulted in type 2 excitations.

It is concluded that cat caudate neurons react to excitatory amino acids by two different mechanisms, one of which (type 2) might involve NMDA receptors as defined by Watkins (1981) because of the very similar pharmacology. Furthermore, the results indicate that NMDA receptors of this type are probably not the receptors mediating cortically evoked excitations.

KEY WORDS:

Caudate neurons; intracellular recordings; microiontophoresis; excitatory amino acid agonists and antagonists.

INTRODUCTION

Evidence from a number of biochemical and lesioning experiments (Divac et al., 1977; Fonnum et al., 1977; Kim et al., 1977; McGeer et al., 1977; Scatton & Lehmann, 1982; Teichberg et al., 1981) and electrophysiological studies (Spencer, 1976; Stone, 1979) has implied a role for an excitatory amino acid in cortico-caudate connections. To date, only two groups have investigated excitatory amino acids in the caudate using intracellular methods (Bernardi et al., 1976; Herrling & Hull, 1980), although both of these were only concerned with glutamate.

The purpose of the experiments described in this report was: 1) to evaluate the effects of excitatory amino acids and some of their recently discovered antago-nists (for review, see Watkins, 1981) on the membrane, action and synaptic poten-tials of cat caudate neurons, and 2) to determine if the classification of ex-citatory amino acid receptors as proposed by Watkins (1981) from evidence ob-tained in other regions of the central nervous system also applies to the caudate.

Some of the results presented here have been published as abstracts (Herrling et al., 1982; Herrling & Salt, 1982).

METHODS

The methods used have been described in detail elsewhere (Herrling & Hull, 1980; Herrling, 1981; Herrling et al., submitted). Briefly, cats of either sex were initially anaesthesized with sodium metohexital (Brietal, Lilly) for the dura-tion of surgical manipulations. They consisted in exposing the dorsal surface of the caudate nuclei, implanting stainless steel stimulation electrodes in the pre-cruciate cortex, performing tracheotomy and pneumothorax as well as cannulation of the femoral artery and vein and opening of the cisterna magna. At the end of surgery, anaesthesia was switched to halothane (Fluothane, ICI) 0.5 - 1.0% in oxygen. The blood pressure was monitored and cells included in the sample only if it exceeded 80 mmHg. The expired CO_2 was measured and kept at 3.5 - 4.2% and the body temperature at 37.8 degrees centigrade.

For recording and drug applications an array of seven pipettes was glued along-side an intracellular recording electrode that was filled with potassium citrate at pH 7.2.

The following drugs were dissolved in water and their pH adjusted to 9 - 9.5 with NaOH: D-alpha-aminoadipic acid (Sigma), 0.5 M; L-aspartic acid (Sigma), 0.5 M; L-glutamic acid (Sigma), 1.0 M, pH 8.0; N-methyl-D,L-aspartic acid (Sigma) 0.2 M; N-methyl-D-aspartic acid (Sandoz), 0.2 M; cis-2,3-piperidine dicarboxilic acid (kindly donated by J. Watkins, Bristol), 0.1 M; quinolinic acid (Sigma), 0.2 M; quisqualic acid (Sigma), 0.1 M.

One lateral pipette of the iontophoretic array was always filled with a physio-logical saline solution at pH 9.8 for current controls and the central barrel with the same solution at neutral pH for current balancing if needed. At the end of each successful experiment the brains were removed for histological localiza-tion of the electrode tracks.

RESULTS

The data presented below was collected from 45 cats that yielded 55 successful cell impalements lasting from 5 to 80 min.

The membrane potential of these cells encountered 400 - 4700 μm below the caudate surface was 50 ± 9 mV (mean ± SD, range 40 - 65 mV). Action potentials had ampli-

tudes of 40 ± 9 mV (range 30 - 70 mV) and durations from 0.5 to 1.5 ms at their
half-maximal amplitude. The cells were usually silent except when excited either
by stimulation of the cortico-caudate pathway, by intracellular current injection
or by the application of drugs. Cortically evoked EPSPs ranged from 5 - 15 mV.
Taken together, these observations suggested that the cells impaled were not
greatly depolarized by electrode penetrations in spite of relatively small action
potential amplitudes. These were possibly due to the high resistances of the
electrodes used here, over 200 megohms in the tissue, and the fact that the iontophoretic array was glued directly alongside the recording electrode. Both of
these factors might have made a complete compensation of stray capacitance impossible (Cornwall & Thomas, 1981).

The iontophoretic application of glutamate (GLU) and quisqualate (QUIS) to 10
and 20 cells, respectively, always resulted in gradual but sometimes relatively
fast depolarizations, i.e. the firing threshold could be reached within 1 s of
the beginning of the iontophoretic current. These depolarizations were accompanied by repetitive firing until increasing amounts of the agonist depolarized
the membrane to the point of total inactivation of action potentials. This type
of excitation was termed type 1. Applications of N-methyl-D,L-aspartate or N-
methyl-D-aspartate (both abbreviated as NMA) also caused type 1 excitations in
13 of 46 cells. In 33 cells, NMA elicited gradual depolarizations, but superimposed on them were abrupt large depolarizations that could reach over 20 mV
and on which most of the drug-induced action potentials occurred. These depolarizations could last up to 500 ms. They were termed plateaus and this type of
excitatory effects type 2 excitations. Examples of type 1 and 2 excitations are
shown in Fig. 1 and 2.

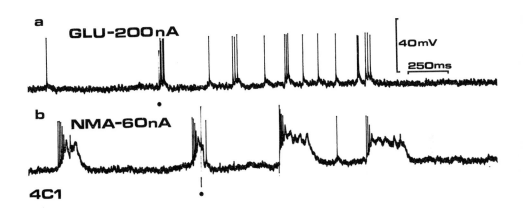

Fig. 1. Excitatory effects of GLU and NMA on the membrane and action
potentials of cat caudate neurons. a) Example of type 1 excitations.
GLU was applied at the indicated current for the whole duration of the
trace. It depolarized the membrane and caused repetitive firing with
action potentials riding on small depolarizations. b) NMA was applied
to the same cell where it also gradually depolarized the membrane but
additionally, it elicited abrupt plateau-like depolarizations on which
most of the action potentials occurred.
In this and all following traces positive is upwards, the dots indicate the time of cortical stimulation and the number at the bottom of
the figures are cell identifications. In some of the traces action
potentials were retouched for clarity.

The endogenous agent quinolinic acid (QUIN, Diem & Lentner, 1971; Stone & Perkins, 1981) caused type 2 excitations in 10 cells on which NMA had done the same (Fig. 2).

In 4 cells, QUIN elicited only type 1 excitations and these were cells on which NMA had done the same.

L-aspartate (ASP) was applied to 10 cells where it caused mixed effects: some plateaus occurred, but they were always less pronounced than those provoked by NMA on the same cells and they were always followed by pronounced type 1 effects. The results obtained with the selective NMDA antagonist D-alpha-aminoadipic acid (DAA; Biscoe et al., 1977; for review, see Watkins, 1981) are summarized in Table 1.

	N cells	Agonist	Type of excitation: 1 or 2	Antagonism by DAA
a)	4	GLU	1	no
		NMA	2	yes
b)	5	QUIS	1	no
		NMA	2	yes
c)	4	QUIS	1	no
		NMA	1	no
d)	2	QUIS	1	no
		NMA	2	yes
		QUIN	2	yes
e)	2	QUIS	1	no
		NMA	1	no
		QUIN	1	no

Table 1. The effects of DAA on type 1 and 2 excitations.
a) - e) the different agonists were applied to each cell in each case.

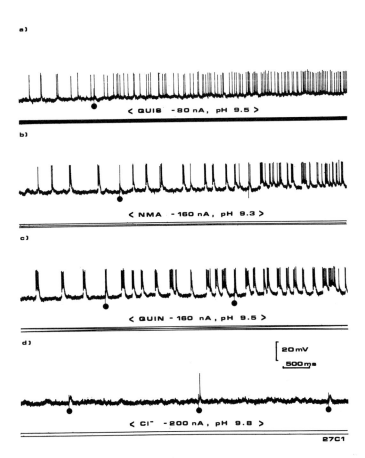

Fig. 2. Comparison of the effects of QUIS, NMA and QUIN on the same cell. a) Type 1 excitation induced by QUIS. b) Type 2 excitation induced by NMA. c) Type 2 excitation induced by QUIN. d) Current and pH control.

DAA selectively inhibited the effects of NMA and QUIN, but only on cells where these agonists elicited type 2 excitations. At low application currents, this antagonist never blocked type 1 effects. At higher currents, DAA occasionally also affected type 1 effects but always distinctly less than type 2 on the same cell. Examples of this selective antagonism are shown in Fig. 3 and 4.

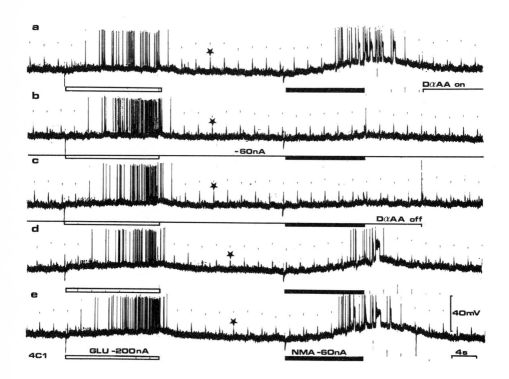

Fig. 3. DAA inhibited NMA-induced type 2 but not GLU-induced type 1 excitations on the same cell. a) Control before the application of DAA. GLU was applied at the time indicated by the white bar, NMA during the black bar. Even at this slow sweep speed type 1 and 2 excitations can be readily distinguished. b) NMA-induced excitations have been totally abolished by DAA applied during the time indicated by the thin bar. d) and e) Progressive recovery of NMA-induced effects. Asterisks indicate examples of cortically induced EPSPs. They are not visibly depressed by DAA (see also below). All traces in this figure are continuous.

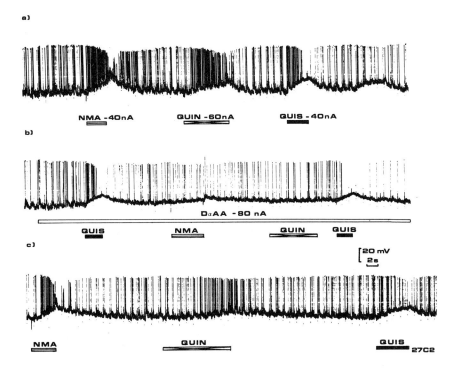

Fig. 4. DAA inhibits NMA- and QUIN-induced type 2 effects while QUIS-induced type 1 effects are much less affected. a) Control where all three agonists were applied. They induced large depolarizations that resulted in an inactivation of action potentials. b) The effects of the same three agonists during the application of DAA. NMA- and QUIN-induced excitations have completely disappeared, those of QUIS only partially. The current used here to expell DAA was twice as large as the one used to expell NMA, this was regarded as a relatively large dose of DAA. c) Partial recovery.

The compound PDA was described in the literature as a broad spectrum antagonist of excitatory amino acids because it inhibited both NMDA and QUIS agonists (Davies et al., 1981; Salt & Hill, 1982). The results of experiments with this substance in the caudate are summarized in Table 2.

	N cells	Agonist	Type of excitation 1 or 2	Effect of PDA on excitations
a)	3	GLU	1	increased
b)	5	GLU	1	increased
		ASP	1 > 2	inhibited first, then increased
		NMA	2	inhibited only

Table 2. The effects of PDA on type 1 and 2 excitations.

PDA applied to caudate cells slightly depolarized their membrane potential but without reaching firing threshold. It selectively inhibited only NMA-induced excitations and increased the excitations caused by GLU, sometimes to the point of total inactivation of action potentials.

ASP was inhibited at low doses of PDA, but its effect was enhanced by higher doses while on the same cells NMA effects remained blocked.

The precruciate cortex (anterior sigmoid gyrus) was stimulated at 0.5 Hz, 100 – 500 µs long pulses and 0.5 – 5 mA intensity, during most of the above described experiments. This resulted as previously described in the literature (Buchwald et al., 1973; Kitai et al., 1976) in monosynaptic EPSPs followed by IPSPs. One peculiarity here was that in most cells, the membrane potential was near the equilibrium potential of the ion responsible for the IPSP so that this synaptic potential became distinctly visible only when the cells were experimentally depolarized. The antagonist DAA did not depress cortically evoked EPSPs in any of 18 cells tested even at currents exceeding those needed on the same cell to abolish NMA-induced excitations completely.

A further experiment was devised in order to determine if NMDA receptors mediating type 2 effects might be involved in the generation of cortically evoked excitations. If this were the case, it should be possible to observe plateaus developing after cortical stimulation at least in some cells. Stimulation at 0.5 Hz never resulted in plateaus even in the rare cases where action potentials were elicited. Excitations with repetitive firing could be obtained if the precruciate cortex was stimulated with 2 – 4 s long trains at 50 Hz. Thus elicited excitations were always similar to type 1 (11 cells) even in those cells where iontophoretic application of NMA or NMDA had resulted in type 2 excitations (5 cells).

DISCUSSION

The present results indicate that cat caudate neurons can be excited by excitatory amino acids applied by microiontophoresis in at least two ways. A type 1 excitation consisting in a depolarization of the membrane and repetitive, relatively regular firing. A type 2 excitation where the gradual depolarizations were associated with superimposed abrupt depolarizations on which most of the drug-induced action potentials occurred (plateaus). The quisqualate receptor preferring agonists GLU and QUIS (Watkins, 1981) elicited type 1 excitations exclusively. These excitations were not antagonized by DAA and increased by PDA. This last finding does not agree with previously published work stating that PDA inhibited both NMDA- and QUIS-induced excitations in spinal neurons (Davies et al., 1981) and in neurons of the caudal trigeminal nucleus (Salt & Hill, 1982). The reason for this discrepancy could be different receptor characteristics in different brain regions. However, because of the relatively small number of cells tested in the caudate nucleus to date, a more definite judgement will have to await further experiments.

The NMDA agonists NMA and QUIN (Watkins, 1981; Stone & Perkins, 1981) elicited type 2 excitations in two thirds of the cells and these were antagonized by DAA and PDA. In the remaining third of the present sample, these agents caused excitations similar to type 1 that were not inhibited by the two antagonists. The receptors responsible for these excitations were probably distinct from the receptors mediating type 1 excitations elicited by the QUIS agonists. If they were the same, it would be expected to see type 2 excitations replaced by type 1 excitations during the application of DAA on cells where NMDA agonists elicit plateaus. During the blockade of NMDA receptors by DAA, NMDA agonists would then have to stimulate QUIS receptors. The data presented shows that this was not the case: during DAA both NMA and QUIN do not elicit any excitations while QUIS or GLU are still active (Figs. 3,4). It must be assumed that on the cells where NMDA agonists provoke excitations without plateaus, they interact with a further entity sensitive to excitatory amino acids. A reasonable candidate is the kainic acid receptor as proposed by Watkins (1981) known to exist in the rat striatum (Teichberg et al., 1981). However, further experiments are needed to test this hypothesis.

The present results with QUIN confirm that this endogenous compound is a NMDA agonist as Stone & Perkins (1981) had concluded from experiments performed in the rat cortex.

The indirect evidence described above indicates that the receptor mediating cortically evoked excitations of cat caudate cells is not a NMDA receptor as defined by Watkins (1981).

ACKNOWLEDGEMENTS

I would like to thank Dr. J.C. Watkins for a generous gift of PDA, Drs. R. Morris and T.E. Salt for their help in some of the experiments and Mrs. B. Misbach-Lesenne for outstanding technical assistance.

REFERENCES

Bernardi, G., Floris, V., Marciani, M.G., Morocutti, C. and Stanzione, P. (1976). Brain Res. 114, 134-138.
Biscoe, T.J., Davies, J., Dray, A., Evans, R.H., Francis, A.A., Martin, M.R. and Watkins, J.C. (1977). Europ. J. Pharmac. 45, 315-316.
Buchwald, N.A., Price, D.D., Vernon, L. and Hull, C.D. (1973). Exp. Neurol. 38, 311-323.
Cornwall, C.M. and Thomas, M.V. (1981). J. Neurosci. Meth. 3, 225-232.
Davies, J., Evans, R.H., Francis, A.A., Jones, A.W. and Watkins, J.C. (1981). J. Neurochem. 36, 1305-1307.
Diem, K. and Lentner, C., eds. (1971). Scientific Tables Ciba-Geigy Ltd., Basle, p. 399.
Divac, I., Fonnum, F. and Storm-Mathisen, J. (1977). Nature 266, 377-378.
Fonnum, F., Storm-Mathisen, J. and Divac, I. (1981). Neurosci. 6, 863-873.
Herrling, P.L. and Hull, C.D. (1980). Brain Res. 192, 441-462.
Herrling, P.L. (1981). Brain Res. 212, 331-343.
Herrling, P.L., Misbach-Lesenne, B. and Salt, T.E. (1982). J. Physiol. 327, 80 P.
Herrling, P.L. and Salt, T.E. (1982). Neurosci. 7 Suppl., 93.

Herrling, P.L., Morris, R. and Salt, T.E. (submitted for publication).
  J. Physiol. (London).
Kim, J.-S., Hassler, R., Haug, P. and Paik, K.S. (1977). Brain Res. 132, 370-374.
Kitai, S.T., Kocsis, J.D., Preston, R.J. and Sugimori, M. (1976). Brain Res. 109,
  601-606.
McGeer, P.L., McGeer, E.G., Scherer, U. and Singh, K. (1977). Brain Res. 128,
  369-373.
Salt, T.E. and Hill, R.G. (1982). Neuropharmac. 21, 385-390.
Scatton, B. and Lehmann, J. (1982). Nature 297, 422-424.
Spencer, H.J. (1976). Brain Res. 102, 91-101.
Stone, T.W. (1979). Br. J. Pharmac. 67, 545-551.
Stone, T.W. and Perkins, M.N. (1981). Europ. J. Pharmac. 72, 411-412.
Teichberg, V.I., Goldberg, O. and Luini, A. (1981). Molec. Cell Biochem. 39,
  289-295.
Watkins, J.C. (1981). In Glutamate: Transmitter in the central nervous system,
  ed. Roberts, P.J., Storm-Mathisen, J. and Johnson, G.A.R., pp. 1-24.
  Chichester, New York, Brisbane: John Wiley & Sons Ltd.

RECENT ADVANCES IN THE PHARMACOLOGY OF EXCITATORY AMINO ACIDS IN THE MAMMALIAN CENTRAL NERVOUS SYSTEM

J. DAVIES*, R. H. EVANS**, A. W. JONES**, K. N. MEWETT**, D. A. S. SMITH**
and J. C. WATKINS***

*Department of Pharmacology, The School of Pharmacy,
Brunswick Square, London WC1N 1AX, England
**Departments of Pharmacology and ***Physiology,
The Medical School, Bristol BS8 1TD, England

ABSTRACT

Current ideas are described on the classification of excitatory amino acid receptors in the mammalian central nervous system. The actions of some new agonists and antagonists for NMA receptors and non-NMA receptors are summarized.

New NMA receptor antagonists include a range of D-aspartyl- and D-glutamyl dipeptides where the second amino acid contains a phosphonic acid moiety. None of these dipeptides is more potent or specific than 2-amino-5-phosphonopentanoic acid or 2-amino-7-phosphonoheptanoic acid.

D-Homocysteine sulphinate is a new selective NMA agonist of high potency. N-Methyl-derivatives of both D- and L-glutamic acid are also highly specific NMA agonists.

γ-D-Glutamylaminomethylsulphonate is a new excitatory amino acid antagonist which depresses agonist-induced responses in the order kainate > quisqualate > N-methyl-D-aspartate > L-glutamate. Other sulphonic peptides have similar, though weaker actions.

The actions of excitatory amino acid antagonists in depressing polysynaptic and monosynaptic excitation in the spinal cord are described.

KEYWORDS

Excitatory amino acid receptors; excitatory amino acid agonists; excitatory amino acid antagonists; spinal cord.

INTRODUCTION

The putative transmitters, L-glutamate and L-aspartate, when exogenously administered to CNS tissue, are considered to have actions at multiple types of receptors (Watkins and Evans, 1981; Davies et al, 1982a). Receptors of one type (NMA receptors) are activated selectively by the agonist N-methyl-D-aspartate (NMDA) and are blocked by a large range of antagonists of which the most potent and specific are the D(-) forms of 2-amino-5-phosphonovalerate and 2-amino-7-phosphonoheptanoate (Evans & Watkins,1981; Perkins et al, 1981; Evans et al, 1982; Davies & Watkins,1982a; McLennan, 1982a,b). Other receptors (non-NMA receptors) are relatively insensitive to NMDA antagonists and appear to be of

43

several sub-types, two of which are probably activated selectively by the agonists kainate and quisqualate (Watkins & Evans, 1981). This paper will briefly describe some of the newer findings relating to the differential activation and blockade of these multiple types of excitatory amino acid receptors.

NMA RECEPTOR ANTAGONISTS

Following the initial recognition of D-α-aminoadipate (DαAA) as an excitatory amino acid antagonist (Hall et al, 1977; McLennan & Hall, 1978), this substance was classified among a growing number of selective NMDA antagonists which also had a differential depressant action on synaptic excitation in the mammalian and amphibian spinal cord (Biscoe et al, 1977, 1978; Evans et al, 1978). Furthermore, this action extended to higher homologues of DαAA (Evans et al, 1979; Davies & Watkins, 1979). The knowledge that 2-amino-4-phosphonobutyrate also had amino acid antagonist and synaptic depressant properties (Cull-Candy et al, 1976; Dudel, 1977; White et al, 1977; Evans et al, 1979; Davies & Watkins, 1979) led naturally to the study of a homologous series of such ω-phosphono α-carboxylic amino acids. Not only did this range of phosphono amino acids show a similar structure-activity profile to that observed with dicarboxylic amino acids but also a considerably higher NMA antagonist and synaptic depressant potency than the corresponding dicarboxylic acids (Evans & Watkins, 1981; Davies et al, 1981a; Evans et al,

Table 1. Homologous series of ω-phosphono α-carboxylic amino acids showing newer and older (square brackets) forms of chemical nomenclature. A simplified abbreviation system is given in the last column.

ω-PHOSPHONO α-CARBOXYLIC AMINO ACIDS

$$H_2O_3P-(CH_2)_n-\overset{\displaystyle COOH}{\underset{\displaystyle NH_2}{\mid}}CH$$

n	Chemical Name(s)	Common Abbrev.	Suggested Abbrev.
1	[PROPIONIC] 2-AMINO-3-PHOSPHONO-PROPANOIC ACID	APP	AP3
2	[BUTYRIC] 2-AMINO-4-PHOSPHONO-BUTANOIC ACID	APB	AP4
3	[VALERIC] 2-AMINO-5-PHOSPHONO-PENTANOIC ACID	APV APP APPent	AP5
4	[CAPROIC] 2-AMINO-6-PHOSPHONO-HEXANOIC ACID	APC APH APX APHex	AP6
5	[HEPTOIC] 2-AMINO-7-PHOSPHONO-HEPTANOIC ACID	APH APHept	AP7
6	[CAPRYLIC] 2-AMINO-8-PHOSPHONO-OCTANOIC ACID	APC APO	AP8

1982).   The two most active compounds, 2-amino-5-phosphonovalerate and 2-amino-7-phosphonoheptanoate showed little difference from one another in either potency or selectivity when tested on neurones of the frog, rat (Evans et al, 1982) or cat (Peet et al, 1982) spinal cord, or rat cerebral cortex (J.Davies and S.E.Johnston, unpublished observations).   Although higher potency and selectivity has been reported in other experiments with the heptanoate compound in the rat cerebral cortex (Perkins et al, 1981), the high iontophoretic currents apparently needed for the valerate (pentanoate) analogue in that work passed from electrode solutions that were not neutralized or diluted with NaCl markedly contrasts with the low currents from NaOH-neutralized NaCl-diluted solutions found very effective in our experiments.   Thus, differences may exist in the activity of phosphonates obtained from different batches or sources, and/or in the iontophoretic conditions used.

At this point it may be worthwhile to discuss nomenclature of phosphono amino acids. Old terminology dies hard, and the familiar names of the members of the ascending series of alkane-1-carboxylic acids, namely, acetic, propionic, butyric, valeric, etc., may yet be with us for some time, especially in the catalogues of chemical suppliers. (The same is probably also true for L and D protein amino acids, now replaced by S and R in current chemical terminology).   Table 1 shows how the phosphono amino acids are named according to modern and earlier terminology, the latter given in square brackets. Such dual nomenclature inevitably leads to confusion not least in the abbreviations to which the two systems give rise. There can be no doubt that it would be preferable to move towards the new chemical nomenclature, but since this introduces difficulties with respect to abbreviations, it is suggested that new abbreviations be used, as given in Table 1. Here the letters A and P stand for the α-amino and ω-phosphono groups, and the numerical suffix for the number of carbons in the alkane carboxylic acid moiety. However, in this paper, we shall retain the use of D and L which are so much more familiar to bioscientists.

The D(-) forms of the phosphono compounds AP5 and AP7, as with their dicarboxylic acid counterparts, carry the major part of the observed NMA receptor antagonist and synaptic depressant properties (Evans & Watkins, 1981; Perkins et al, 1981; Evans et al, 1982; Davies & Watkins, 1982a; McLennan, 1982a,b). With AP4 the situation is more complex. The D form (D-AP4) has only weak NMA antagonist and synaptic depressant properties compared with the higher homologues D-AP5 and D-AP7, and is less selective (Evans et al, 1982; Davies & Watkins, 1982a). Thus, D-AP4 antagonizes kainate responses equally as effectively as NMDA responses.   On the other hand, L-AP4 is a relatively potent depressant of some forms of synaptic excitation in the hippocampus (Koerner & Cotman, 1981) and spinal cord (Evans et al, 1982; Davies & Watkins, 1982a) but is apparently devoid of amino acid antagonist properties (Evans et al, 1982; Davies & Watkins, 1982a). It may act by inhibiting the release of an excitatory amino acid or by antagonizing the effects of an unknown transmitter. At concentrations above that required for depression of synaptic excitation, L-AP4 is an excitant with a selective action at NMA receptors (Evans et al, 1982), and this action is antagonized by the D form.   This mixture of actions of the different isomers of AP4 probably explains the varied effects reported for the racemic form of this substance (e.g. Watkins et al, 1977; Evans et al, 1979; Davies & Watkins, 1979; Slaughter & Miller, 1981; Hori et al, 1982).

AP6 and AP3 have not yet been resolved into separate D and L forms.   However, in analogy with dicarboxylic amino acids, it would be expected that D-AP6 would carry the NMDA antagonist activity, but that it would be considerably less potent than D-AP5 or D-AP7.   AP3 has been reported to have both amino acid agonist (Curtis & Watkins, 1965; Evans et al, 1982) and synaptic depressant (White et al, 1979) properties, which, like those of AP4 may be a reflection of different actions of D and L forms.

Preliminary results have been reported on a range of dipeptides with chain lengths analogous to those in AP6, AP7 and AP8 (Davies et al, 1982a). These substances include peptides of D-aspartic acid and D-glutamic acid in which the second amino acid contains a phosphonic acid group.   Such dipeptides have proved to be very effective NMA antagonists, as predicted by analogy with γ-D-glutamylglycine (Francis et al, 1980; Davies & Watkins, 1981a); however, they are more specific in this regard than the dicarboxylic peptides which also depress kainate- (especially) and quisqualate- induced responses in addition to NMDA responses (Francis et al, 1980; Davies & Watkins, 1981a, 1982b; Davies et al, 1982a; Peet et al, 1982).   The structures of two of these phosphono peptides, and their potencies relative to AP5 and AP7 as NMA antagonists, are given in Fig. 1.

SELECTIVE NMA RECEPTOR AGONISTS

Fig.2 shows the structures of a range of compounds, the actions of which can be abolished by specific NMA receptor antagonists.   This range includes the N-monomethyl derivatives not only of D-aspartate (i.e. NMDA) but also of L-aspartate and of both D- and L-glutamic acids.   NMDA is the most potent of these agonists, the order being NMDA > N-methyl-L-aspartate > N-methyl-L-glutamate > N-methyl-D-glutamate (Davies et al, 1982a).   It is interesting that the introduction of a methyl group confers marked NMA receptor selectivity on substances that, without this N-substituent, produce their actions substantially via non-NMA receptors.   This is particularly evident in the case of L-glutamate.

A generalization that seems to be emerging (Davies et al, 1982a) is that with some important exceptions, a secondary amino group favours interaction with NMA receptors. Thus, trans-2,3- and trans-2,4-piperidine dicarboxylate (Fig. 2), which are N-alkylated

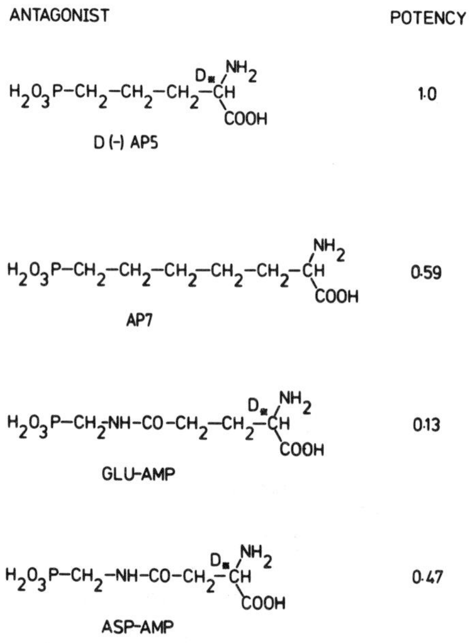

ANTAGONIST	POTENCY
$H_2O_3P-CH_2-CH_2-CH_2-\overset{D_\bullet}{\underset{\backslash COOH}{CH}}\overset{NH_2}{/}$ D (-) AP5	1.0
$H_2O_3P-CH_2-CH_2-CH_2-CH_2-CH_2-\overset{NH_2}{\underset{\backslash COOH}{CH}}$ AP7	0.59
$H_2O_3P-CH_2NH-CO-CH_2-CH_2-\overset{D_\bullet}{\underset{\backslash COOH}{CH}}\overset{NH_2}{/}$ GLU-AMP	0.13
$H_2O_3P-CH_2-NH-CO-CH_2-\overset{D_\bullet}{\underset{\backslash COOH}{CH}}\overset{NH_2}{/}$ ASP-AMP	0.47

Fig. 1.   Chemical structures and relative potencies of some NMA receptor antagonists.   The relative potencies shown are the reciprocals of the equi-effective molar ratios required to produce the same degree of reversal of NMDA-induced depolarization of frog spinal moto-neurones in vitro.   AP5, 2-amino-5-phosphonovalerate; AP7, 2-amino-7-phosphonoheptanoate; GLU-AMP, γ -D-glutamylaminomethylphosphonate; ASP-AMP, β-D-aspartylaminomethylphosphonate.

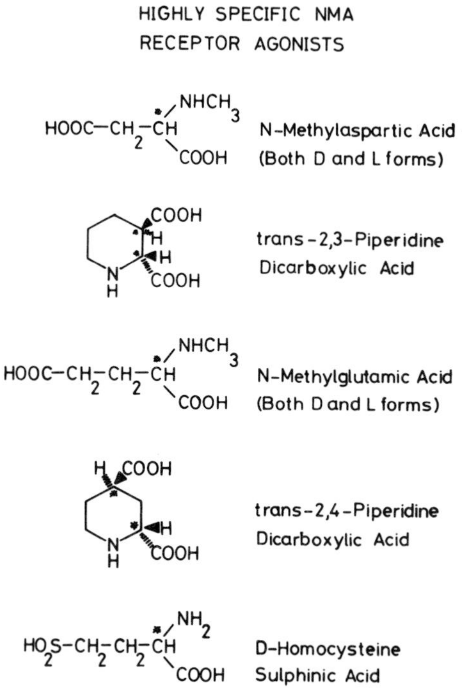

HIGHLY SPECIFIC NMA
RECEPTOR AGONISTS

$$HOOC{-}CH_2{-}\overset{\overset{\displaystyle NHCH_3}{\diagup}}{\underset{\diagdown}{CH}}{\diagdown}COOH$$

N-Methylaspartic Acid
(Both D and L forms)

trans-2,3-Piperidine
Dicarboxylic Acid

$$HOOC{-}CH_2{-}CH_2{-}\overset{\overset{\displaystyle NHCH_3}{\diagup}}{\underset{\diagdown}{CH}}{\diagdown}COOH$$

N-Methylglutamic Acid
(Both D and L forms)

trans-2,4-Piperidine
Dicarboxylic Acid

$$HO_2S{-}CH_2{-}CH_2{-}\overset{\overset{\displaystyle NH_2}{\diagup}}{\underset{\diagdown}{CH}}{\diagdown}COOH$$

D-Homocysteine
Sulphinic Acid

Fig. 2. The structures of some highly specific agonists for NMA receptors.

aspartic and glutamic acids, respectively, have potent and selective actions at NMA receptors (Davies et al, 1982b).   A related substance, quinolinic acid, the excitatory action of which was first reported without reference to receptor selectivity (Watkins, 1978) was recently classified as NMA-like by Stone and Perkins (1981).

As exemplified by kainate and domoate however (Davies et al, 1982a), not all substances having a secondary α-amino group are selective NMA receptor agonists. Moreover, some potent NMA receptor agonists have primary α-amino groups.   Thus, D-homocysteine sulphinate (Fig. 2) is a highly selective NMA agonist with a potency in the isolated spinal cord of the immature rat equal to or greater than that of NMDA and comparable with that of the non-NMA receptor agonists quisqualate and kainate (K.N. Mewett, D.A.S. Smith and J.C. Watkins, unpublished observations.).

MIXED AGONISTS

A large range of agonists have actions which may be suppressed partially but not completely by concentrations of specific NMA receptor antagonists sufficient to abolish equal magnitude responses produced by NMDA and other selective NMA agonists. Different proportions of responses produced by such mixed agonists are resistant to the action of D(-)AP5 and other potent NMA receptor antagonists depending on the agonist in question. The magnitude of the resistant component in each case, as a proportion of the total response, gives an indication of the relative involvement of NMA and non-NMA receptors in producing the total response. An example is shown in Fig.3.

Table 2 lists some of these mixed agonists in approximate deceasing order of sensitivity to selective NMA receptor antagonists as determined on the isolated spinal cord of the frog. Among these compounds is S-sulpho-L-cysteine (Watkins, 1978). This amino acid occurs in mammalian tissues in sulphite oxidase deficiency (Irreverre et al, 1967) and produces lesions of the excitotoxic type (Olney et al, 1975). The potent excitatory action of S-sulpho-L-cysteine (approximately one-half that of NMDA) is predominantly mediated by NMA receptors and this is one of the few amino acids yet known where the L form appears to be more selective for NMA receptors than is the D form (Fig. 3). In this respect S-sulphocysteine resembles homocysteate, from which it differs structurally only by having a sulphur atom instead of a methylene group in the chain linking the acidic groups.

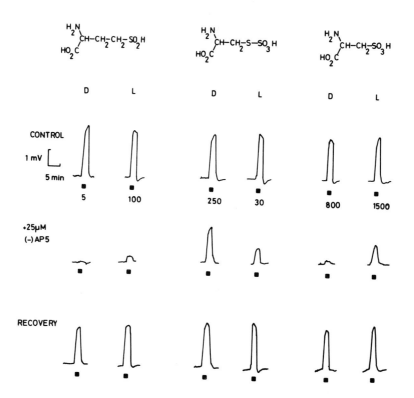

Fig. 3. Differential antagonism by D(-)-2-amino-5-phosphonopentanoate (AP5) of the depolarizing responses produced by a range of sulphur-containing amino acids in the frog spinal cord *in vitro*. Approximately equal magnitude responses of motoneurones, measured in ventral roots (for Methods, see Evans, et al.,1982), were produced by the D and L forms, as shown, of: left panel, homocysteine sulphinic acid; middle panel, S-sulphocysteine; right panel, cysteic acid (concentrations, μm). The superfusion medium contained tetrodotoxin (10^{-7}M). Note that the response to D-homocysteine sulphinate was abolished by D(-)AP5, but that a varying proportion of the other responses was resistant to the action of the antagonist, the response to S-sulpho-D-cysteine being only slightly antagonized.

TABLE 2.   Amino acids with mixed NMA and non-NMA receptor agonist activity in frog spinal cord.

D-Cysteate[1]	L-Homocysteate[2]	L-Cysteate[2][2]
Ibotenate[2]	L-S-Sulphocysteine[2][2]	D-Aspartate[2]
Aminomalonate[3]	L-Homocysteine sulphinate[2][2]	L-Aspartate[2]
D-Glutamate[2]	D-Homocysteate[1]	D-S-Sulphocysteine[1]
	L-Cysteine sulphinate[2]	L-Glutamate[2]
	D-Cysteine sulphinate[1]	

The amino acids are listed in three indistinctly delineated groups according to the magnitude of the non-NMA receptor component in the responses they produce, this being smallest in the left hand group and largest in the right hand group. References: 1, R.H. Evans, K.N. Mewett, D.A.S. Smith & J.C. Watkins, unpublished observations; 2, Evans et al., 1979;   3, Davies et al., 1982.

'NON-NMA' RECEPTOR AGONISTS

Where the separate isomers of enantiomeric pairs of α-amino acids have been tested, those excitants with actions that are relatively insensitive to the most specific NMA antagonists have all been found to have the L configuration at the aminated carbon atom; such non-NMA agonists also seem generally to possess a chain length between the two acidic groups which is equal to or greater than that present in the maximally or near-maximally extended glutamate molecule. With the exception of kainate and domoate, which may act at a specific sub-type of receptors (see Watkins & Evans, 1981), the most potent non-NMA agonists also appear to have a bulky ω-acidic group in which the negative charge may be distributed over several atoms within delocalized electron systems (Watkins, 1978; Krogsgaard-Larsen et al, 1980).

A selection of non-NMA agonists is shown in Table 3. The first three amino acids shown are relatively weak excitants and are included only to show the structure activity relations of a series of dicarboxylic amino acids from the shortest member, aminomalonate (Table 2) which has pronounced action at NMA receptors, through L-aspartate and L-glutamate (Table 2), which show decreasing action at NMA receptors and a predominant action in both cases at non-NMA receptors (Davies et al 1982a), to L-α - amino-adipate, L-α-amino pimelate and L-α-aminosuberate (Table 3) which show little or no NMA agonist activity (Davies, et al, 1982a). The most potent non-NMA receptor agonists are quisqualate AMPA, ODAP and 5-bromowillardiine while 1-H-2-oxo-6-pyridylalanine and L-DOPA (both relatively weak) and 6-hydroxy DOPA (moderately potent and long acting) are also included in Table 3 to indicate the variability of the terminal acidic moity found in such agonists (Davies. et al, 1982a). Fig.4 gives the structures of some of the most potent non-NMA agonists.

NEW KAINATE ANTAGONISTS

Even the most effective antagonists at non-NMA receptors, for example, (±)-cis-2,3-piperidine dicarboxylate (PDA) and γ-D-glutamylglycine (γ DGG) (see Watkins & Evans, 1981) are considerably less potent than most of the NMA receptor antagonists in current use. Thus, in the isolated spinal cord of the frog or immature rat, effective depression of kainate or quisqualate- induced responses require concentrations of cis-2,3-PDA (Davies et al, 1981b) or γDGG (Francis et al, 1980) that are 2 to 3 orders of magnitude greater

TABLE 3. Amino acid excitants without significant action at NMA receptors in
frog spinal cord.

L-α-Aminoadipate[1]   Quisqualate (L)[2]   Kainate[2]
L-α-Aminopimelate[3]   AMPA[3,4]   Domoate[1]
L-α-Aminosuberate[1]   4-Bromohomoibotenate[4]
                             ODAP (L)[5]
                             Willardiine[6]
                             5-Bromowillardiine[3]
                             L-DOPA[3]
                             6-Hydroxy-DOPA[3]
                             1-H-2-Oxo-6-pyridylalanine[3]

References

1-3, as in Legend of Table 2;   4. Krogsgaard-Larsen et al. 1980;
5 Pearson and Nunn, 1981;   6. Evans et al. 1980.

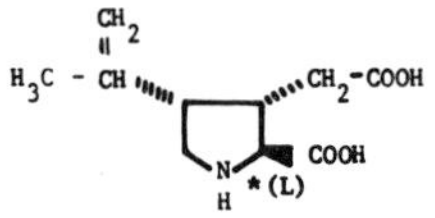

Kainic Acid

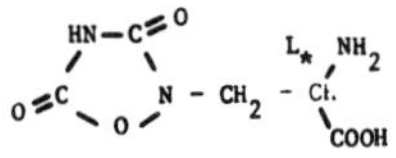

Quisqualic Acid

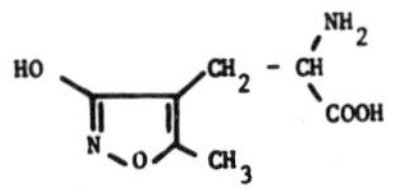

AMPA
((±)-2'-Amino-3-hydroxy-
5-methylisoxazole-4-
propionic acid)

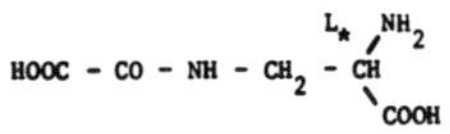

ODAP
(L-β-N-Oxalyl-α,β-diamino-
propionic acid)

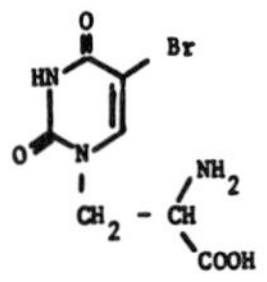

5BW
((±)-5-Bromowillardiine)

Fig. 4. Structures of some excitatory amino acids that produce their actions
mainly at non-NMA receptors.

than those required of AP5 or AP7 to produce comparable depression of NMDA induced responses (Evans et al, 1982). A further disadvantage of cis-2,3-PDA and γDGG is that both these compounds are more effective as NMDA antagonists than as kainate or quisqualate antagonists. The dipeptides γ-D-glutamyl- β alanine, β-D-aspartylglycine, and β-D-aspartyl- β-alanine (Fig. 5) have actions which are qualitatively similar to though somewhat weaker than those of γDGG (Davies etal,1982a). However, sulphonic acid analogues of these dipeptides (Fig.6) possess kainate/quisqualate antagonist activity that is similar to, or slightly higher than, that of the corresponding carboxylic peptides, while showing a very much reduced antagonist activity at NMA receptors (Davies et al, 1982a). Indeed the most potent of these substances, γ-D-glutamylaminomethyl sulphonate (GAMS) antagonizes responses in the cat spinal cord in vivo clearly in the order kainate > quisqualate > NMDA (Davies & Watkins, 1982c). A further point of difference between GAMS and γDGG is that, whereas the latter dipeptide usually depresses quisqualate- and L-glutamate-induced responses in parallel (Davies & Watkins, 1981a) GAMS usually has a considerably greater effect on responses to quisqualate than on those produced by L-glutamate (Davies & Watkins, 1982c). This raises the possibility that quisqualate receptors are distinct from those activated by exogenous L-glutamate, supporting the idea (Luini et al, 1981) of yet further multiplicity with respect to the various sub-types of non NMA receptors that may exist. An example of the action of GAMS on cat spinal neurones is illustrated in Fig.7.

DEPRESSION OF SPINAL SYNAPTIC EXCITATION BY AMINO ACID ANTAGONISTS

The use of excitatory amino acids for characterizing sites of synaptic excitation in the mammalian CNS were recently reviewed (Watkins & Evans, 1981) and are also discussed elsewhere in this symposium. Here some recent observations relating to the differential effects of excitatory amino acid antagonists on mono- and polysynaptic excitation in the spinal cord will be presented.

All NMA antagonists also depress polysynaptic excitation evoked by stimulation of dorsal root fibres in the amphibian and mammalian spinal cords, and, for several series of substances, the relative potencies of the substances are parallel for both antagonism of NMDA-induced and synaptic excitation (Evans et al, 1982). When tested on single cells in the cat spinal cord, NMA receptor antagonists depress the polysynaptic excitation of Renshaw cells and dorsal horn neurones evoked by stimulation of low threshold primary afferent fibres. Thus, NMA receptors seem to mediate the effects of a transmitter liberated from excitatory spinal interneurones. Since L-aspartate-induced responses are often depressed by NMA antagonists in parallel with depression of polysynaptic excitation and in the absence of depression of L-glutamate-induced responses of the same cells, L-aspartate has been considered more likely than L-glutamate to be a transmitter released by spinal interneurones in response to impulses in low threshold primary afferent fibres (Davies & Watkins, 1982b).

The most specific NMA receptor antagonists generally have little or no effect on monosynaptically-evoked excitation of dorsal or ventral horn cells following stimulation of low threshold primary afferent fibres (Evans et al, 1981, 1982; Davies & Watkins, 1981b, 1982a,b). In particular, levels of antagonists that depress responses to NMDA and L-aspartate, but not L-glutamate, usually have no effect on monosynaptic excitation. However, many such monosynaptically-evoked responses are depressed by levels of antagonists that depress kainate, quisqualate and L-glutamate-induced responses in addition to NMDA- and L-aspartate-induced responses of the same cells.(Davies & Watkins, 1981b, 1982b). This has tended to support the view, initially based mainly on neurochemical evidence (Davidoff et al, 1967) that L-glutamate is a likely transmitter to be released by primary afferent terminals in the spinal cord. On the other hand, the newly discovered antagonist GAMS has been found in several instances to depress monosynaptic excitation in the absence of effect on L-glutamate-induced responses (Davies & Watkins, 1982c). An example of this action of GAMS is illustrated in Fig.7.

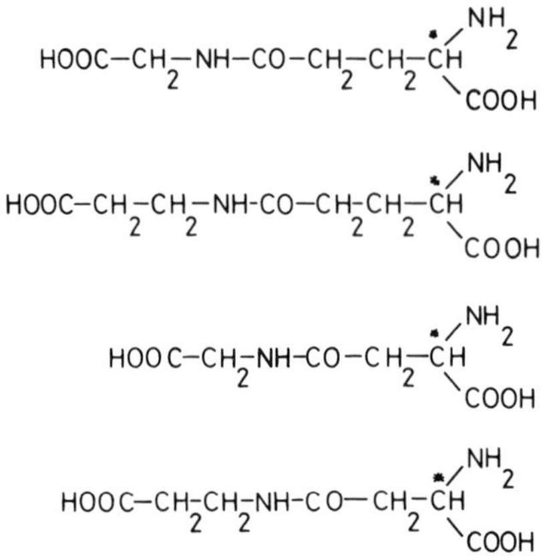

$$\text{HOOC-CH}_2\text{-NH-CO-CH}_2\text{-CH}_2\text{-CH} \underset{\text{COOH}}{\overset{\text{NH}_2}{<}}$$ ɣ-D-GLU-GLY (ɣDGG)

$$\text{HOOC-CH}_2\text{-CH}_2\text{-NH-CO-CH}_2\text{-CH}_2\text{-CH} \underset{\text{COOH}}{\overset{\text{NH}_2}{<}}$$ ɣ-D-GLU-ß-ALA

$$\text{HOOC-CH}_2\text{-NH-CO-CH}_2\text{-CH} \underset{\text{COOH}}{\overset{\text{NH}_2}{<}}$$ ß-D-ASP-GLY

$$\text{HOOC-CH}_2\text{CH}_2\text{-NH-CO-CH}_2\text{-CH} \underset{\text{COOH}}{\overset{\text{NH}_2}{<}}$$ ß-D-ASP-ß-ALA

Fig. 5.   Structures of some dicarboxylic peptides related to γ-D-glutamylglycine. γ-D-GLU-GLY, γ-D-glutamylglycine; γ-D-GLU-β-ALA,
γ-D-glutamyl-β-alanine; β-D-ASP-GLY, β-D-aspartylglycine;
β-D-ASP-β-ALA, β-D-aspartyl-β-alanine.

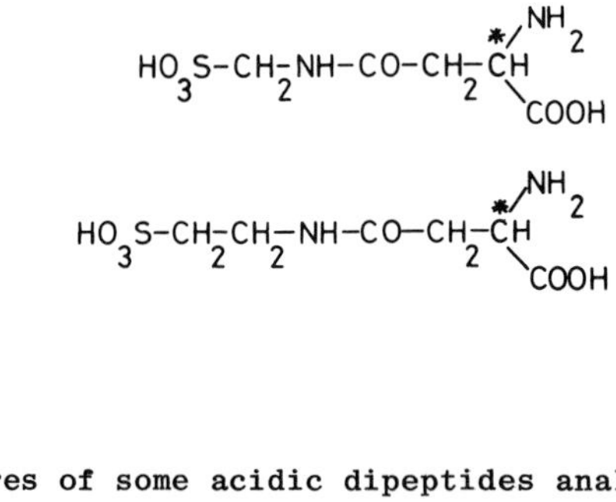

$$\text{HO}_3\text{S-CH}_2\text{-NH-CO-CH}_2\text{-CH}_2\text{-CH} \underset{\text{COOH}}{\overset{\text{NH}_2}{<}}$$ ɣ-D-GLU-AMS (GAMS)

$$\text{HO}_3\text{S-CH}_2\text{-CH}_2\text{-NH-CO-CH}_2\text{-CH}_2\text{-CH} \underset{\text{COOH}}{\overset{\text{NH}_2}{<}}$$ ɣ-D-GLU-TAU

$$\text{HO}_3\text{S-CH}_2\text{-NH-CO-CH}_2\text{-CH} \underset{\text{COOH}}{\overset{\text{NH}_2}{<}}$$ ß-D-ASP-AMS

$$\text{HO}_3\text{S-CH}_2\text{CH}_2\text{-NH-CO-CH}_2\text{-CH} \underset{\text{COOH}}{\overset{\text{NH}_2}{<}}$$ ß-D-ASP-TAU

Fig. 6.   Structures of some acidic dipeptides analogous to those shown in
Fig. 5, but containing a terminal sulphonic acid residue instead
of a carboxylic group. γ-D-GLU-AMS, γ-D-glutamylaminomethylsulphonate; γ-D-GLU-TAU, γ-D-glutamyltaurine; β-D-ASP-AMS,
β-D-aspartylaminomethylsulphonate, β-D-ASP-TAU, β-D-aspartyltaurine.

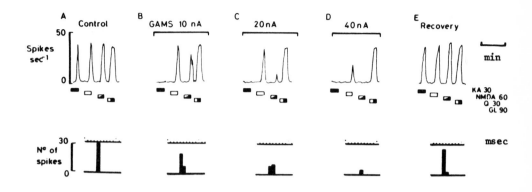

Fig. 7. Action of γ-D-glutamylaminomethylsulphonate (GAMS) on amino acid-
         induced and monosynaptic excitation of a cat dorsal horn neurone.
         Note (upper sequence) selective depression of kainate responses with
         the lowest ejection current of GAMS used (10 nA), with successive
         antagonism of quisqualate and NMDA-induced responses with higher
         ejection currents of the antagonist. The L-glutamate-induced
         response was resistant to the action of GAMS in this cell. Lower
         series shows peristimulus time histograms (64 successive stimuli)
         for the monosynaptic excitation of the same cell following stimula-
         tion of the gastrocnemius soleus nerve. Note that depression of
         this response correlates with the antagonism of kainate and quisqua-
         late but not NMDA or L-glutamate-induced responses.

This raises questions as to the identity of the transmitter released from primary afferent
endings at GAMS-sensitive sites, though it should be emphasized that endogenous and
exogenous L-glutamate may activate different receptors.

ACKNOWLEDGEMENT

This work was supported by the Medical Research Council.

REFERENCES

Biscoe, T.J., R.H. Evans, A.A. Francis, M.R.Martin, J.C.Watkins, J. Davies and A. Dray
     (1977). Nature (Lond) 270, 743-745.
Biscoe, T.J., J.Davies, A.Dray, R.H.Evans, M.R.Martin and J.C.Watkins (1978). Brain
     Res. 148, 543-548.
Cull-Candy, S.G., J.F.Donellan, R.W. James and G.G. Lunt (1976). Nature (Lond), 262,
     408-409.
Curtis, D.R. and J.C.Watkins (1960). J. Neurochem, 6, 117-141.
Curtis, D.R. and J.C.Watkins (1965). Pharmacol. Rev. 17, 347-391.
Davidoff, R.A., R.T.Graham, R.P.Shank, R. Werman and M.H. Aprison (1967). J.
     Neurochem. 14, 1025-1031.

54 J. Davies, R. H. Evans, A. W. Jones, *et al.*

Davies, J., A.A. Francis, A.W. Jones and J.C. Watkins (1981a). Neurosci. Lett., 21, 77-81.

Davies, J., R.H. Evans, A.A. Francis, A.W.Jones and J.C. Watkins. (1981b). J. Neurochem., 36, 1305-1307.

Davies, J., R.H. Evans, A.W. Jones, D.A.S.Smith and J.C. Watkins (1982a). Comp. Biochem. Physiol. 72C, 211-224.

Davies, J., R.H. Evans, A.W. Jones, D.A.S. Smith and J.C. Watkins (1982b). J. Neurochem. Res., in press.

Davies, J. and J.C. Watkins (1979). J.Physiol. (Lond) 297, 621-635.

Davies, J. and J.C. Watkins (1981a). Brain Res. 206, 172-177.

Davies, J. ad J.C. Watkins (1981b). In P.L.Morselli et al., eds. Neurotransmitters, Seizures and Epilepsy. Raven Press, New York, pp 141-149.

Davies, J. and J.C.Watkins (1982a). Brain Res. 235, 378-386.

Davies J. and J.C.Watkins (1982b). Exp. Brain Res., in press.

Davies, J. and J.C.Watkins (1982c). J. Physiol. (Lond), abstr., in press.

Dudel, J. (1977). Pflugers Arch. 369, 7-16.

Evans, R.H., A.A. Francis, K. Hunt, D.J. Oakes and J.C.Watkins (1979). Br. J. Pharmac. 67, 591-603.

Evans, R.H., A.A. Francis, A.W. Jones, D.A.S. Smith and J.C. Watkins (1982). Br. J. Pharmac. 75, 65-75.

Evans, R.H., D.A.S.Smith and J.C.Watkins (1981). J. Physiol. (Lond) 320, 55P.

Evans, R.H., and J.C.Watkins (1981). Life Sci., 28, 1303-1308.

Francis, A.A., A.W.Jones and J.C.Watkins (1980). J. Neurochem. 35, 1458-1460.

Hall, J.G., H. McLennan and H.C. Wheal, (1977).. J. Physiol. (Lond), 272, 52-53P.

Hori, N., C.R.Auker, D.J. Braitman and D.O. Carpenter (1981). Cell Molec. Biol. 1, 115-120.

Irreverre, F., S.H. Mudd, W.D. Heizer and L. Laster (1967). Biochem. Med, 1, 187-217.

Koerner, J.F. and C.W. Cotman (1981). Brain Res., 216, 192-198.

Krogsgaard-Larsen, P., T. Honoré, J.J. Hansen, D.R.Curtis and D. Lodge (1980). Nature (Lond), 284, 64-66.

Luini, A., O. Goldberg and V.I. Teichberg (1981). Proc. Natl. Acad. Sci. 78, 3250-3254.

McLennan, H. (1982a). Eur. J. Pharmacol. 79, 135-137.

McLennan, H. (1982b). Can.J. Physiol. Pharmacol., 60, 91-94.

McLennan, H. and J.G. Hall (1978). Brain Res. 149, 541-545.

Olney, J.W., C.H. Misra, and T. de Gubareff (1975). J. Neuropathol. Exp. Neurol. 34, 166-177.

Perkins, M.N., T.W.Stone, J.F.Collins and K. Curry (1981). Neurosci. Lett., 23, 333-336.

Peet, M.J., J.D. Leah and D.R. Curtis (1982). Brain Res. in press.

Slaughter, M.M. and R.F. Miller (1981). Science, 211, 182-185.

Stone, T.W. and M.N. Perkins (1981). Eur. J. Pharmacol. 72, 411-412.

Watkins, J.C. (1978). In McGeer E.G. et al., eds., Kainic Acid as a Tool in Neurobiology Raven Press, New York, pp 37-69.

Watkins, J.C. (1981). In Roberts, P.J. et al., eds., Glutamate: Transmitter in the Central Nervous System. Wiley, Chichester, England. pp 1-23.

Watkins, J.C. and R.H. Evans (1981). Ann. Rev. Pharmacol. Toxicol. 21, 165-204.

Watkins, J.C., D.R. Curtis and S.S. Brand (1977). J. Pharm. Pharmacol. 29, 324.

White, W.F., J.V. Nadler and C.W. Cotman(1979). Brain Res. 164, 177-194.

White, W.F., J.V. Nalder, A. Hamberger, C.W. Cotman and J.T.Cummins (1977). Nature (Lond), 270, 356-357.

ALTERATION BY KAINATE OF ENERGY STORES AND NEURONAL-GLIAL METABOLISM OF GLUTAMATE *IN VITRO*

WILLIAM J. NICKLAS

Department of Neurology, Rutgers Medical School-UMDNJ,
Piscataway, N. J. 08854, U.S.A.

ABSTRACT

Kainate was found to decrease the energy charge of cerebellar slices and increase inosine monophosphate levels. In addition, it caused leakage of glutamate and aspartate from the tissue and decreased the synthesis of glutamine from a variety of radioactive precursors. These effects were attributed to alterations in glial cells secondary to massive depolarization of neurons. These results and those of others are discussed in terms of their implication for the mechanism of neurotoxicity of excitatory substances.

KEYWORDS

Kainate; glutamate; glutamine; metabolic compartmentation; excitotoxins; neuronal-glial interactions; adenine nucleotides.

INTRODUCTION

Evidence has rapidly accumulated during the past few years that glial cells, as well as neurons, contribute to the metabolism and, therefore, the regulation of the neuroactivity of the amino acids glutamate/aspartate and GABA (see Schoffeniels et al., 1978; Hertz, 1979; Nicklas and Krespan, 1982). These conclusions are, for the most part, consistent with earlier biochemical studies which demonstrated the compartmentation of glutamate metabolism in brain (Van den Berg et al., 1975). Studies on the disparate distribution of key enzymes of glutamate and GABA metabolism (Van den Berg, et al. 1975; Nicklas et al., 1979; Hertz, 1979) as well as those showing active uptake of these amino acids by isolated neuronal and glial cells and tissue culture preparations of these cell types (see Hertz, 1979 for review) indicate that glial cells may play a role in maintaining the extracellular homeostasis of these neuroactive substances (Schrier and Thompson, 1974; Nicklas and Browning, 1978; Hertz, 1979). In a variety of in vivo and in vitro brain preparations exogenous glutamate, aspartate and GABA appear to be metabolized in a "small" metabolic compartment (Berl and Clarke, 1969) which has been associated with glial cells. Central to these concepts, and consistent with the experimentally observed rapid conversion of exogenous glutamate and ammonia to glutamine in brain, is the demonstration of the astrocytic localization of glutamine synthetase (Norenberg and Martinez-Hernandez, 1979) and its coupling to the high affinity, high capacity glial uptake system.

55

An understanding of the metabolism of glutamine, therefore, in the various "compartments" of CNS tissue is probably pivotal to elaborating the regulation of the metabolism of transmitter glutamate/aspartate and GABA. Glutamine has been postulated to be a major precursor of transmitter pools of these neuro-active amino acids (Benjamin and Quastel, 1976; Van den Berg et al., 1975; Bradford and Ward, 1976; Benjamin, 1981). In this way, transmitter glutamate and GABA levels within their respective nerve endings can be maintained by glutamine derived from the extracellular space, which in turn can be replenished by synthesis in the glial cells via glutamine synthetase.

This push-pull hypothesis by which glutamine can be metabolized to glutamate in synapses (presumably, by the enzyme glutaminase) is not dependent on a singular localization of this enzyme to nerve endings. The activity of this highly regulated enzyme is dependent on a number of factors, including the concentration of glutamate which demonstrates product inhibition. Thus, depletion of glutamate in the synapse (by release or decarboxylation to GABA) might, in itself, turn on glutaminase activity (Bradford and Ward, 1976; Benjamin, 1981). Therefore, a control of these systems may depend not merely on the differential distribution of glutaminase between neurons and glia but rather upon a delicate poising of glutamate: glutamine ratios within these cells. A great deal of experimental evidence on the metabolic compart-mentation of amino acid metabolism in brain has shown that labeled precursors such as acetate are preferentially metabolized in the small compartment, i.e., glial cells whereas, others, e.g., glucose, are more ubiquitously metabolized (see Nicklas et al., 1979). Using these substances in dual-labeling experiments coupled with the use of glutaminase or glutamine synthetase inhibitors has recently enabled us to demonstrate directly that glutamine synthesized in glial cells does indeed contribute to transmitter pools of glutamate and GABA according to the above hypothesis (Nicklas and Krespan, 1982; Nicklas, 1982).

Glutamate itself can be neurotoxic (Olney, 1978). Thus, maintenance of low extracellular levels of glutamate via glial uptake and metabolism to glutamine also serves the purpose of deactivating this neurotoxic potential. It was with these thoughts in mind that we undertook several years ago to examine the metabolic effects of excitotoxic amino acid analogues such as kainate. The in vivo complexity of the CNS makes a quantitative determination of the relative contribution of metabolic compartments difficult and, therefore, we have chosen to use the intact rat cerebellar slice in these investigations. The results of these studies have shown numerous deleterious sequelae of kainate treatment of slices, some of which are initially reversible. These changes indicate a disruption of the normal neuronal-glial homeostatic regulation of glutamate metabolism and are compatible with the extreme potency of kainate as a neurotoxin.

STUDIES ON EFFECTS OF KAINATE

As this volume attests, kainate when injected into various brain areas is a potent neurotoxin. However, despite much study the mechanism of its toxicity is not understood. Current theories suggest that interactions between specific receptors for excitatory substances and an altered synaptic input combine to initiate a massive depolarization which leads eventually to neuronal death (McGeer et al., 1978a). For example, lesion of the corticostriatal glutamergic pathway protects against the neurotoxic action of kainate in the striatum (Biziere and Coyle, 1978a; McGeer et al., 1978b). The good correlation which exists between the neurotoxic and excitatory potencies of various glutamate analogues (Olney et al., 1978) also suggests that the neurotoxic activity may be related to changes in ion permeability thereby increasing membrane ATPase activities which decreases stores of creatine phosphate and ATP necessary for maintenance of cellular integrity (Olney et al., 1971; Biziere and Coyle, 1978b). Retz and Coyle (1982) recently showed that kainate injected into mouse striatum caused significant decreases in creatine phosphate and ATP within 30 min after injection; prior decortication protected against these effects. Biziere and Coyle (1978b) had previously shown that high exogenous levels of glutamate or a combination of glutamate and kainate decrease ATP levels in striatal slices. However, the striatal slice is, in a sense, decorticated, and so we thought a better in vitro preparation might be the rat cerebellar slice which contains an intact glutamergic neuron, the granule cell (Tran and Snyder, 1979).

Effects of kainate on nucleotides. It was found that kainate incubated with cerebellar slices altered ATP levels at concentrations (<1 mM) which had no effect on striatal slices. In the experiments described in Table 1, after a preincubation period in normal Krebs-Ringer bicarbonate medium (Nicklas et al., 1980) the slices were incubated for 30 min with the excitotoxic compounds indicated. Maximal decreases of approximately 35% were obtained at 0.4 - 0.7 mM kainate; incubation of up to 10 mM kainate gave no further decrement. Glutamate showed a lesser ATP decrease. Racemate homocysteate was more potent than glutamate but less so than the kainate. The dihydrokainate was included not because it is neurotoxic-it is not-but rather because it is a kainate analogue which is as good (if not better) a glutamate uptake blocker as is kainate (Johnston et al., 1979). The data with N-methyl-aspartate is interesting in that it is a fairly potent toxin in vivo but had no effects in vitro in cerebellar slices even when dihydrokainate was present. This may be because the adult rat cerebellum, unlike newborn cerebellum, may not have an NMA receptor (Schmidt et al., 1977; Foster and Roberts, 1980).

TABLE 1. EFFECT OF VARIOUS AMINO ACIDS OR ANALOGUES ON ATP LEVELS IN ADULT RAT CEREBELLAR SLICES

ADDITIONS	% CONTROL ATP ± S.E.	(N)
10 mM Glutamate	82 ± 3**	(6)
0.01 mM Kainate	102 ± 2	(4)
0.10 mM Kainate	80 ± 3**	(4)
0.50 mM Kainate	65 ± 4*	(3)
1.0 mM Kainate	64 ± 6*	(4)
1 mM D,L-homocysteate	82 ± 6**	(4)
10 mM D,L-homocysteate	67 ± 3*	(4)
1 mM Dihydrokainate	97 ± 7	(6)
1 mM N-methyl-D-aspartate	98 ± 2	(4)
10 mM N-methyl-D,L-aspartate	89 ± 6	(4)

*p <.005   **p< 0.05 from control levels of ATP which were 11.2 ± 0.2 nmol·mg prot^{-1} (N=29). Tissue slices were incubated in Krebs-Ringer bicarbonate medium containing 5.5 mM glucose for 20 min and then transferred to the same medium but with the above additions and incubated a further 30 min. Some of the data are taken from Nicklas et al., 1980; a portion are previously unpublished observations of Krespan and Nicklas.

Preliminary experiments indicate that both kainate and NMA are active in altering nucleotides in cerebellar slices from 12 day old rats (Table 2). In Table 2 the data are expressed in terms of ATP/ADP ratio which is a more sensitive parameter and, in addition, the inosine monophosphate levels are given. The latter reflect the adenosine deaminase activity of the tissue, i.e., the deamination of AMP. It should be noted that kainate in the adult slices and NMA and kainate in the 12-day old slices decrease the ATP/ADP ratio and increase the IMP levels significantly. The effects of an oxidative phosphorylation uncoupling agent (FCCP) and the synaptic depolarizing agent, veratridine are given for comparison. The veratridine-induced changes but not those from kainate, were not observed when the slices were pretreated with tetrodotoxin indicating a fundamental difference between the two phenomena.

TABLE 2.   NUCLEOTIDE CHANGES IN CEREBELLAR SLICES

	ATP/ADP RATIO	IMP nmol·mg protein^{-1}
Adult Rats		
Control	8.22	0.39
10 μM FCCP	0.74*	1.25*
10 μM Veratridine	1.50*	1.40*
1 mM Kainate	3.96*	1.15*
2 mM N-methylaspartate	7.72	0.41
12-Day Old Rats		
Control	13.9	0.23
1 mM Kainate	6.50*	1.04*
2 mM N-methylaspartate	6.72*	0.72*

* $p < .01$ from corresponding control slices

The kainate-induced nucleotide changes were, to some extent, reversible. If the slices were removed to fresh, kainate-free, medium, further incubation increased the ATP levels toward normal (Nicklas et al., 1980). This dose-dependent alteration in nucleotides can be seen within 10 min of incubation time and may correspond to the changes observed in vivo by Retz and Coyle (1982). The concentrations of kainate used - 0.1 to 1 mM - are not unphysiological. Most studies, in which in vivo kainate injections are made, use concentrations of 5 to 10 mM in the injection volume of 0.3 to 1 μl. The local dilutions at the site of injection are probably no more than 10 to 100-fold and, therefore, the acute concentration acting on the cells are within the range in these in vitro studies. Although this pressure on ATP levels is partially reversible, it is likely that continuation of this phenomenon could indeed lead to sufficient cellular damage to cause its demise.

Effects of kainate on amino acids.   There have been several alternative hypotheses proposed concerning the mechanism of kainate toxicity of which two are most tenable:

   1. Direct action on specific dicarboxylic amino acid receptors which induce massive depolarization and eventual cell death (Olney, 1978).

   2. Stimulation of the neurotoxicity of glutamate itself by causing

release of glutamate or inhibition of its reuptake (McGeer et al., 1978a).

To this, I should like to add the following hypothesis, which is, in some ways, a combination of the above.

3. Complex interactions of various sequelae which disrupt the homeostatic systems which normally protect against glutamate toxicity (Nicklas et al., 1980; Krespan et al., 1982).

McGeer et al., (1978a) have discussed the reasons why the first hypothesis cannot completely account for the toxicity of kainate. This group has opted for the second hypothesis by which the toxicity would be indirect and be due to abnormally high levels of glutamate in the synaptic cleft. But this proposal also has difficulties. Kainate has been found to be a moderately potent inhibitor of glutamate uptake both in tissue slices (Johnston et al., 1979) and synaptosomal preparations (McGeer et al., 1978a). The latter point has been disputed (Cox and Bradford, 1978). In our hands, kainate is an inhibitor of the uptake of glutamate by purified synaptosomal preparations with no appreciable effect on that of GABA (Table 3). However, there is no effect of kainate on the veratridine-stimulated release of glutamate, either when kainate was present during the uptake phase (Table 3) or when the synaptosomes were preloaded with radioactive glutamate prior to incubation with kainate (Nicklas and Krespan, 1982). This data, coupled with the observations that dihydrokainate-an equipotent glutamate uptake blocker-is not neurotoxic, seems to argue against the arguments of proposal 2. However, since kainate did have effects on nucleotide metabolism in cerebellar slices, whereas dihydrokainate did not, we decided to look at the possibility of amino acid release from the slices anyway.

TABLE 3. UPTAKE AND STIMULATED RELEASE OF ^{14}C-GLUTAMATE AND ^{3}H-GABA FROM CORTICAL SYNAPTOSOMES.

	GLUTAMATE	GABA
	Uptake, nmole·mg prot^{-1}·5 min^{-1}	
Control	2.40 ± 0.21	0.99 ± 0.09
+ 1 mM Kainate	0.66 ± 0.08*	0.55 ± 0.10
	% VERATRIDINE-RELEASABLE	
Control	35.4 ± 3.8	32.4 ± 2.7
+ 1 mM Kainate	32.9 ± 2.5	31.5 ± 0.3

p <.01 significantly different from control, t test. Synaptosomes were prepared by method of Booth and Clark (1979). After a 5 min preincubation, an aliquot of the preparation in Krebs-Ringer bicarbonate medium with 3 mM glucose was incubated for 5 min with a mixture of 10 μM each ^{3}H-GABA and ^{14}C-glutamate. Tissue and medium were separated by filtration through a Millipore filter. To release prelabeled stores, 10 μM veratridine was added and after 3 min tissue and medium separated by ultrafiltration. Results are average ± S.D. of 3 experiments.

TABLE 4. THE EFFECTS OF KAINATE (KA), N-METHYL-D-ASPARTATE (NMA) AND
DIHYDROKAINATE (DHK) ON LEVELS OF AMINO ACIDS IN CEREBELLAR
SLICES AND INCUBATION MEDIUM.

	TISSUE LEVEL μmol·100 mg prot^{-1}	ADDITIONS TO MEDIUM		
		KA	NMA	DHK
		% Control		
Glutamate	7.15 ± 0.22	80 ± 3*	97 ± 6	97 ± 13
Aspartate	1.71 ± 0.05	64 ± 4*	107 ± 7	113 ± 9
Glutamine	3.16 ± 0.20	35 ± 9*	98 ± 11	101 ± 15
	MEDIUM LEVEL μmol·100 mg prot^{-1} ·2.5 ml^{-1}			
Glutamate	1.58 ± 0.20	243 ± 5*	112 ± 17	147 ± 26
Aspartate	0.35 ± 0.05	334 ±12*	123 ± 7	103 ± 25
Glutamine	6.55 ± 0.49	96 ± 6	102 ± 5	104 ± 12

*p <.005 significantly different from control, t test. After 15 min
preincubation at 37°, cerebellar slices were incubated a further 30 min with
no additions or 1 mM KA, NMA or DHK. The results are average ± S.D. of 8
slices for controls and 4 each for other conditions. Data taken from Nicklas
et al, 1980.

When adult rat cerebellar slices were incubated with kainate, glutamate was
released into the medium (Table 4) (Nicklas et al., 1980; Krespan et al.,
1982). There was a 15-30% decrease in tissue levels of glutamate and aspartate
with two-to-three-fold increases in the medium concentrations. The actual
glutamate concentration reached in the medium in these experiments was about
70 μM. Similar to the ATP results, dihydrokainate or N-methyl-D-aspartate had
minimal effects on amino acids. The time and kainate concentration-dependen-
cies were also similar to those found for the nucleotides. Thus, there was a
lag period of about 10 min and with 0.3 mM kainate the glutamate efflux was
about 60% of that observed with 0.6 mM or above. Neither GABA levels in the
tissue nor in the medium were appreciably altered by any concentration of
kainate (Nicklas et al., 1980; Krespan et al., 1982). The alterations in
glutamate/aspartate were not totally unexpected, but the large (60-70%)
decrease in glutamine tissue levels were surprising. These slices normally
synthesize and accumulate glutamine because this neutral amino acid is easily
diffused into the medium (Krespan et al., 1982); this accumulation was
completely inhibited by 1 mM kainate. Other experiments indicated that
kainate had no direct effects on the enzyme activities of either glutamine
synthetase or glutaminase nor did it interfere with glutamine transport
(Krespan and Nicklas, unpublished observations). The kainate-induced
alterations in glutamate efflux and glutamine synthesis were not observed with
striatal slices. These results are consistent with the hypothesis of McGeer
et al., (1978a) that an enhanced synaptic activity of glutamate is responsible
for the actual neurotoxicity of kainate. However, the negative experiments
cited above for direct involvement of uptake/release mechanisms caused us to
examine further the nature of glutamate efflux, especially the site(s) from
which the glutamate is released.
As discussed earlier, studies of amino acids in brain have demonstrated that

the metabolism of glutamate, glutamine and GABA are compartmentalized and that some of these metabolic compartments have been proposed to be localized to certain cellular types. The use of radioactive precursors to label one or more of these "pools" preferentially has proven a most useful tool. For example, because of its avid labeling of glutamine, acetate is thought to be preferentially metabolized in glia, whereas glucose is more ubiquitously metabolized (Van den Berg and Garfinkel, 1971; Baláẑs et al., 1973; Nicklas et al., 1979). These hypotheses have been used to elaborate the cellular basis of action of a number of substances with CNS activity. For example, one can determine whether a given agent causes a preferential release of amino acids from glia or nerve endings. Minchin (1977) showed that in spinal cord slices veratridine enhanced the efflux of glucose-labeled glutamate, but not of acetate-labeled glutamate. This was consistent with studies in which it was shown that synaptosomal preparations can form, and are stimulated to release glucose-but not acetate-labeled glutamate (de Belleroche and Bradford, 1972; Bradford et al., 1978). In addition, glucose-labeled glutamate is released from slices in a Ca^{2+}-dependent manner (Potashner, 1978; Hamberger et al., 1979). Therefore, experiments were carried out using various radio-active precursors with cerebellar slices either prior to or after treatment with kainate (Nicklas et al., 1979; Nicklas et al., 1980; Krespan et al., 1982).

The labeling data corroborates those obtained on level changes of amino acids. Since glutamine synthetase is present in glial cells in high levels compared to neurons, precursors which are primarily metabolized extraneuronally give rise to the so-called "compartmentation effect." With such compounds, the specific radioactivity of glutamine isolated from the tissue is usually much greater than that of glutamate from the same tissue (Berl and Clarke, 1969; Van den Berg et al., 1975). This ratio is, therefore, very sensitive to agents which interfere with the metabolism of this "small" compartment in which glutamine is synthesized (Clarke et al., 1970).

TABLE 5. EFFECT OF KAINATE (KA) ON THE RELATIVE LABELING OF AMINO ACIDS FROM VARIOUS RADIOACTIVE PRECURSORS.

PRECURSOR		RELATIVE SPECIFIC ACTIVITY (Glutamate=1)	
		GLUTAMINE	ASPARTATE
[^{3}H] acetate	Control	7.93 ± 1.85	0.15 ± 0.02
	1 mM KA	2.87 ± 0.28*	0.23 ± 0.04**
[2-^{14}C] glucose	Control	0.90 ± 0.18	0.57 ± 0.07
	1 mM KA	0.68 ± 0.15**	0.46 ± 0.06
[U-^{14}C] GABA	Control	1.74 ± 0.33	10.5 ± 1.9
	1 mM KA	0.36 ± 0.13*	11.2 ± 2.8
[U-^{14}C] Glutamate	Control	4.43 ± 0.22	0.57 ± 0.03
	1 mM KA	3.21 ± 0.92**	0.49 ± 0.07
[U-^{14}C] Glutamine	Control	10.1 ± 0.6	0.48 ± 0.04
	1 mM KA	20.3 ± 5.6**	0.34 ± 0.05*

*$p < .005$; ** $p < 0.05$ different from control, t test. Cerebellar slices were preincubated 15 min then transferred to fresh medium with and without 1 mM KA. After 30 min incubation, one of the above labeled precursors was added for 10 min. Data taken from Krespan et al., 1982.

As is evident from Table 5, the synthesis of glutamine was indeed impaired by

preincubation of the slice with kainate. The data with ^{3}H-acetate and ^{14}C-GABA
are especially illustrative in this regard. In fact, with GABA, the only
radioactivity change seen in the tissue slice was the decreased labeling of
glutamine. It should be noted that labeling of glutamate itself from
^{3}H-acetate was decreased by kainate pretreatment (Krespan et al., 1982).
Interestingly, Watkins (1971) found that the in vivo labeling in mouse brain
of glutamate and glutamine from ^{14}C-acetate was decreased by injection of
N-methyl-D-aspartate or glutamate. To determine the origin of the released
glutamate, tissue slices were preincubated with radioactive precursors prior
to incubation with kainate (Table 6). Under control conditions, <10% or <2%
of the total radioactivity present in acetate-or glucose-labeled glutamate,
respectively, was spontaneously leaked into the medium. In the presence of
kainate the effluxes of both species were enhanced six-to-seven-fold with no
apparent differences between the two precursors. Measurement of the specific
radioactivities of glutamate in the tissue and medium indicated that kainate
released the more newly-synthesized glutamate.

TABLE 6.   RELEASE OF LABELED GLUTAMATE FROM CEREBELLAR SLICES PREVIOUSLY
INCUBATED WITH D-[2-^{14}C]-GLUCOSE AND [^{3}H] ACETATE.

PRECURSOR	FRACTION RELEASED[a]	
	[2-^{14}C] GLUCOSE	[^{3}H] ACETATE
Control	0.017 ± 0.002	0.079 ± 0.007
1 mM KA	0.126 ± 0.012*	0.475 ± 0.034*
Control	0.014 ± 0.003	0.046 ± 0.015
10 μM Veratridine	0.051 ± 0.007*	0.049 ± 0.010

*p <.005, different from control, t test. Cerebellar slices were incubated
with a mixture of [^{14}C] glucose and [^{3}H] acetate for 20 min. The slices were
then transferred to fresh medium to which was added either KA, veratridine or
their respective control vehicles. Data taken from Krespan et al., 1982.
[a] Fraction released = (dpm glutamate in medium)/(total glutamate dpm).

In contrast, veratridine did not alter the fraction of acetate-labeled
glutamate released into the medium but preferentially released the glucose-
labeled glutamate (Table 6). The veratridine-, but not the kainate-induced
efflux of glutamate, was completely blocked by 3 μM tetrodotoxin. Therefore,
if tetrodotoxin-blocked veratridine release of glutamate reflects synaptic
pools, it would appear that kainate also releases another from compartment,
probably glial. Minchin (1977) similarly argued in his experiments that,
whereas veratridine released from nerve endings preferentially, 50 mM K$^+$
released glutamate from both neurons and glia. Therefore, the proposal of
McGeer et al., (1978a) that kainate causes increased extracellular levels of
glutamate appears to be true, at least in cerebellum, in vitro. However, the
source of this glutamate is extrasynaptic, probably glial.

Mechanistic implications of cerebellar slice data. The third proposal for the
mechanism of toxicity of kainate seems to be most compatible with all the
data. The initiating factor is probably an interaction with a "kainate"
receptor, one of the dicarboxylate amino acid receptor sites. This triggers a
potent depolarization of the neuron—whether this is dendritic, somal or axonal

is not completely clear. But the data would seem to indicate that a primary effect on synaptic endings does not occur. The disruption of ionic fluxes which ensues probably effects the astrocytes. Neuronal depolarization causes a depolarization of surrounding glial processes which may be linked to K^+ currents (Hösli et al., 1979). Evans (1980) showed that excitatory amino acids cause dose-dependent, large increases of extracellular $[K^+]$ in the dorsal horn of hemisected frog spinal cords; prolonged treatment causes an irreversible loss of synaptic activity. High extracellular $[K^+]$ would be expected to swell astrocytes accompanied by an enhanced influx of Na^+, Cl^{-1} and H_2O (Bourke et al., 1981). This would put pressure on the Na^+, K^+-ATPase to restore the membrane potential and lower ATP levels in the glia. This is probably the cause of the astrocytic swelling seen after kainate injection in vivo (Herndon et al., 1980). Both sequelae are also consistent with the labeling data especially that using acetate. ATP depletion would decrease acetate activation via acetate thiokinase as well as decrease glutamine synthetase activity. In addition, high $[Na^+]$ was found to be inhibitory to acetate activation both in studies with enzyme preparations (Von Korff, 1953) as well as in metabolic studies with cortical slices (Chan and Quastel, 1967). The secondary swelling of astrocytes might also alter their ability to retain the normally high levels of intracellular glutamate and it is this glutamate which is released into the medium by kainate. In studies with glioma cultures, it was found that kainate had no direct effect on glutamate uptake or retention but increasing $[K^+]$ caused a 50% decrease in maximal glutamate uptake (Browning and Nicklas, 1982).

TABLE 7.   EFFECT OF VERATRIDINE OR KAINATE PRETREATMENT ON RELEASABILITY OF GLUTAMATE FROM CEREBELLAR SLICES.

ADDITIONS TO MEDIUM		MEDIUM GLUTAMATE
PREINCUBATION	INCUBATION	μmol$\cdot$100 mg prot$^{-1}\cdot$2$\cdot$5 ml^{-1}
None	None	0.30
Veratridine	None	0.36
None	Veratridine	0.67[a]
Veratridine	Veratridine	0.49
Kainate	None	0.39
None	Kainate	0.99[a]
Veratridine	Kainate	1.45[a,b]
Kainate	Veratridine	1.28[a,b]

[a] p <.005 significantly different from no addition to incubation medium.
[b] p< .005 significantly different from corresponding no addition to preincubation medium.
Cerebellar slices were preincubated for 15 min then to this preincubation medium was added either nothing, 10 μM veratridine or 1 mM kainate for 10 min. The drugs were then washed away and the slices reincubated with and without drugs for 20 min. Results are average for 3-4 slices. Data are taken from unpublished work of Krespan and Nicklas.

All of these sequelae would be deleterious to neurons. Not only is the neuron depolarized but extracellular glutamate levels increase and the role of the glial cell in maintaining glutamate homeostasis via uptake and glutamine synthesis is severely impaired. However, the apparent necessity for the integrity of an excitatory (presumptively glutamergic) input (McGeer et al.,

1978a; Biziere and Coyle, 1978a) remains somewhat puzzling. Perhaps the members of the super-compartment consisting of synapse, post-synapse and surrounding glial cells are "clamped" into given potentials by the intact innervation which renders them more susceptible to massive depolarization by kainate. Some support for this hypothesis is shown in the experiment illustrated in Table 7. As stated earlier, both kainate and veratridine cause glutamate release into the medium with kainate-induced release being somewhat greater (Table 7). However, if the tissues are preincubated with veratridine and then transferred to a medium with kainate, the glutamate release is even more enhanced. Similar results are seen with pretreatment with kainate followed by veratridine. In contrast, veratridine pretreatment followed by a second incubation with veratridine showed no such increased release. Thus, the normal state of electrical activity in a tissue may be sufficient to predispose that tissue to kainate neurotoxicity. Intact excitatory inputs would, therefore, be necessary to demonstrate the phenomenon.

In any case, the actions of kainate, and probably the other excitotoxic amino acids as well, are much more complex than originally thought. Our data, as well as that of others, suggest that biochemical and morphological alterations of glia occur acutely after exposure of the tissue to kainate. These effects are suggested to be causally related to the eventual neuronal degeneration. This interpretation raises other possibilities in investigating the general problem of neuronal death in degenerative neuronal disorders.

ACKNOWLEDGEMENT

Portions of this work were supported by U.S.P.H.S. grants MH 25505 and NS 17360. The author wishes to thank Dr. Graham Johnston for providing the dihydrokainate and N-methyl-D-aspartate.

REFERENCES

Baláazs, R., A.J. Patel and D. Richter (1973). In: Metabolic Compartmentation in the Brain, (R. Balazs and J. Cremer, eds.) pp. 167-184, MacMillan Press, London.
Benjamin, A.M. (1981). Brain Res., 208, 363-377.
Benjamin, A.M. and J.H. Quastel (1976). J. Neurochem., 26, 431-441.
Berl, S. and D.D. Clarke (1969). In: Handbook of Neurochemistry, Vol. 2, (A. Lajtha, ed.), pp. 447-472, Plenum Press, New York.
Biziere, K. and J.T. Coyle (1978a). Neurosci. Lett., 8, 303-310.
Biziere, K. and J.T. Coyle (1978b). J. Neurochem., 31, 513-520.
Booth, R. and J.B. Clark (1979). FEBS Lett., 107, 387-392.
Bourke, R.S., H.K. Kimelberg, M.A. Daze et al., (1979). In: Neural Trauma, (A.J. Popp, R.S. Bourke and L.R. Nelson, eds.) pp. 95-113, Raven Press, New York.
Bradford, H. and H.K. Ward (1976). Brain Res., 110, 115-125.
Bradford, H.F., J.S. de Belleroche and H.K. Ward (1978). In: Amino Acids as Chemical Transmitters, (F. Fonnum, ed.) pp. 367-377, Plenum Press, New York.
Browning, E.T. and W.J. Nicklas (1982). Trans. Am. Soc. Neurochem., 13, 264.
Chan, S.L. and J.H. Quastel (1967). Science, 156, 1752-1753.
Clarke, D.D., W.J. Nicklas and S. Berl. (1970). Biochem. J., 120, 345-351.
Cox, D.W.G. and H.F. Bradford (1978). In: Kainic Acid as a Tool in Neurobiology, (E.G. McGeer, J.W. Olney and P.L. McGeer, eds.) pp. 71-93, Raven Press, New York.
de Belleroche, J.S. and H.F. Bradford (1972). J. Neurochem., 19, 585-602.
Foster, G.A. and P.J. Roberts (1980). Life Sci., 27, 215-221.
Evans, R.H. (1980). J. Physiol., 298, 25-35.

Hamberger, A., G.H. Chiang, E.S. Nylen, S.W. Scheff and C.W. Cotman (1979). Brain Res., 168, 513-530.

Herndon, R.M., E. Addicks and J.T. Coyle (1980). Neuroscience, 5, 1015-1026.

Hertz, L. (1979). Prog. Neurobiol., 13, 177-223.

Hösli, L., P.F. Andres and E. Hösli (1979). J. Physiol. (Paris) 75, 655-659.

Johnston, G.A.R., S.M.E. Kennedy and B. Twitchin (1979). J. Neurochem., 32, 121-127.

Krespan, B., S. Berl and W.J. Nicklas (1981). Trans. Am. Soc. Neurochem., 12, 150.

Krespan, B., S. Berl and W.J. Nicklas (1982). J. Neurochem., 38, 509-518.

McGeer, P.L., E.G. McGeer and T. Hattori (1978a). In: Kainic Acid as a Tool in Neurobiology, (E.G. McGeer, J.W. Olney and P.L. McGeer, eds.) pp. 123-138, Raven Press, New York.

McGeer, E.G., P.L. McGeer and K. Singh (1978b). Brain Res., 139, 381-383.

Minchin, M.C.W. (1977). Exp. Brain Res., 29, 515-526.

Nicklas, W.J. (1982). Trans. Am. Soc. Neurochem., 13, 221.

Nicklas, W.J. and E.T. Browning (1978). J. Neurochem., 30, 955-963.

Nicklas, W.J., R. Nunez, S. Berl and R.C. Duvoisin (1979). J. Neurochem., 33, 839-844.

Nicklas, W.J., B. Krespan and S. Berl (1980). Eur. J. Pharmacol., 62, 209-213.

Nicklas, W.J. and B. Krespan (1982). In: Neurotransmitter Interaction and Compartmentation, (H.F. Bradford, ed.) Plenum Press, New York and London.

Norenberg, M.D. and A. Martinez-Hernandez (1979). Brain Res., 161, 303-310.

Olney, J.W. (1978). In: Kainic Acid as a Tool in Neurobiology, (E.G. McGeer, J.W. Olney and P.L. McGeer, eds.) pp. 95-122, Raven Press, New York.

Olney, J.W., O.L. Ho and V. Rhee (1971). Exp. Brain Res., 14, 61-76.

Potashner, S.J. (1978). J. Neurochem. 31, 187-195.

Retz, K.C. and J.T. Coyle (1982). J. Neurochem., 38, 196-203.

Schmidt, M.J., J. Thornberry and B.B. Molley (1977). Brain Res., 121, 182-189.

Schoffeniels, E., G. Franck, L. Hertz and D.B. Tower, eds. (1978). Dynamic Properties of Glial Cells., Pergamon Press, Oxford.

Schrier, B.K. and E.J. Thompson (1974). J. Biol. Chem., 249, 1769-1780.

Tran, V.T. and S.H. Snyder (1979). Brain Res., 167, 345-353.

Van den Berg, C.J. and D.A. Garfinkel (1971). Biochem. J., 123, 211-218.

Van den Berg, C.J., A. Reijnierse, G.G.D. Blockhuis, M.C. Kroan, G. Ronda, D.D. Clarke and D. Garfinkel (1975). In: Metabolic Compartmentation and Neurotransmission, (S. Berl, D.D. Clarke and D. Schneider, eds.) pp. 515-543, Plenum Press, New York.

Von Korff, R.W. (1953). J. Biol. Chem., 203, 265-271.

Watkins, J.C. (1971). J. Neurochem., 18, 1733-1739.

RECEPTORS FOR EXCITOTOXINS

PETER J. ROBERTS and GEORGE A. FOSTER

Department of Physiology and Pharmacology, University of Southampton,
Southampton, SO9 3TU, U.K.

I. INTRODUCTION

"Excitotoxins" represent a very special group of neurotoxic substances, in that they act upon specific somatic and dendritic receptors such that if the excitation produced is of sufficient magnitude, the neurones die.

In general, each of the excitotoxins (the prototype being kainate, KA) is an agonist of close structural similarity to L-glutamate and other potential excitatory amino acid neurotransmitters. Olney and his colleagues were the first to evaluate the relationship between excitatory potency and neurotoxic potential (see Olney, 1978) and reported that each of the agents investigated produced an acute, axon-sparing, neurotoxicity; the severity of which was directly proportional to the iontophoretic potency of the excitotoxin under examination. Table 1. indicates the major substances which have been shown to possess axon-sparing excitotoxic properties and other, endogenous substances of expected neurotoxic potential.

TABLE 1.   EXCITOTOXINS

A. Exogenous Excitotoxins:	
kainate	N-methyl-D-aspartate (NMDA)
quisqualate	cyclopentylglutamate
(±) ibotenate	cis-piperidine dicarboxylate
α-amino-3-hydroxy-5-methylisoxazole-4-propionate (AMPA)	
dipiperidinoethane	
B. Putative Endogenous Excitotoxins:	
L-glutamate	S-sulphocysteine*
L-aspartate	N-acetylaspartyl glutamate
L-cysteine sulphinate	DL-β-hydroxybutyryl-asp-asp-glu
L-homocysteate*	folates
L-homocysteine sulphinate*	quinolinic acid
	acetylcholine

* Not yet identified in brain.

Because of the close structural similarities between these substances, it has been widely proposed that their neurotoxicity is mediated through postsynaptic receptors, possibly those activated physiologically by the neurotransmitter candidates,

glutamate or aspartate. Recently however, it has been reported that dipiperidino-
ethane, an agent which resembles the potent cholinergic agonist, oxotremorine,
mimics the convulsant and neurotoxic actions of KA (Olney et al., 1980). Further
studies with several cholinergic agonists, and the anticholinesterases, physostigmine and neostigmine (Olney et al., 1982), suggest that acetylcholine may play
a role in at least seizure-linked neurotoxic mechanisms.

In the peripheral nervous system, there is certainly a precedent for acetylcholine
-induced neurotoxicity. At the mouse neuromuscular junction, anticholinesterases
and carbachol produce cellular damage which may be prevented by α-bungarotoxin
(Salpeter,1981; Salpeter et al., 1979). In addition, removal of calcium from the
medium results in full protection against toxicity. In dystrophic mice, which have
high levels of calcium-activated proteases, exposure to carbachol results in a
greater toxicity, which is again preventable by zero calcium.

II. EXCITOTOXIN RECEPTORS AND THEIR SIGNIFICANCE IN RELATION TO NEUROTOXICITY

It is still far from clear how excitotoxic agents produce cell death. For example,
do each of the agents listed in table 1. act in a similar manner ? While the
actual molecular mechanisms involving the receptors may differ, it seems likely
that a final common process is involved. Implicit to the term "excitotoxic" cell
death, is the concept that these substances by virtue of their great excitatory
potency (eg. KA), or by swamping the perikaryal or dendritic neuronal membranes
(eg. glutamate) effect a state of continuous depolarization. A distinction has to
be made here between increased firing of neurones and prolonged depolarization.
In the latter state, the homeostatic mechanisms of the cell become strained,with
eventual shutting down of Ca^{2+} extrusion mechanisms. The sustained increases in
intracellular Na^+ may cause release of intracellular bound Ca^{2+} pools. Calcium
might then represent the common pathway in toxic cell death by activation of intra
-cellular proteases (Schanne et al., 1979; Farber, 1981), following increased
plasma membrane Ca^{2+} permeability, increased intracellular mobilisation from SER
and a loss of mitochondrial buffering capacity. It is noteworthy for example,
that the most vulnerable neurones in the hippocampus have a high Ca^{2+} influx. On
the other hand, KA toxicity appears not to be blocked by EDTA, EGTA or by verapamil and other calcium channel blockers (Roberts, unpublished). This does not
discount the theory however, because calcium may enter down its very large concentration gradient, irrespective of specific channels.

Thus, excitotoxicity is an event occurring beyond the formation of the initial
excitotoxin-receptor complex. What then may studies of their receptors tell us
about the mechanisms of excitotoxicity ?

(i)   The possible nature of the natural endogenous (excitotoxic) transmitter
        with whose receptors the excitotoxin is interacting.
(ii)   The possibility of cooperative interactions between excitotoxins and
        endogenous excitatory transmitters.
(iii)   The ionic and enzymatic (eg activation of guanylate cyclase) consequences
        of receptor activation.
(iv)   The possibility of interfering with excitotoxic actions by pharmacological
        agents. In the case of putative endogenous excitotoxins where their aberr-
        ant behaviour may possibly result in neurodegenerative disorders (eg.
        Huntington's disease, olivopontocerebellar atrophy etc.), new pharmacol-
        ogical antagonists may provide new strategies for the therapy of these
        diseases.

III.   APPROACHES FOR THE INVESTIGATION OF EXCITOTOXIN RECEPTORS

Here, discussion will be limited to the excitotoxic amino acids and congeners.

A. Neurophysiological Studies

Approximately 100 α-amino acids have been found to have excitatory actions at
vertebrate central neurones (Watkins, 1978). Almost without exception, these
compounds have one cationic and two anionic groups. One of the latter is a carbox-
ylate group, and the cationic group is a primary or secondary amino group. The
most potent excitatory amino acids include KA, quisqualate and N-methyl-D-aspartate (NMDA), which have been widely used for receptor characterisation; their
rigid or restricted cyclical structures offer major advantages over the prototype
compounds, such as glutamate or aspartate. Many of these studies have been carried
out employing the technique of microiontophoresis combined with extracellular
recording. However, there are major limitations inherent to the approach, eg
localisation of receptors compared with sites of application and recording; avid
uptake sites for natural amino acids etc.

Systematic studies over many years by Watkins and his colleagues have suggested
that there are at least three types of excitatory amino acid receptor. The development of selective and reasonably potent antagonists has strengthened this view
(Watkins, 1981a); divalent metal ions (Mg^{2+}, Co^{2+}, Mn^{2+}), long chain aminodicarbox
-ylic acids (D-α-aminoadipate, DL-α-aminosuberate), the phosphonoaminoacids
(2-amino-5-phosphonovalerate and 2-amino-7-phosphonoheptanoate), cyclic compounds
(cis-2,3-piperidinedicarboxylate) and dipeptides (eg. γ -D-glutamylglycine)
exhibited selective actions against NMDA-type receptors while affecting the responses to KA, glu/asp or quisqualate variably, and generally weakly. While NMDA
was originally proposed as an analogue acting at physiological aspartate receptors
(Johnston et al., 1974), the pharmacological data would suggest that NMDA acts at
receptors for some other excitatory agent. While NMDA receptor pharmacology has
been reasonably well characterised, this cannot be said for the other postulated
receptor types, largely because of the lack to date, of suitable antagonists. It
is still unclear how many types, or sub-types of receptor are represented by the
non-NMDA category. L-glutamate diethylester (GDEE) has been reported to antagonise
quisqualate and glutamate, but not KA-induced responses in cat spinal neurones
(Davies and Watkins, 1979; McLennan and Lodge, 1979). However, this compound is a
rather unreliable antagonist, with an uncertain mode of action. However, γ-D-
glutamyl glycine will discriminate between quisqualate and KA receptors, selectively depressing spinal responses elicited by the latter compound (Watkins, 1981b).
The most potent antagonist at quisqualate receptors is cis -2,3-PDA. However,
this substance also blocks NMDA and KA receptors.

L-glutamate and L-aspartate can be considered as mixed agonists, since the actions
of both of these substances are susceptible to each of the antagonists currently
available. This point indicates therefore, that glu and asp should not be used in
isolation in any study to investigate receptor characteristics, unless there is
other a priori evidence (eg neurochemical) that glu or asp is likely to be the
transmitter at a particular synapse. As yet, it is not possible to identify excitatory amino acid transmitters acting at specified synapses from the sensitivity
of cells to agonists and antagonists.

B. Binding Studies

Over the last few years there has been an explosive development in the application of binding studies to the investigation of receptors. Binding studies per se
probably represent one end of the spectrum, with iontophoresis, patch-clamping
and intracellular recording at the other. While the electrophysiologist must live
with the uncertainty of the site of drug application and recording of responses,
in drug binding studies, the problem is much greater. In the general situation
where a crude synaptic membrane preparation is being employed, to what receptors
(and other binding sites) is the labelled ligand likely to be exposed ? Clearly,
there are quite a number of possibilities:

(i)   Postsynaptic receptors; i.e. the receptors it is hoped to label.
(ii)   Subpopulations or different classes of receptor with which the ligand may
           interact in a similar manner.
(iii)   Extrajunctional and non physiologically-active (vestigial) receptors.
(iv)   Presynaptic receptors; e.g. a glu receptor present on say a DA or ACh
           nerve terminal, possibly involved in the regulation (modulation) of trans-
           mitter release.
(v)   Presynaptic autoreceptors.
(vi)   Receptor/ionophore complex.
(vii)   Neurotransmitter uptake sites (not necessarily Na^+-dependent) on neuronal
           and glial elements.
(viii)   Synthetic and degradative enzymes

Thus, the ability to detect specific binding of an excitotoxin may allow us to
discern very little about the receptor involved. For the excitatory amino acids,
which play major roles in cellular biochemistry, it is evident that the possibility of interactions with an array of binding sites is of prime importance. In
addition to this problem of site heterogeneity (and, as we have seen, within
the receptors themselves - we have the likelihood of 3 or 4 receptor populations
at least), we are faced with a present lack of suitable labelled probes. The
ligands currently available include: agonists - KA, AMPA, NMDA, glutamate,
aspartate and quinolinic acid, and antagonists - 2-APV, 2-APH, 2-APB and D-α-am-
inoadipate (largely directed against NMDA-type receptors). Finally, the lack of
suitably selective (with a few exceptions) and potent pharmacological agents for
displacement studies, renders the definition of specific sites problematical. It
is to be expected that although Scatchard analysis of agonist binding may yield
linear plots, inhibition curves obtained with the current antagonists may reveal a
complex heterogeneity of sites.

Notwithstanding these inherent problems, a number of laboratories have carried out
studies on the binding of the available ligands to membranes prepared from the
mammalian CNS, and a large family of binding sites has emerged, with affinities
ranging from nanomolar to millimolar. Additionally, the distribution of the sites
and their pharmacological characteristics, support the concept that at least some
of these sites may represent excitatory receptors. Direct comparisons with electrophysiologically derived data are always tenuous, since "binding" is essentially
an uncoupled event, whereas the firing of a cell is dependent upon a number of
subsequent integrated processes.

B(i) Specific binding of L-glutamate -   The earliest experiments aimed at investigating glutamate receptors, involved studies with the invertebrate neuromuscular junction, where glutamate is almost certainly the natural transmitter.
Hydrophobic proteins were extracted, and were found to bind glutamate specifically
(Lunt, 1973; De Plazas and De Robertis, 1974). Extension of this approach to the
mammalian CNS (DeRobertis and De Plazas, 1976) involving chloroform-methanol extraction of rat cerebral cortex, revealed three binding sites for glutamate. However
apart from the high-affinity site (K_D= 0.3 μM) which was stereoselective for
L-glutamate, they were of such high capacity that it would seem unlikely that
they represented physiological receptors.

Utilizing a different strategy, Michaelis et al., (1974) and Roberts (1974) described independently, the specific sodium-independent binding of L-glutamate to
synaptic membrane fractions. More recently, Foster and Roberts (1978) have characterised extensively the binding of L-glutamate to freshly-prepared cerebellar
synaptic membranes. Binding occurred to an apparently homogeneous population of
sites and was saturable with a K_D = 744nM and a max. capacity of 73 pmol/mg
protein. Binding was enriched in synaptic membranes and occurred optimally under
physiological conditions of temperature, pH etc. Pharmacological agents used as

inhibitors of glutamate binding, provided the best evidence that this cerebellar glutamate binding site may be equivalent to the receptor in this tissue (Table 2).

TABLE 2.   INHIBITION OF L-^{3}H-GLUTAMATE (0.8 μM) BINDING TO RAT CEREBELLAR SYNAPTIC MEMBRANES

Agonist	K_i (μM)	Hill Coefficient*
L-glutamate	2.3	0.97
D-glutamate	13.9	0.92
L-aspartate	20.3	0.66
D-aspartate	66.4	1.06
(±)-ibotenate	3.9	0.62
quisqualate	3.2	0.83
DL-homocysteate	5.3	-
cis-cyclopentylglutamate	8.6	0.52
L-cysteine sulphinate	10.4	0.86
∝-ketokainate	120.6	0.60

* From Slevin et al., (1982). The following were inactive: KA, ∝-allo-KA, dihydrokainate, NMDA, AMPA and quinolinic acid.

L-glutamate was the most potent inhibitor, followed by quisqualate and ibotenate. 1-amino-1,3-dicarboxycyclopentane (cis-cyclopentylglutamate) was approx. 3.5 times less active than L-glutamate, suggesting that glu interacts with its binding site in an extended form. Thus, D- and L-aspartate and particularly NMDA, were poor inhibitors of binding. Binding was unaffected by threo-3-hydroxy-β-aspartate and by DL-aspartate-β-hydroxamate; thus binding was unlikely to have been to uptake sites (Roberts and Watkins, 1975). As can be seen in table 2. quisqualate, cyclopentylglutamate, L-cysteine sulphinate and ∝-ketokainate had Hill coeffs. significantly less than unity, providing evidence of receptor site heterogeneity (Slevin et al., 1982).

TABLE 3.   INHIBITION OF GLUTAMATE BINDING TO CEREBELLAR SYNAPTIC MEMBRANES BY EXCITATORY AMINO ACID ANTAGONISTS

Antagonist	K_i (μM)	Hill coefficient *
D-∝-aminoadipate	6.3	-
(±)-2APB	5.5	0.58
(±)-2APV	15.9	0.54
(±)-2APH	17.5	-

* From Slevin et al., (1982). Inactive: GDEE, HA-966, γ-D-glutamyl-glycine, L-methionine-DL-sulphoximine.

In relation to the proposed antagonists of glutamate-induced depolarization, D-∝-aminoadipate (Biscoe et al., 1977) and 2-amino-4-phosphonobutyrate (2APB) (Cull-Candy et al., 1976) were the most potent (Table 3.). The higher phosphonate analogues, 2APV and 2APH both exhibited activity as expected, but their Hill coefficients were again less than unity, indicating site heterogeneity. A number of other pharmacologically active agents, GABA, glycine, baclofen, N-acetyl-asp, pentobarbitone, substance P, diazepam, were all inactive.

The binding of L-glutamate has recently been shown to be capable of modification by ions, in particular calcium (Baudry and Lynch, 1979,1980; Fagg et al., 1982) and chloride (Mena et al., 1982; Fagg et al., 1982). Calcium enhances glutamate binding, although Cl^- is a requirement for this effect to be manifest. Inhibition of glutamate binding in the presence of Ca^{2+} and Cl^- is similar to the inhibitory effects observed electrophysiologically at the perforant path-granule cell synapse of hippocampus. Fagg et al (1982) suggest that there are two distinct populations of sodium-independent glutamate binding sites on synaptic membranes, distinguishable on the basis of their Ca^{2+}/Cl^- -dependence. Further evidence for a major role of calcium at the glutamate receptor comes from the finding of a modulatory effect of concentrations of calmodulin, likely to be encountered in the synaptic cleft (Bardsley and Roberts, unpublished).

It therefore seems likely that a variety of factors are involved in the regulation of the glutamate receptor system (for a discussion of this topic, see Roberts, 1981). Michaelis et al., (1981) have proposed a major role for brain gangliosides; more recently, Foster et al. (1982) have shown that the phospholipid, phosphatidyl serine is a good inhibitor of 2-APB -sensitive L-glutamate binding.

The glutamate-binding macromolecule from synaptic membranes has been solubilised and purified by Michaelis and his colleagues (Michaelis et al., 1981) and it is a small molecular weight glycoprotein (M_r approx=13,000). The protein was found to form aggregates which have higher specific activity at low (nanomolar)concentrations of glutamate. While the overall affinity of the purified protein was lower than that of the membrane high-affinity sites, the pharmacological characteristics of the solubilised binding sites were very similar to those encountered in the membranes. The glutamate binding glycoprotein is an iron-containing metalloprotein whose activity is dependent on the integrity of its metallic centre (this contrasts with properties of glutamate transport carriers).

In summary, the binding of L-glutamate to synaptic membranes probably involves several sites, which may be discriminated on the basis of the actions of agonists and antagonists. The pharmacological specificity of binding is consistent with labelling of a specific excitatory receptor. It is pertinent to note that several of the most potent excitotoxins listed in Table 1. (eg. KA, NMDA, AMPA,quinolinic acid) do not influence glutamate binding.

B (ii) Binding of L-aspartate   -   Characterisation of binding sites for L-aspartate is at a very preliminary stage. Fiszer de Plazas and De Robertis (1976) investigated binding to proteolipids and identified three sites. For the high-affinity site (K_D = 0.2 μM), L-aspartate and NMDA were potent inhibitors of binding, while L-glutamate and D-aspartate were only weakly active. D-aspartate did however inhibit binding to the medium affinity site. We have recently begun to investigate the binding of $L-^3H$-aspartate to freshly prepared (binding of glu and asp is lost with freezing), sonicated, and extensively-washed synaptic membranes (Sharif and Roberts, 1981). The binding characteristics were rather similar to those observed with glutamate with regard to affinity (K_D=874 nM) and effects of ions, temperature, pH etc. However, the density of sites was less, and the pharmacological specificity of binding was different in several respects from the glutamate system (Table 4.)

Quisqualate and 2-APB, which were good inhibitors of glutamate binding were only weakly active on the aspartate system. Similarly, the potent excitotoxins, KA and NMDA and quinolinic acid were inactive. Ibotenate, which appears from electrophysiological experiments to interact preferentially with NMDA-preferring receptors, was active, as were the NMDA antagonists, HA-966 , 2-amino-5-phosphonovalerate (2APV) and 2-amino-7-phosphonoheptanoate (2APH). DiLauro et al. (1982) have reported the binding of L-aspartate to whole brain membranes and their results are insubstantial agreement with our own. Again, NMDA (the proposed aspartate receptor preferring agonist) was totally devoid of any inhibitory activity on binding.

TABLE 4.   INHIBITION OF SPECIFIC L-^{3}H-ASPARTATE BINDING TO RAT CEREBELLAR
SYNAPTIC MEMBRANES

Compound	K_i (μM)
L-glutamate	1.3
L-aspartate	3.3
(+)-ibotenate	6.6
DL-α-aminosuberate	6.6
HA-966	6.9
(-)-2APV	25.2
(+)-2APV	40.6
(+)-2APH	49.4
L-cysteine sulphinate	82.4
D-α-aminoadipate	237
D-aspartate	301

Inactive: KA, quisqualate, NMDA, DL-homocysteate, 2-APB, GDEE,
quinolinic acid, DL-threo-3-hydroxyaspartate.

Since electrophysiological studies on NMDA receptors have largely been carried out
in spinal cord, we have recently (Butcher and Roberts, in preparation) examined
aspartate binding to spinal cord synaptic membranes. Complex binding patterns were
observed, with the apparent presence of at least 3 sites of K_D's= 10 nM, 800 nM
and 40 μM.At all labelled aspartate concentrations investigated, L-asp, L-glu,
(+)-ibotenate, L-cysteate and cysteine sulphinate were potent displacers. NMDA
could also inhibit binding to some degree, but this was totally unrelated to
concentration.

Thus, at the present time we can say that there are sites for L-aspartate quite
distinct from those for glutamate. Whether they are relevant to a physiological
aspartate receptor is as yet uncertain.However, it is striking that binding is
not inhibited by NMDA to any significant degree, which is in accord with current
ideas of the nature of the NMDA receptor, deduced from electrophysiological studies.

B (iii)   NMDA receptors and the possible endogenous NMDA-like excitotoxic
transmitter   -   NMDA exhibits high activity when applied iontophoretically to
spinal neurones (McCulloch et al., 1974). A single brief abstract has appeared
(Snodgrass, 1979) describing the binding of ^{3}H-NMDA to cerebellar membranes,with
a K_D = 9.8nM. Binding was antagonised effectively by aspartate, DL-homocysteate
and DL-α-aminoadipate, while L-glutamate was a weak displacer. However, our
laboratory and others (eg Ramirez et al, 1981; Olverman and Watkins; Johnston,
personal communications) have not found it possible to replicate these initial
findings. It may be that the affinity of NMDA for its (low density of) receptors
is too low. Several groups (unpublished) are currently investigating the binding
of ^{3}H-DL-2APV and 2APH to brain membranes, and have found that these ligands are
bound specifically and are sensitive to inhibition by NMDA.

Since it is apparent that L-aspartate is a relatively poor candidate for the natural ligand acting at the NMDA recptor, one might propose that either NMDA interacts with a specific site associated with the receptor and/or ionophore, distinct
from the transmitter recognition site, or that there is an alternative endogenous
ligand. Discovery of such a natural ligand would be of major importance considering the potent excitotoxic properties of both NMDA and ibotenate, which appear to
act through the same receptor mechanism. To this end, Stone and Perkins (1981)
reported that the endogenous compound, quinolinic acid (2,3-pyridine dicarboxylic

acid) is a potent excitant, possibly acting preferentially on NMDA receptors, since its actions were antagonised by 2-APV. Injected intra-striatally or into the hippocampus, quinolinic acid has pronounced neurotoxic properties which are antag- onised by 2-APV and 2-APH (Schwarcz et al., 1982). Thus the possible availability of labelled quinolinic acid and its readily available structural analogues, may facilitate the investigation of NMDA receptors, and NMDA receptor-mediated excitotoxicity.

B (iv) Kainic acid binding -   Because glutamate may interact with an array of binding sites, the binding of KA, a conformationally-restricted analogue was originally studied (Simon et al., 1976) following the assumption (not now accept- ed generally) that KA is a specific agonist for glutamate receptors. Although glu- tamate is an effective inhibitor of KA binding, the converse is not true, with only 10% or less of specific glutamate binding being susceptible to inhibition by KA (Foster and Roberts, 1978). Michaelis et al, (1980) have reported a dissociat- ion of KA and glutamate binding sites, following mild treatment of membranes with cholate (Table 5.)

TABLE 5.   EFFECTS OF CHOLATE TREATMENT OF SYNAPTIC MEMBRANES ON ^{3}H-KAINATE AND ^{3}H-GLUTAMATE BINDING

Preparation	kainate binding	Glutamate binding
	pmol/mg protein	
Control membranes	0.173 ± 0.057	5.26 ± 0.9
0.5% cholate-treated membranes	0.084 ± 0.055	17.08 ± 2.17
0.5% cholate soluble supernatant	0.065 ± 0.026	0.10 ± 0.02

From Michaelis et al., 1980.

Since the original study by Simon et al (1976), several other workers have confir- med and expanded upon these findings (Johnston et al., 1979; Beaumont et al., 1979; London and Coyle, 1979a,b; Schwarcz and Fuxe, 1979; Vincent and McGeer, 1979). In the detailed study of binding characteristics by London and Coyle (1979a), two apparent populations of KA binding site were identified in rat fore- brain membranes, with K_D's of 7.8 and 37.6 nM. In the cerebellum (where KA has powerful neurotoxic actions) only a single, low affinity (K_D=50nM) population of sites was detected. Binding exhibited a highly selective susceptibility to inhib- ition (Table 6). Determination of Hill coefficients for L-glutamate, dihydro- kainate and D-glutamate, yielded values substantially less than 1.0, indicating a negative cooperativity between these substances, or alternatively, multiple site interactions. This again reinforces the idea that KA does not act at the bulk of glutamate receptors. The electrophysiological evidence also suggests disc- rete but interacting receptor populations. KA potentiates the neuroexcitatory actions of glutamate (Shinozaki and Konishi, 1970) and also the stimulation of cyclic GMP production by glutamate (Foster and Roberts,1980, and see later).

It appears that the ^{3}H-KA binding sites do represent the receptors mediating the compound's neurophysiological and excitotoxic actions, since KA lesions are accompanied by a loss of KA binding sites (Beaumont et al., 1979). Of interest in relation to this observation is the finding that the regional distribution of KA binding sites correlates only very roughly with the regional neurotoxicity of kainate (Schwarcz and Fuxe, 1979). However, since the neurotoxic action of KA is dependent upon the "permissive effect" of an intact excitatory innervation (McGeer et al., 1978), this lack of correlation is not unexpected.

TABLE 6.   INHIBITION OF SPECIFIC 3H-KAINATE BINDING TO CEREBELLAR MEMBRANES

Compound	K_i (μM)	Hill Coefficient
kainate	0.023	0.98
ketokainate	0.40	0.91
L-glutamate	0.44	0.61
quisqualate	0.65	0.90
D-glutamate	49.0	0.63
dihydrokainate	59.0	0.38

Weak or inactive: allokainate, ibotenate, cyclopentylglu, DL-homocysteate, NMDA, 2-APB, D-α-aminoadipate, GDEE (from Coyle et al., 1981)

Thus, if KA does not interact with the major glutamate receptor, is it therefore a substrate for a subset of glutamate receptors (eg. 5-10% of the total glutamate sites), or are KA receptors for an as yet unidentified endogenous substance, such as one of the sulphur-containing amino acids, or perhaps a small, glutamate-containing peptide? A number of workers have examined the latter possibility, and Ruck et al. (1980) reported that methyltetrahydrofolate (MTHF) and other folate derivatives were potent inhibitors of 3H-KA binding to cerebellar membranes. Folate and derivatives do have convulsive properties in experimental animals (Spector, 1971; Hommes and Obbens, 1972) and are therefore reasonable theoretical candidates for an endogenous ligand. However, it was reported recently that the MTHF has no direct excitatory effects on spinal neurones, but produces some inhibitory effects (McLennan, 1982). Following from the initial observations of Ruck et al., Olney et al. (1981) and Roberts et al (1981), demonstrated that MTHF and other folates possessed minimal direct neurotoxic properties; also, the latter workers failed to find any evidence for an interaction of MTHF with KA receptors as determined by their lack of ability to increase levels of cyclic GMP. Thus the status of folates as possible endogenous KA-mimetics remains uncertain at present.

B (v) Binding of other potential endogenous excitotoxic substances   - As is evident from Table I., there are a large number of other potent excitants which may interact with one or more of the excitatory amino acid receptors so far classified. To date, the majority of these substances have not been investigated in binding studies. L-cysteine sulphinate has recently been subject to study, since this substance satisfies many of the criteria required of a neurotransmitter. It is an excitant (Curtis et al., 1972), is present with its synthetic enzymes in nerve terminals (Recasens and DeLaunoy, 1981; 1982a) and there exist transport and binding sites for this substance (Recasens et al., 1982a,b). Specific L-3H-cysteine sulphinate (CSA) binding was enriched in synaptic membranes. CSA was the most potent displacer of binding, with L-glutamate being the next most active. There appeared to be several binding sites invoved, some of which were common to both CSA and glutamate, and others which were separate. CSA binding was not inhibited by KA or NMDA, or by D-glutamate, and only weakly by L-aspartate. Other substances recently subject to investigation, include an endogenous peptide (N-acetyl-aspartyl-glu), which possesses high affinity for L-glutamate, but not for KA receptors (Zaczek et al., 1982). After intra-hippocampal injection, this dipeptide caused a prolonged seizure disorder, similar to that produced by the selective agonist, quisqualate.

B (vi) Summary of binding studies -   In comparison with "traditional" neuro-transmitters and many drug receptors, there is still a very long way to go in the characterisation of the binding sites for excitatory amino acids and their excitotoxic analogues. The KA receptor(s) is probably the best understood from binding studies at this stage (cf. the NMDA receptor from electrophysiological approaches), although its relationship to glutamate or other endogenous excitants is not known. While the information accumulated for the glutamate binding site is totally consistent with its being linked to the receptor(s), that for aspartate is not yet so convincing. The NMDA receptor, which, as mentioned above, has been so well characterised by electrophysiological studies, so far, remains largely inaccessible by the binding approach.

Because of the inherent limitations of binding studies, which become particularly acute with regard to the excitatory amino acids, it is useful to develop other strategies as adjuncts to investigation of their receptors solely by the former approach.

C. Cyclic Nucleotides and Excitatory Amino Acid Receptors

The chief disadvantage of the binding approach, is that no information is gained as to a pharmacological response. The ability of a transmitter to activate or inhibit adenylate, or guanylate cyclases, or to modify ion fluxes, permits the possibility of a more direct approach. However, in relation to _physiological_ responses, one is faced with the uncertainty as to whether the interaction of the transmitter with its receptor does indeed produce that effect, at physiological concentrations _in vivo_.

C (i)   Agonists   -   L-glutamate and related substances were reported to produce a Ca^{2+}-independent activation of adenylate cyclase (Shimizu et al.,1974),although there were a number of anomalies concerning the pharmacological specificity. Our own particular interest has been directed towards the ability of excitatory amino acids to increase the concentrations of cyclic GMP, particularly in cerebellum. This area of the CNS contains unusually high concentrations of cyclic GMP and L-glutamate produces small increases in this nucleotide in slices of mouse (Ferrendelli et al., 1974) or rat (Schmidt et al., 1974,1977) cerebellum incubated _in vitro_, and to cause larger increases after i.c.v. injection (Briley et al.,1979).

TABLE 7.   STRUCTURE-ACTIVITY RELATIONSHIPS FOR THE STIMULATION OF CYCLIC GMP
CONCENTRATIONS BY EXCITATORY AMINO ACIDS

Compound	EC_{50} (mM)	Potency relative to glutamate	
		cyclic GMP	Excitation*
L-glutamate	1.2	1	1
D-glutamate	0.7	1.7	0.5
L-aspartate	1.4	0.9	1
D-aspartate	1.4	0.9	0.5
cis-cyclopentylglu	0.05	24	10
trans-cyclopentylglu	0.86	1.4	-
NMDA	0.06	22	7-18
(±)-ibotenate	0.17	6.5	2-7
4-fluoroglutamate	0.16	8.0	1
Kainate	1.0	1.2	8-80
DL-homocysteate	0.3	4	3-6
α-ketokainate	3.0	<1	-
dihydrokainate	>3	≪1	0.06
L-cysteate	0.6	2	1
L-cysteine sulphinate	0.51	2.4	1

* Data from Watkins (1978)

Recently, it was demonstrated that during a short period of postnatal development, (days 8-14 after birth), glutamate was able to elicit very large increases in cyclic GMP in rat cerebellar slices (Garthwaite and Balázs, 1978). In our pharmacological studies, we have investigated the effects of glutamate and related amino acids in cerebella from young animals.

L-glutamate produced a dose-related increase in cyclic GMP levels in 0.5x0.5 mm cerebellar slices from 8-day old rats, with an EC_{50} of 1.2mM (Foster and Roberts, 1980). The maximum stimulation occurred at 10mM, and gave a peak concentration of approximately 100 pmol cGMP/mg protein, which was an almost 200 fold increase over basal levels. A large number of excitatory amino acids have been examined in this system, and in general, their potencies were close to those for excitation of mammalian neurones (Table.7). Where comparative electrophysiological data have been available, the potencies of these compounds, both in absolute terms, and relative to glutamate, are very similar to those we have observed in vitro. The only exception to this was KA, which despite being substantially more potent than glutamate in depolarizing spinal neurones, was only equipotent with glutamate in stimulating cyclic GMP. However, the peak of KA's efficacy in increasing cyclic GMP, occurs at postnatal days 15-20; some 7-12 days later than that for glutamate. It may be that the variation in its ontogeny can account for this discrepancy.

C (ii) Antagonists   -   A number of excitatory amino acid antagonists have been investigated for ability to inhibit the cyclic GMP response to either glutamate, NMDA, or KA. Each of these agonists possessed a different pharmacological profile (Table 8.)

TABLE 8.   INHIBITION OF THE STIMULATION OF CYCLIC GMP LEVELS BY EXCITANT AMINO ACIDS

Antagonist	Agonist				
	L-glu (1mM)	L-asp (1mM)	NMDA (0.3mM)	($\pm$)ibo (1mM)	KA (1mM)
GDEE	0.25	1.0	>1.0	>3	0.1
($\pm$)-2APB	2.9	>3	>3	>3	>3
D-α-aminoadipate	>3	>3	>3	2.0	-
2-APV	3.2	0.25	0.054	0.08	0.01
γ-DGG	>3	0.25	0.55	1.0	0.074
cis-PDA	>3	3.0	1.2	0.3	0.3
HA-966	>3	1.3	0.19	0.95	0.25
(+)-2APH	-	-	0.45	-	-
(-)-2APH	-	-	0.06	-	-

Results are concentrations of antagonist producing 50% inhibition of response to respective agonist. - = Not tested.

The most potent inhibitor of glutamate stimulation of cyclic GMP, was L-glutamate diethylester (GDEE) with an apparent K_i = 1 mM. In contrast, the effects of NMDA were antagonised most effectively by 2-APV, with an apparent K_i of 15 μM, and the phosphonoheptanoate. KA however, showed an exceptional sensitivity to inhibition by nearly all the antagonists tested, and detailed analysis revealed that this effect was totally non-competitive (Foster and Roberts, 1981). Ca^{2+} ions are able to overcome this antagonism of the KA response, although it is uncertain whether these drugs are acting at or near a calcium-binding site, or are able to induce a membrane conformational change which subsequently inhibits calcium binding. However, it is clear that KA does not act at NMDA, or glu-type receptors. Of the other agonists, aspartate ressembled glutamate in its sensitivity to antagonists, and ibotenate was like NMDA.

C (iii)   Ionic effects   - Tetrodotoxin (TTX), which blocks sodium channels was
without effect at concentrations up to 0.3mM, whereas the Ca^{2+} channel antagonist,
verapamil (0.01-1 mM), or calcium-free medium, completely abolished the response.
Mg^{2+} (2mM) however, was almost inactive, and Mn^{2+} (10 mM) produced only a 50%
reduction in the stimulation by glutamate. Merely raising the intracellular Ca^{2+}
by using the ionophore, A23187, or the mitochondrial Ca^{2+} uptake inhibitor, ruth-
enium red, was an insufficient stimulus alone, to cause a major increase in cyclic
GMP. For example, the maximal effect of A23187, which occurred at 10 μM, was less
than one tenth of that seen with glutamate. Thus the dependence on Ca^{2+} would
appear to be at the membrane, rather than involving an intracellular location.

It has been suggested (Watkins and Evans, 1981) that stimulation of cyclic GMP
production may be secondary to depolarisation and the concomitant release of K^{+}.
However, protoveratrine (PTV) which prevents the closing of voltage-dependent
Na^{+} channels existing in neuronal, but not in glial membranes, and which produces
selective release of transmitter substances, was ineffective in 8 day old animals
in enhancing cyclic GMP production. By 16 days of age, it produced a stimulation
as high as that caused by glutamate (Foster and Roberts, 1981). It is pertinent
that the depolarisation-evoked, Ca^{2+}-dependent release of endogenous glutamate
from cerebellar slices, only becomes apparent by this age. The response to PTV
is markedly attenuated by the antagonist GDEE, but not by the NMDA receptor-type
antagonists, 2-APV or DL-α-aminosuberate.

C (iv).   Localization of excitotoxin receptors and cyclic GMP response   -
In the rat cerebellum, KA produces potent neurotoxic effects on all inhibitory
cell types (Purkinje cells, Basket, Golgi II and stellate cells) while largely
sparing the excitatory granule cells (Herndon and Coyle, 1977; Foster and Roberts
1980). The Purkinje cells which receive a glutamatergic input from the granule
cells and a probable glutamate/aspartate innervation from the climbing fibres, are
for a number of reasons considered to be the major location of the enhanced cyclic
GMP activity. Several workers have localised cyclic GMP itself (Chan-Palay and
Palay, 1979; Cumming et al., 1979), its synthetic enzyme, guanylate cyclase (Ariano et al., 1982; Zwiller et al., 1981), or the protein kinase, for which it is a
selective cofactor (Lohmann et al., 1981), utilising immunocytochemical techniques
in fixed tissue. Data obtained in these studies have differed substantially and
furthermore, suffer from the major disadvantage of not discriminating between
those sites sensitive to excitatory amino acids, and those exhibiting merely basal
activity.

We have utilised alternative approaches, producing specific lesions to individual
cerebellar cell types. X-irradiation of rat cerebellum 8-15 days postnatally results in a large reduction in granule cell population (70%) accompanied by a small
reduction in synaptosomal D-^{3}H-aspartate uptake, and a 60% attenuation of Ca^{2+}-
dependent glutamate release from superfused cerebellar slices. Cyclic GMP levels
were not altered by either glutamate or KA. However, there was a consistent major
reduction in the ability of PTV to stimulate cyclic GMP production. Thus this diminution of the response via the endogenous substance released by PTV indicates
that this substance originates from the parallel fibre terminals.

Rather similar data have been obtained by using 3-acetylpyridine (3-AP) for effec-
ting complete destruction of the inferior olive, the sole source of climbing fibres (Foster and Roberts, 1982). Within 3 days of treatment, D-^{3}H-aspartate uptake
was reduced by 40%; however, no change in the release of either endogenous glutamate or aspartate was observed. The loss of the climbing fibre input did result in
a 40% decrease in the maximal effect of PTV in stimulating cyclic GMP, with no
change in the EC_{50} for this substance. Again, no difference was observed in the
dose-response curves for either glutamate or KA, indicating that the CF's themselves do not possess receptors for these compounds. It does appear though, that

PTV is releasing an endogenous glutamate-like substance from the CF terminals, which interacts with the only target structure, the Purkinje cell dendrites.

C(v) Kainate - glutamate interactions - As discussed earlier, not only in young animals was KA less potent than either glutamate or NMDA, but it produced a max- imum stimulation of cyclic GMP formation only 50% of that of either of the latter compounds. When KA was however combined with glutamate, a synergistic effect on cyclic GMP formation was observed, and the KA dose-response curve was shifted to the left of either glutamate or NMDA. Neither NMDA nor aspartate produce more than additive effects with KA (Foster and Roberts, 1981). Thus these data demonstrate a major interaction at the cellular level (probably postsynaptic) between KA and glutamate.

C(vi) Summary - At present, the role of excitatory amino acid-stimulated cyclic GMP in the central nervous system, and cerebellum in particular, is unknown. It is not likely that it mediates the fast depolarisation associated with afferent act- ivation; rather, it might fulfil a role in mediating changes in neuronal sensitiv- ity by regulating various intra-membrane, or intracellular events.

Whatever the function of cyclic GMP in this system, its measurement does provide a most valuable model for assessing the stimulation of excitatory amino acid recept- ors, and as such, it has already provided us with clues as to the mode of action of KA and other excitotoxins.

IV. OTHER POSSIBLE RECEPTOR SYSTEMS AND THEIR USE AS MODELS FOR EXCITOTOXIN
RECEPTOR INVESTIGATION

A. Presynaptic Amino Acid Receptors

In the rat striatum, glutamate and analogues, including KA and NMDA, are potent stimulants of ^{3}H-dopamine release from tissue slices (Sharif and Roberts,1978; Roberts and Anderson, 1979), while NMDA congeners evoke a TTX- and Mg^{2+}-sensitive release of acetylcholine. The precise localisation of these receptors is unknown, although in the former case, KA lesions of the striatum effectively abolished the response, implicating interneuronal involvement.

In the hippocampus, we have recently reported (McBean and Roberts, 1981) that glu- tamate and several other neuroactive analogues inhibited the calcium-dependent, K^+-evoked release of D-^{3}H-aspartate from mini-slices. This effect was abolished by selective amino acid antagonists (GDEE, APV, and DL-α-aminosuberate) and, as it was TTX-insensitive, may be mediated through presynaptic autoreceptors. In this study, KA was without effect. However, when it was extended to the release of end- ogenous glutamate, KA (50-100 μM) was found to possess a marked releasing action (Roberts and Holden-Dye, unpublished). This is in accord with a recent report by Ferkany et al. (1982) who have reported that in several areas of brain, KA causes a significant release of both aspartate and glutamate by a calcium-dependent process. These findings of a further type of interaction, in addition to at the postsynaptic site, between glutamate and KA, are of important significance for excitotoxic mechanisms.

B. Postsynaptic systems

Michaelis and his colleagues (1981) have documented the presence of functional glutamate receptors in synaptosomes and resealed synaptic membranes, by the demonstration of activated Na^+ fluxes across these membranes. More recently, Teichberg et al. (1981) have preloaded tissue slices with Na^+ and have then inves- tigated the efflux of this ion during exposure to amino acids and other depolar- ising stimuli . In the striatum for example (Table 9.), NMDA was the most potent

TABLE 9.   RELATIVE POTENCY OF EXCITATORY AMINO ACIDS IN INDUCING ^{22}Na$^+$ EFFLUX
FROM PRELOADED RAT STRIATAL SLICES

NMDA	80.0	D-glutamate	1.2
DL-homocysteate	11.6	L-glutamate	1.0
kainate	6.6	L-aspartate	0.6
quisqualate	6.4	dihydrokainate	0.6
KA methyl ketone	5.2	DL-α-aminoadipate	0.2
carboxy kainate	2.5		

After Teichberg et al., 1981

agonist in stimulating ^{22}Na$^+$ efflux. Also, when slices were exposed to a depolarising concentration (40 mM) of K$^+$, the efflux rate was increased, presumably due to
an indirect action through release of endogenous excitatory transmitter. Striking-
ly, this effect was antagonised by NMDA antagonists (2-APV, DL-α-aminoadipate,
γ-D-glutamylglycine etc.), suggesting that the natural transmitter is an NMDA-
like substance. However, these results are somewhat difficult to reconcile with
the now very substantial evidence in support of glutamate's candidature as the
major cortico-striatal excitatory transmitter, and the glutamate-KA interactions
occurring in striatal neurotoxic mechanisms. However, using this technically
simple Na$^+$ efflux assay system, Teichberg has provided most interesting data, and
recently has attempted to categorize the natural transmitter of several areas of
the CNS, viz. striatum, NMDA-like; cortex, NMDA-like; hippocampus, glutamate-like;
cerebellum, glutamate-like, and substantia nigra, kainate-like. Whether this syst-
proves to have a major predictive value for identifying excitatory transmitters/
potent excitotoxins remains to be elucidated. Bearing in mind the complexity of
excitatory amino acid receptor systems, answers concerning the mechanisms of
action of the excitotoxins which appear to be so closely related to glutamate
and aspartate in particular, are likely to come only from a diversity of model
systems - binding, cyclic GMP systems, ion flux measurements, and transmitter
interactions, when investigated at the neurochemical level.

ACKNOWLEDGEMENTS

This work was supported by grants to P.J.R. from the Wellcome Trust, the Science
and Engineering ResearchCouncil, and the Nuffield Foundation. G.A.F. was an
S.E.R.C. Research Student.

REFERENCES

Ariano, M.A., J.A. Lewicki, H.J. Brandwein and F. Murad (1982). Proc. Natl. Acad.
    Sci. USA., 79, 1316-1320.
Baudry, M., and G. Lynch (1979). Nature, Lond., 282, 748-750.
Baudry, M., and G. Lynch (1980). Proc. Natl. Acad. Sci. USA., 77, 2298-2302.
Beaumont, K., Y. Murrin, T.D. Reisine, J.Z. Fields, E. Spokes, E.D. Bird and H.I.
    Yamamura (1979). Life Sci.,24, 809-816.
Biscoe, T.J., R.H. Evans, A.A. Francis, M.R. Martin, J.C. Watkins, J. Davies and
    A. Dray (1977). Nature, Lond., 270, 743-745.
Briley, P.A., J.C. Kouyoumdjian, M. Haidamous and P. Gonnard (1979). Eur. J.
    Pharmacol., 54, 181-184.
Chan-Palay, V., and S.L. Palay (1979). Proc. Natl. Acad. Sci. USA., 76, 1485-1488.
Coyle, J.T., R. Zaczek, J. Slevin and J. Collins (1981). In Glutamate as a Neuro-
    Transmitter, Eds: G. DiChiara and G.L. Gessa, Raven Press, N.Y. pp 337-346.
Cull-Candy, S.G., J.F. Donnellan, R.W. James and G.G. Lunt (1976). Nature, Lond.,
    262, 408-409.

Cumming, R., G. Arbuthnott and A.L. Steiner (1979). J. Cycl.Nucl.Res., 5, 463-467.
Curtis, D.R., A.W. Duggan, D. Felix, G.A.R. Johnston, A.K. Tebēcis and J.C. Watkins (1972). Brain Res, 41, 283-301.
Davies, J., and J.C. Watkins (1979). J. Physiol.(Lond),297, 621-635.
De Robertis, E., and S.F. De Plazas (1976). J. Neurochem.,26, 1237-1243.
De Plazas, S.F., and E. De Robertis (1976). J. Neurochem., 23, 1115-1120.
Di Lauro, A., J.L. Meek, and E. Costa (1982). J. Neurochem., 38, 1261-1267.
Fagg, G.E., A.C. Foster, E.E. Mena and C.W. Cotman (1982). J. Neurosci., in press.
Farber, J.L. (1981). Life Sci., 29, 1289-1295.
Ferkany, J.W., R. Zaczek and J.T. Coyle (1982). Nature, Lond., 298, 757-759.
Ferrendelli, J.A., M.-M. Chang and D.A. Kinscherf (1974). J. Neurochem., 22, 535-540.
Fiszer de Plazas, S., and E. De Robertis (1976). J. Neurochem., 27, 889-894.
Foster, A.C., G.E. Fagg, E.W. Harris and C.W. Cotman (1982). Brain Res, in press.
Foster, A.C., and P.J. Roberts (1980) J. Neurochem., 34, 1191-1200.
Foster, G.A., and P.J. Roberts (1980). Life Sci., 27, 215-221.
Foster, G.A., and P.J. Roberts (1981). Br. J. Pharmacol., 74, 723-729.
Foster, G.A., and P.J. Roberts (1981). Neurosci. Lett., 23, 67-70.
Foster, G.A., and P.J. Roberts (1982). Neuroscience, in press.
Herndon, R.M., and J.T. Coyle (1977). Science, 198, 71-72.
Hommes, O.R., and E.A.M.T. Obbens (1972). J. neurol. Sci., 16, 271-281.
Johnston, G.A.R., D.R. Curtis, J. Davies and R.M. McCulloch (1974). Nature, Lond., 248, 804-805.
Johnston, G.A.R., S.M.E. Kennedy and B. Twitchin (1979). J. Neurochem., 32, 121-127.
Lohmann, S.M., U. Walter, P.E. Miller, P. Greengard and P. de Camilli (1981). Proc. Natl. Acad. Sci. USA., 78, 653-657.
London, E.D., and J.T. Coyle (1979a). Mol. Pharmacol., 15, 492-505.
London, E.D., and J.T. Coyle (1979b). Eur. J. Pharmacol., 56, 287-290.
Lunt, G.G. (1973). Comp. Gen. Pharmacol., 4, 75-79.
McBean, G.J. and P.J. Roberts (1981). Nature, Lond., 291, 593-594.
McLennan, H. (1982). Eur. J. Pharmacol., 79, 307-310.
McLennan, H., and D. Lodge (1979). Brain Res., 169, 83-90.
McCulloch, R.M., G.A.R. Johnston, C.J.A. Game and D.R. Curtis (1974). Exp. Brain Res., 21, 515-518.
McGeer, E.G., P.L. McGeer and K. Singh (1978). Brain Res., 139, 381-383.
Mena, E.E., G.E. Fagg and C.W. Cotman (1982). Brain Res., 243, 378-381.
Michaelis, E.K., M.L. Michaelis, H.H. Chang, R.D. Grubbs and D.R. Kuonen (1981). Molec. Cell Biochem., 38, 163-179.
Michaelis, E.K., M.L. Michaelis and L.L. Boyarsky (1974). Biochim. Biophys. Res. Comm., 87, 106-112.
Michaelis, E.K., M.L. Michaelis and R.D. Grubbs (1980). Febs Letts., 118, 55-57.
Olney, J.W. (1978). In Kainic Acid as a Tool in Neurobiology, Eds, E.G. McGeer, J.W. Olney and P.L. McGeer, Raven Press, N.Y., pp 95-122.
Olney, J.W., T. de Gubareff and J. Labruyere (1982). Nature, in press.
Olney, J.W., T.A. Fuller, R.C. Collins and T. de Gubareff (1980). Brain Res., 200, 231-235.
Olney, J.W., T.A. Fuller and T. de Gubareff (1981). Nature, Lond., 292, 165-167.
Ramirez, G., J. Gómez-Barriocanal, E. Escudero, S. Fernández-Quero and A. Barat (1981). In, Amino Acid Transmitters, Eds, F.V. DeFeudis and P. Mandel, Raven Press, N.Y., pp 467-474.
Recasens, M., and J.P. Delaunoy (1981). Brain Res., 205, 351-361.
Recasens, M., V. Varga., F. Saadoun, F.V. DeFeudis, P. Mandel, G. Lynch and G. Vincendon (1982). Neurochem. International., in press.
Recasens, M., V. Varga, D. Nanopoulos, F. Saadoun, G. Vincendon and J. Benavides (1982). Brain Res., in press.
Roberts, P.J. (1974). Nature, Lond., 252, 399-401.
Roberts, P.J. (1981). In, Glutamate: Transmitter in the Central Nervous System,

Eds, P.J. Roberts, J. Storm-Mathisen and G.A.R. Johnston, John Wiley & Sons Ltd Chichester, pp. 35-54.

Roberts, P.J., and S.D. Anderson (1979). J. Neurochem., 32, 1539-1545.

Roberts, P.J., Foster, G.A. and E.M. Thomas (1981). Nature, Lond., 293,654-655.

Roberts, P.J., and J.C. Watkins (1975). Brain Res, 85, 120-125.

Ruck, A., S. Kramer, J. Metz and M.J.W. Brennan (1980). Nature, Lond., 287, 852-853.

Salpeter, M.M. (1982). Report on workshop on Huntington's Disease, Hereditary Disease Foundation, Baltimore, August 1-2.

Salpeter, M.M., H. Kasprzak, H. Feng and H. Fentuck (1979). J. Neurocytol., 8, 95-115.

Schanne, F.A.X., A.B. Kane, E.E. Young and J.L. Farber (1979). Science, 206, 700-702.

Schmidt, M.J., J.J. Ryan and B.B. Molloy (1974). Brain Res., 112, 113-126.

Schmidt, M.J., J.F. Thornberry and B.B. Molloy (1977). Brain Res., 121, 182-189.

Schwarcz, R., and K. Fuxe (1979). Life Sci., 24, 1471-1480.

Schwarcz, R., C. Köhler and R.M. Mangano (1982). Neurosci. Suppl.7, 188

Sharif, N.A., and P.J. Roberts (1978). Brain Res, 157, 391-395.

Sharif, N.A., and P.J. Roberts (1981). Brain Res., 211, 293-303.

Shimizu, H., H. Ichishita and H. Odagiri (1974). J. biol. Chem., 249, 5955-5962.

Shinozaki, H., and S. Konishi (1970). Brain Res., 24, 368-371.

Simon, J.R., Contrera, J.F. and M.J. Kuhar (1976). J. Neurochem, 26, 141-147.

Slevin, J., J. Collins, K. Lindsley and J.T. Coyle (1982). Brain Res., in press.

Snodgrass, S.R. (1979). Soc. Neurosci. Abst., 5, 572.

Spector, R.G., (1971). Biochem. Pharmacol., 20, 1730-1732.

Stone, T.W., and Perkins, M.N. (1981). Eur. J. Pharmacol., 72, 411-412.

Teichberg, V.I., O. Goldberg and A. Luini (1981). Mol. Cell Biol., 39, 281-295.

Vincent, S.R., and E.G. McGeer (1979). Life Sci., 24, 265-270.

Watkins, J.C. (1978).In, Kainic Acid as a Tool in Neurobiology, Eds, E.G. McGeer, J.W. Olney and P.L. McGeer, Raven Press, N.Y., pp. 37-69.

Watkins, J.C. (1981a). In Glutamate: Transmitter in the Central Nervous System, Eds, P.J. Roberts, J. Storm-Mathisen and G.A.R. Johnston, John Wiley & Sons Ltd, Chichester, pp.1-24.

Watkins, J.C., and R.H. Evans (1981). Ann. Rev. Pharmacol. Toxicol., 21, 165-204.

Zaczek, R., Koller, K. R. Cotter, D. Heller and J.T. Coyle (1982). Nature, Lond., in press.

Zwiller, J., M.S. Ghandour, M.O. Revel and P. Basset (1981). Neurosci. Lett., 23, 31-36.

EXCITOTOXINS: AN OVERVIEW

JOHN W. OLNEY

Department of Psychiatry, Washington University, St. Louis, Missouri

The theme of this conference--excitotoxins (ET)--is a fascinating one that poses many intriguing research challenges and promises substantial rewards for the effort spent in pursuing these challenges. If we are right in suspecting that endogenous excitotoxins--glutamate (Glu), aspartate (Asp) and perhaps others--are the neurotransmitters released at the majority of excitatory synapses in the mammalian CNS, this is reason enough for our intrigue with these agents. If these transmitter candidates, which are distributed abundantly throughout the CNS, can attack and destroy central neurons, this suggests they might be involved in human neuropathological processes, a prospect that certainly enhances one's level of interest. If by harnessing the powerful neurotoxic activities of ET, we can use them as tools to explore the magnificent organization and functions of the CNS, this is a splendid bonus for which we must indeed be grateful. But there are many gaps in our understanding of these agents, gaps which can only be filled by years of methodical research, but gaps which must be filled if we are to decipher the roles of ET in the physiology and pathology of the CNS and realize their full potential as tools in neuroscience research. In this overview on ET lesions, I will not attempt a comprehensive review of the burgeoning literature on ET--a task that would be impossible within the time constraints--but rather will focus on a few key issues which I consider fundamental to our understanding of these agents and the lesions they induce.

Foundations of the Excitotoxic Concept

The quest for an understanding of the toxic properties of Glu, Asp and related compounds has revolved closely around the working hypothesis that receptors specialized for excitatory neurotransmission mediate their neurotoxic activities. The original evidence supporting the ET concept derives from molecular specificity studies (Curtis & Watkins, 1960; Watkins, 1978; Olney et al.,1971; Olney, 1978; Schwarcz et al.,1978) conducted in the 1960s and 1970s showing that certain analogs of Glu and Asp mimic both their excitatory and toxic properties and do so with a similar order of potencies for the two phenomena. Reinforcing the concept is ultrastructural evidence (Olney, 1971, 1978; Hattori & McGeer, 1977) that the toxic process impinges focally upon postsynaptic dendritic or somal membranes where excitatory synaptic receptors are located but does not disturb presynaptic axonal elements (Fig. 1). Because of the dendrosomal locus of toxic action it was originally predicted (Olney et al.,1975; Coyle & Schwarcz, 1976) that ET might prove useful as lesioning tools for destroying neurons in a given brain region while sparing axons of passage. Considerable evidence, primarily neurochemical and morphological, is now available confirming that ET do produce dendrosomatotoxic/axon-sparing lesions (Coyle et al., 1978; Heggli et al., 1981; Olney & deGubareff, 1978a). It is noteworthy that neurons throughout the CNS are susceptible to both the excitatory and toxic actions of these agents. This implies--if ET phenomena are mediated through Glu/Asp receptors --that the vast majority of CNS neurons have such receptors, a conclusion which is tenable provided one views Glu and Asp, not as minor transmitters, but as the workhorse excitatory transmitters throughout the CNS. That the excitatory and toxic activities of these agents are tightly linked and probably receptor-mediated is illustrated most dramatically by the findings of Colonnier et al.(1979) and DeMontigny and Lund (1980) that certain neurons--those of the mesencephalic trigeminal nucleus--are not depolarized by liberal iontophoretic application of Glu or kainic acid (KA) nor are they harmed by local injection of KA in doses sufficient to destroy neurons throughout the midbrain and overlying cerebellum.

The most recent evidence supporting the ET concept--evidence which I consider rather compelling--comes from experiments focusing on the N-methyl-D-aspartate (NMDA) receptor. Several years ago, when electrophysiological studies largely spearheaded by Watkins and Colleagues (Biscoe et al.,1977; Watkins et al., 1981; Hall et al.,1977) began showing that certain agents such as DL-α-aminoadipate (αAA) and DL-aminophosphonovalerate (APV) antagonize excitations induced by various ET, especially NMDA, we began exploring the ability of these agents to prevent systemically administered ET agents from destroying neurons in the *in vivo* mouse hypothalamus. Initially we found (Olney et al.,1979a) that DL-αAA blocks the toxic action of NMA on arcuate hypothalamic (AH) neurons,although even very high doses did not completely abolish NMA toxicity. Subsequent experiments with the separate isomers of αAA revealed the D isomer to be the antagonist and the L isomer to be an ET

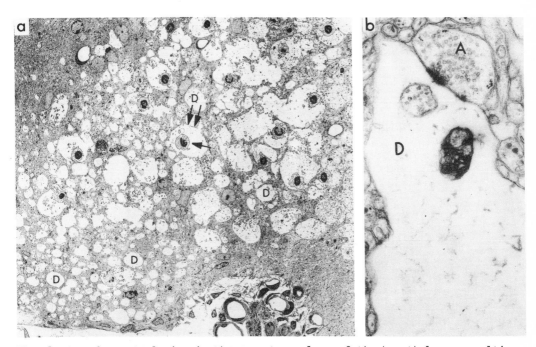

Fig. 1. a. An acute lesion in the arcuate nucleus of the hypothalamus resulting from oral administration of Glu to an infant mouse 5 h previously. Note edematous swelling of dendrites (D) and neuronal cell bodies (double arrows) and pyknotic nuclear changes (single arrow). b. A magnified view from mouse hypothalamus of a normal axon (A) in synaptic contact with a swollen degenerating dendrite (D) 30min after systemic Glu injection (Olney, 1978).

TABLE I

Relative antagonist potencies of D-αAA and D-APV

n	Agents	Dose (mg/kg)	Lesion severity[a]
24	NMA	50	23.8 ± 1.2
10	NMA + D-αAA	50 + 250	13.3 ± 2.1[c]
5	NMA + D-αAA	50 + 500	1.5 ± 0.7[c]
3	NMA + D-αAA	50 + 750	0.7 ± 0.6[c]
6	NMA + D-APV	50 + 2.5	17.0 ± 3.0[b]
6	NMA + D-APV	50 + 5.0	5.5 ± 2.1[c]
6	NMA + D-APV	50 + 7.5	0.5 ± 0.2[c]
9	NMA + D-APV	50 + >7.5	0.0 ± 0.0[c]

[a] AH is a bilateral nucleus. Counts given here are mean (± S.E.M.) number of necrotic AH neurons (per hemi nucleus) per transverse section at point of maximal damage to AH. A typical lesion is depicted in Fig. 2; [b] $P < 0.05$ compared to NMA control; [c] $P < 0.001$ compared to NMA control.

agonist which destroys AH neurons, and when mixed with the D isomer, weakens its blocking activity (Olney et al.,1980a). This, of course, correlates well with the findings of McLennan and Hall (1978) that D-αAA antagonizes whereas L-αAA stimulates firing of thalamic neurons. More recently we tested the D isomer of APV and found it 100 times more potent than D-αAA in blocking NMA neurotoxicity (Olney et al., 1981c). Also we have observed that the D isomer of aminophosphonoheptanoate (APHep), the higher homolog of APV, is approximately equipotent with D-APV in preventing NMA from destroying AH neurons or in blocking NMA neurotoxicity when both NMA and antagonist are coinjected into specific brain regions such as the amygdala or striatum (Olney et al., unpublished). Previously we demonstrated (Price et al.,1978) in adult male rats that low (subtoxic) doses of NMA cause release of luteinizing hormone (LH), presumably secondary to NMA-induced

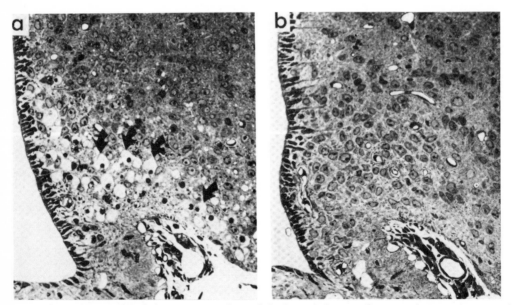

Fig. 2. Light micrographs of the arcuate nucleus of the hypothalamus of a control mouse (a) treated with NMA (50 mg/kg) and an experimental (b) treated with NMA (50 mg/kg) plus D-APV (5 mg/kg). Note the acutely necrotic neurons (arrows) in a which are not present in b ($\times$ 150).

stimulation of Glu/Asp excitatory receptors on AH neurons, and that this LH-releas-
ing action is blocked by αAA (Olney & Price, 1980). Stone and colleagues (1981),
applying D-APV and D-APHep microelectrophoretically to rat cerebrocortical neurons,
recently demonstrated the extreme potency of these agents in blocking NMA excitations. Comparing their findings with ours, it is clear that agents such as D-αAA,
D-APV and D-APHep have a similar order of potencies for antagonizing the excitatory and toxic actions of NMA. An important stimulus for these recent studies, of
course, was the prior work by Watkins and Colleagues (Evans et al.,1979; Watkins et
al.,1981) showing that DL-APV powerfully blocks both the excitations induced by
exogenous NMA and by natural transmitter at NMA-type synapses. From their DL-APV
findings, these authors predicted that D-APV would be an extremely powerful antagonist of the excitatory action of NMA and today we can say without reservation
that this prophecy has been fulfilled not only for the excitatory but the toxic
half of the ET equation.

Taxonomic Considerations

NMDA-type ET. Efforts to establish subclasses of ET amino acid receptors have met
with mixed success (see Roberts, this volume). Although an NMDA receptor through
which ET exert both their excitatory (Watkins et al.,1981) and toxic (Olney et al.,
1981c) actions and through which synaptic transmission is mediated (Evans et al.,
1979; Watkins, this volume) seems well established, little progress has been made
in identifying the natural transmitter released at the NMDA-type of synapse. Moreover, interpretation becomes complicated by new evidence (Herrling, this volume)
that cat caudate neurons display two types of response to iontophoretically
applied NMDA, one of which is Glu-like but neither of which seems related to corticostriatal synaptic transmission. Interpretation of electrophysiological studies
pertaining to the receptor interactions of ET agonists is confounded by poorly
controlled and poorly understood variables such as the presence on a given neuron
of more than one ET receptor subtype and the lack of absolute specificity of a
given agonist molecule for a particular receptor subtype. Specific antagonists
for each receptor subtype, when such become available, will undoubtedly play an
important role in resolving this interpretational conundrum.

KA-type ET. In addition to the relatively unambiguous evidence for NMDA receptors,
there is more tentative electrophysiological and receptor binding data (Watkins et
al.,1981; McLennan, 1981; Simon et al.,1976; London & Coyle, 1979) suggesting that
neural membranes have multiple non-NMDA receptor sites, those for KA and quisqualate (Quis) being the additional sites most frequently proposed. Indeed, such a
puzzling array of findings have recently been accumulating, especially with respect
to the KA receptor, that one might be tempted to postulate as many as three separate types of KA receptors (e.g., see McLennan, this volume). Approaching the
classification problem from a toxicological standpoint, we have compared certain
cyclic molecules (KA, Quis, and the ibotenate analog, AMPA) with one another and
with NMDA-type ET for their toxic effects when injected into the adult rat amygdala.
We chose the amygdala as our testing ground after introducing various ET into
several brain regions, including the hippocampus, and finding that our results from
intraamygdaloid injection were more consistent and easily interpreted. By this mode
of testing, all agents fall into two broad groups which I shall refer to as typical
(NMDA-type) and atypical (KA-type) ET. The typical group (DL-NMA, L-Glu, L-Asp, DL-
homocysteic acid) caused local neuronal necrosis without other toxic effects. The
atypical group (KA, Quis, AMPA) caused, in addition to local neuronal necrosis, sustained
limbic seizures and a pattern of disseminated distant lesions. Comparing our toxicological classification with that derived from electrophysiological data (Watkins
et al.,1981; McLennan, 1981), the major difference is that we find no basis for
placing AMPA and Quis in a spearate category from KA. Tentatively, we would
ascribe this difference to the poor resolution of our toxicological testing approach.

Quinolinic acid, an ambivalent molecule. Years ago we tested the pyridine Glu
analog quinolinic acid (Quin) by subcutaneous (sc) administration and found that it
does not damage AH neurons of either the infant or adult rodent (Olney et al, unpublished). This was consistent with the observation by Evans and colleagues
(cited in Watkins, 1978) that Quin, when applied to the isolated frog spinal cord,
has very little excitatory action. After Stone and Perkins (1981) recently reported that Quin is approximately as potent as Glu in exciting rat cerebrocortical
neurons, we injected Quin into various brain regions (amygdala, striatum, hippocampus) and were surprised to find that it is roughly as potent as DL-NMA in
destroying local neurons (Fuller & Olney, unpublished). Moreover, it behaves like
NMA in causing only local lesions without sustained seizures or distant brain
damage. At this point, therefore, Quin seems difficult to classify. By direct
injection it has NMA-type neurotoxic properties but resembles KA in being dispro-
portionately more powerful as a neurotoxin than excitant. By sc administration
Quin resembles KA more than NMA since NMA destroys AH neurons at least as potently
as neurons elsewhere in brain whereas KA and Quin are both weak in their toxic
actions against AH compared with other CNS neurons.

        The Seizure-Related Brain Damage Enigma

By electron microscopy, the local lesions induced by either the NMDA-type or KA-
type of ET have the dendrosomatotoxic/axon-sparing feature that has traditionally
been identified with ET lesions (Olney et al.,1971; Hattori & McGeer,1977; Olney,
1981); therefore,the distant pattern of seizure-related brain damage (SRBD) induced
by atypical (KA-type) ET appears to be the major toxicological characteristic that
differentiates the two groups. It is a fascinating feature of the distant seizure-
related lesions, however, that they differ only in pattern, not in cytopathological
detail, i.e., they too have the dendrosomatotoxic/axon-sparing characteristics of
an ET lesion (Olney & deGubareff, 1978b; Olney et al.,1979) (Fig. 3). Is this just

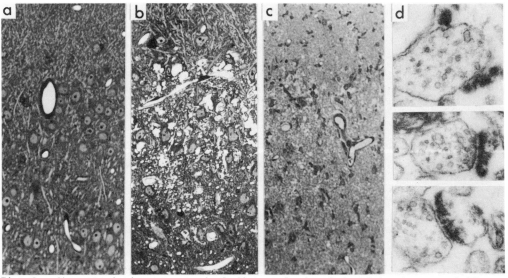

Fig. 3. Characteristics of a typical distant lesion induced in the rat piriform
cortex by KA injection into the diencephalon. a. Saline control. b. Acute reaction (primarily dendritic and glial swelling) 4 h after KA. c. Loss of piriform
cortical neurons and replacement by glia 1 wk after KA. d. Axon terminals of the
lateral olfactory tract 1 wk after KA with adherent postsynaptic receptor densities
but absence of the dendrites that previously housed these receptors (a-c = X280;
d = X50,000) (Olney & deGubareff, 1978).

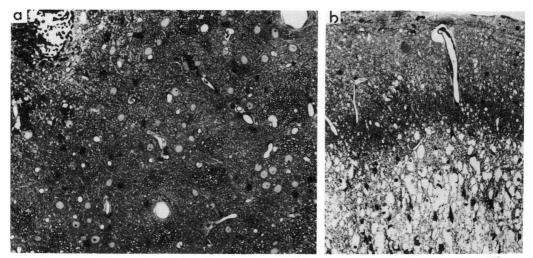

Fig. 4. Distant lesion in the rat piriform cortex (b) 22 h after injection of folic acid (150 nmol) into the striatum (a). Note that striatal neurons in (a) close to the injection site (upper left corner) appear normal, whereas piriform cortical neurons in (b) are acutely necrotic (X240) (from Olney et al., 1981b).

a coincidence or does it imply that an ET mechanism is involved? In a series of recent studies, we have been intensively examining this and related questions.

Folates reproduce SRBD syndrome. Prompted by the recent report of Ruck et al. (1980) that methyltetrahydrofolate (MTHF) competes powerfully for KA binding, we injected folate molecules into the rat amygdala or striatum and found that although MTHF was rather weak, certain other folates, including folic acid itself, were very effective in causing KA-like limbic seizure activity and a KA-like pattern of SRBD without inducing local lesions (Olney et al., 1981a, 1981b) (Fig. 4). Diazepam pretreatment blocks the seizures and SRBD induced by folates (Fuller et al., 1981) just as it is known to block the SRBD syndrome induced by KA (Ben-Ari et al.,1979; Fuller & Olney, 1981). Our folate findings do not provide any basis for believing that a folate receptor mediates the typical ET activity of KA (local neuron-necro-tizing activity) but they do raise the question whether the atypical features of KA neurotoxicity might involve a folate receptor or at least some receptor with which both KA and folates interact. It is of interest that folic acid, when injected into the striatum, mimics not only the sustained seizures but other important acute behavioral effects of KA, including stereotypic turning behaviors. Thus, folates may represent useful tools for reproducing most if not all of the atypical facets of KA neurotoxicity separately from its typical ET activity.

Cholinomimetics reproduce SRBD syndrome. To further investigate the SRBD syndrome, we recently followed-up our previous observation (Olney et al., 1980b) that dipipe-ridinoethane (DPE), an agent not structurally related to KA, mimics the SRBD effects of KA when administered subcutaneously to adult rats. Since DPE did not reproduce this syndrome when injected in very high doses into the amygdala, we initially proposed that a metabolite generated peripherally might be responsible for the central toxicity. Synthesis of several DPE analogs by J.F. Collins recent-ly enabled us to explore this possibility. We found that an oxidized derivative, DPE-di-N-oxide which structurally resembles the cholinergic agonist oxotremorine, does induce a KA-like SRBD syndrome when injected into the amygdala (Olney et al., 1982a). In other related studies, we found that both cholinergic agonists and

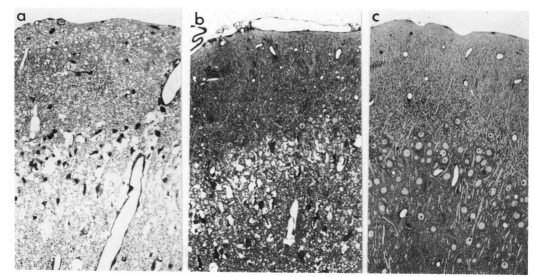

Fig. 5. Seizure-related damage to rat piriform cortex following cholinomimetic
treatment. a. Physostigmine (25 nmol) injected into basolateral amygdala 24 h
previously; compare this seizure-related distant lesion at 24 h with that induced
by intrastriatal folic acid (Fig. 4b). b. Appearance of the piriform cortex 4 h
after pilocarpine (30 mg/kg) administered subcutaneously to a rat treated 24 h
previously with lithium chloride (3 meq/kg). Compare this acute (4 h) lesion with
the distant lesion induced by intradiencephalic KA (Fig. 3b). c. Normal appearance of piriform cortex from a rat treated with lithium and pilocarpine as in (b)
but protected from seizures and brain damage by atropine, 150 mg/kg given 30 min
prior to pilocarpine (X240) (from Honchar et al., 1982 and Olney et al., 1982b).

cholinesterase inhibitors, when injected into the rat amygdala, also cause a KA-
like SRBD syndrome (Olney et al., 1982b) (Fig. 5). Strictly speaking, the syndrome
induced by DPE-di-N-oxide or known cholinomimetics is folate-like, in that it consists of seizures and a distant disseminated pattern of brain damage in the absence
of local lesions. The most consistently effective and potent cholinergic agent we
have tested is the cholinesterase inhibitor neostigmine which causes a well developed SRBD syndrome in 100% of animals receiving 3-4 nmol by microinjection into
the basolateral amygdala. Thus, neostigmine has approximately the same potency
as KA for inducing the SRBD component of KA neurotoxicity and it achieves this
without inducing local damage at the injection site.

In a more recent series of experiments we have learned that certain cholinergic
agonists or cholinesterase inhibitors, when administered sc, faithfully reproduce
all features of the SRBD syndrome that KA induces by sc administration, provided
the rat is pre-treated with lithium (Honchar et al., 1982) (Fig. 5). This Li/
cholinotoxic syndrome is blocked by atropine and also by diazepam. Our cholinergic
findings signify that increased activity at central cholinergic receptors is
sufficient in itself to cause a SRBD syndrome resembling that caused by KA or
folic acid. Thus, the possibility that a cholinergic mechanism could underlie the
seizure-linked pathology induced by either KA or folic acid warrants consideration.

Persistent focal motor seizures and distant lesions. In collaborative experiments
with Dr. Robert Collins we recently observed that topical application of various
convulsants to the sensorimotor cortex of the adult rat results in persistent

focal motor seizure activity for several hours and Glu-type local lesions in specific thalamic nuclei that receive glutamergic projections from cortical neurons involved in the seizure process (Collins & Olney, 1982; Labruyere et al., 1982) (Fig. 6). Hypoxia is not a likely explanation for the thalamic lesions since the focal seizure activity is restricted behaviorally to repetitive unilateral forearm jerking and respiratory function is not compromised. Moreover, the cytopathology is of the typical ET type (dendrosomatotoxic/axon-sparing) and one would not expect hypoxia to spare metabolically active presynaptic terminals while destroying postsynaptic dendrosomal structures.

Sustained perforant path stimulation and distant lesions. In an innovative set of experiments, Sloviter and Damiano (1981) recently demonstrated that persistent electrical stimulation of the perforant path (putative glutamergic excitatory input to the hippocampus) causes KA-like electrophysiological and light microscopic histopathological changes in the rat hippocampus. Dr. Sloviter sent the brains of his rats to my laboratory for electron microscopic examination and we found that the acute hippocampal cytopathology induced by perforant path stimulation is indistinguishable from the distant seizure-linked cytopathology induced by KA, folates, or cholinergic agents (Olney & Sloviter, 1981), which in turn has the dendrosomatotoxic/axon-sparing characteristic of the lesions that typical ET such as Glu or Asp induce locally when injected into brain. An explanation for these several correlations is suggested by the fact that persistent hippocampal discharge activity, a common denominator linking perforant path stimulation with KA, folate or cholinergic drug treatment, probably entails excessive release of endogenous ET such as Glu or Asp at many hippocampal synapses. The pattern of dendrosomal damage in each case follows a laminar distribution corresponding fairly well with putative Glu/Asp innervation patterns in the hippocampus (Olney et al., 1979b, 1980b).

SRBD: an excitotoxic process? The above findings collectively suggest that distant brain damage associated with seizures induced by a wide range of treatments may be both seizure-mediated and excitotoxin-mediated in the sense that it may be the toxic consequence of seizure-induced release of endogenous ET (Glu, Asp or unidentified endogenous ET) at distant receptor sites. Thus, we propose that KA induces local lesions by acting directly as an exogenous ET on local neurons and causes distant lesions by releasing endogenous ET on distant neurons. An ET process is involved in either case but to avoid confusion it may be useful to call the former an exo-ET lesion and the latter an endo-ET lesion. Thus it may be appropriate to refer to the neurotoxic process unleashed by many different types of treatment-- folates, DPE, cholinergic agents, perforant path stimulation or topical application of convulsants to the sensorimotor cortex--as an endo-ET process. It would confuse the issue to call the agents themselves (e.g., folates, DPE or cholinergic agents) ET but they could be called ET-mimetics. Applying this terminology to the toxic process induced by cholinesterase inhibitors one would ascribe the sustained seizure activity to a cholinomimetic mechanism and the resultant brain damage to an ET-mimetic or endo-ET mechanism. If this interpretation is correct, the most important implication may be that an endo-ET process may play a role in the brain damage that occurs in human epilepsy.

It may be questioned whether excessive release of Glu or Asp would destroy postsynaptic neurons, considering the exceedingly efficient uptake processes in axon terminals and glia for inactivating Glu or Asp. We propose that continuous discharge activity through Glu/Asp axon terminals may represent a condition which compromises these homeostatic mechanisms, i.e., repetitive depolarization and repolarization of the axonal membrane may usurp so much energy from the terminal that its reuptake process founders for want of energy to drive it. This might impair the uptake capacity enough to allow toxic concentrations of Glu to accumulate in the synaptic cleft. While glial uptake might be expected to function as

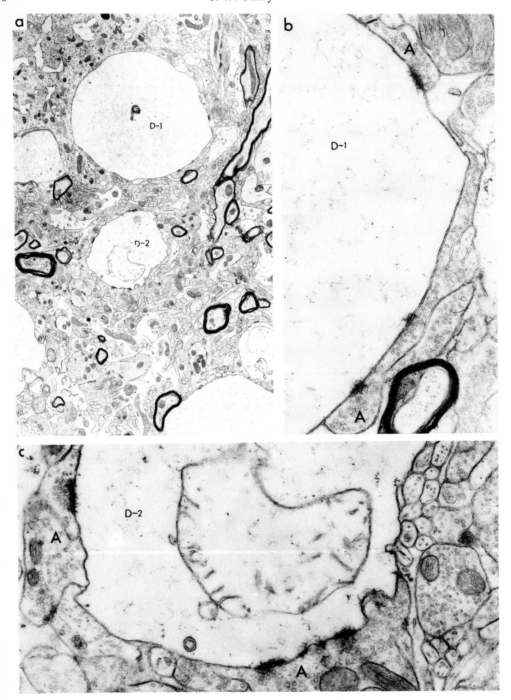

Fig. 6. a. Survey view of ventrolateral thalamic lesion resulting from focal
cortical seizure activity (X2h) induced by topical application of folic acid to
the dura. Massively swollen dendrites (D-1 and D-2) are shown at higher magnification in (b) and (c). Note the normal appearance of presynaptic axons (A).
(a = X5000; b and c = X45000) (from Collins and Olney, 1982).

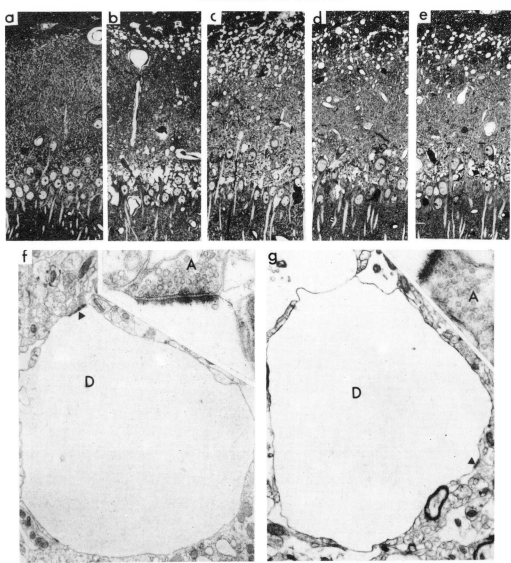

Fig. 7. Panels a-e are from the CA-1 region of rat hippocampus; the pyramidal
cells are at bottom, alveus at top and stratum oriens (basilar dendritic field) in
between. Treatment conditions were: a. Control; b. KA (12 mg/kg sc) 4h previously;
c. Perforant path stimulation for 2h; d. Intraamygdaloid folic acid (25 nmol) 4h
previously; e. LiCl (3 meq/kg sc) 1 day previously, then physostigmine (40 mg/kg
sc) 4h prior to sacrifice. A characteristic acute SRBD reaction consisting of two
laminar bands of edematous swollen structures is evident. Swollen elements in the
pyramidal cell layer are glia and those in the stratum oriens are massively dilated
distal dendrites of CA-1 pyramids. The swollen dendrites in the electron micrographs (f and g) are from the CA-1 distal basilar dendritic field of the brains
shown in (b) and (c) following KA and perforant path stimulation, respectively.
In each case, the postsynaptic dendrite (D) displays conspicuous edematous degenerative changes while the presynaptic axon (A) appears normal (a-e = X200; f and
g = X8000, insets X45,000) (from Olney et al., 1979b; Olney and Sloviter, 1981);
Olney et al., 1981a; Honchar et al., 1982).

an auxiliary protective mechanism, glial uptake may also be impaired since glia in the region of injury are grossly edematous and swollen--a pathological state possibly reflecting the deleterious effects on glia of large amounts of K+ released by repetitively firing neurons (Hosli et al., 1979; Evans, 1980; Krespan et al., 1982).

Other Challenging Issues

Mechanistic considerations. It is clear that there is a close relationship between the excitatory and toxic actions of ET but we need to decipher in more detailed pathophysiological terms what that relationship is. We know that all ET, when applied to neurons in excess, cause the same sequence of events--initial acceleration of firing followed by depolarization block, electrical silence and neuronal death. However, until we learn what kind of specific membrane changes and trans-membrane ionic or molecular movements are induced by different classes of ET, both in the interval prior to depolarization block and the electrical silence period thereafter, we can only guess how the excitatory actions of ET lead to neuronal destruction. In this volume Meldrum proposes that excessive entry of Ca^{++} into the neuron may explain the type of brain damage associated either with seizures or local injection of ET into brain. This is consistent with the hypothesis (see above) that either type of brain damage is ET mediated since excessive extra- to intracellular movement of Ca^{++} might occur as a consequence of membrane permeability changes induced by exogenous ET following local injection or by endogenous ET released in the course of seizures.

What is the relationship, if any, between the excitatory process by which all ET exert rapidly lethal toxic action upon neurons and the excitatory process by which KA-type ET initiate and maintain seizure activity for hours? If one assumes that KA, when injected directly into brain, acts through a single population of local neurons to effect both of these excitatory processes, is this not a contradiction? How can a cell which has succumbed to depolarization block and electrical silence simultaneously serve as generator of sustained seizure activity for several hours? Do different cell types separately mediate these seemingly dissimilar excitatory processes?

Anyone who has worked with KA is probably impressed with the complexity of this neurotoxin. There is risk that readings obtained by testing KA may represent an uninterpretable composite of multiple interacting effects perhaps superimposed upon one another. One way around this problem is to study partial KA-mimetics, i.e., agents that reproduce specific facets of KA neurotoxicity separately from other facets. Folates and cholinomimetics qualify as selective mimics of the SRBD facet of KA neurotoxicity. NMA-type ET qualify as selective mimics of the local neuron-necrotizing activity. Quin perhaps qualifies as a compound mimic which has both the latter activity and a KA-like disproportionality between its toxic and excitatory potencies. One multi-mechanism hypothesis proposes that the extreme toxic potency of KA stems from its ability to act not only as a direct Glu-like excitant but as an augmentor of Glu release (see Coyle, this volume) and/or inhibitor of Glu reuptake. Since Quin mimics KA in being a more potent toxin than excitant, tests might be performed to determine whether Quin has KA-like effects on Glu uptake and/or release. By focusing on agents that mimic separate components of KA neurotoxicity it is possible that one will be studying in isolation the very mechanism underlying the KA effect, but if not, the information acquired will nevertheless be of heuristic value.

We need, of course, to obtain more definitive information regarding the distribution and types of receptors with which ET interact. Since the main obstacle to progress here is the lack of specific antagonists, research aimed at the development of specific antagonists is of the highest priority. If KA-type ET act by more than one excitatory mechanism, it may be possible with appropriate antagonists to block one mechanism at a time. If KA acts by a combination of several mechanisms, and KA binding data identify a specific KA-type receptor, which of the KA mechanisms does this receptor pertain to? If there are multiple subtypes of ET receptors, how are these distributed over CNS neurons? If they are unevenly distributed, and a given agonist is relatively specific for a given receptor type, it should be possible to demonstrate differential sensitivity of specific neuronal populations to specific ET. While there is evidence that ET spare some neurons at a given lesion site, there has been no systematic attempt to determine whether a given ET spares the same neurons as another ET at a given site. We need studies comparing in many brain regions the cytotoxic specificities of representative ET from each proposed receptor class (NMA, KA and Quis).

ET as lesioning tools. It is essential that we learn more about ET mechanisms if we are to use ET successfully as research tools. As mentioned above, it must be ascertained whether there is a useful degree of cytospecificity in the toxic actions of particular classes of ET, e.g., do the local lesions induced by KA, NMA, and Quis in any particular brain region exactly duplicate one another or is each agent at least partially selective for certain cell types?

Since KA is the ET currently used most widely for lesioning studies, it is important to resolve the problem of distant lesions. It has been suggested that diazepam be used to block the distant lesions induced by KA without interfering with its local lesioning action. The status of this proposal, however, is tentative. Recent evidence suggests that diazepam may also interfere with local KA toxicity (Di Chiara et al., 1981) and it remains unknown whether diazepam is consistent in its protective actions regardless of the CNS region in which KA is injected.

Ibotenate does not induce distant lesions (Schwarcz et al., 1979) and therefore has been proposed as a useful alternative to KA; however, ibotenate has the disadvantage of being potentially unstable, difficult to synthesize and commercially unavailable except at exorbitant cost. Fortunately, DL-NMA, which also is without distant lesioning potential, has the same cytospecificity as ibotenate, is nearly as potent and is readily available at reasonable cost. Although information on Quin is currently very preliminary, it may prove to be a valuable lesioning tool as it is even less expensive than NMA, appears to have the same cytotoxic specificity and potency as NMA and does not cause distant lesions (Fuller & Olney, unpublished; Schwarcz, this volume).

It should be noted that both folates and cholinomimetics have excellent potential as tools for studying mechanisms of epilepsy and epilepsy-related brain damage. Since both classes of agent are naturally present in brain, either could have complicity in human seizure-related neuropathology. Cholinomimetics are especially versatile and valuable tools for epilepsy research since they act by well understood mechanisms related to a specific central transmitter system and are effective as SRBD agents when injected either directly into brain or systemically. Moreover, for studying epilepsy-related brain damage they may prove more useful than KA since they do not have the confounding property of destroying neurons by seizure-unrelated as well as seizure-related mechanisms. As discussed above, folates and cholinomimetics are not ET but if, as we postulate, the SRBD they induce has an Endo-ET mechanism, they qualify as neuroscience ET tools, i.e., tools that act by an ET mechanism.

ET in human neurodegenerative diseases. It has been speculated that Glu or a more potent KA-like endo-ET might have complicity in Huntington's disease (Coyle et al., 1978; Olney, 1979). Elsewhere in this volume Shoulson reviews evidence for this proposal and describes a well designed ongoing study aimed at testing the possibility that baclofen, a putative inhibitor of Glu release, may retard the progression of neuronal degeneration in patients with Huntington's disease. We all await eagerly the outcome of this important study.

Recently we have been examining the possible role of an ET mechanism in neurolep-tic-induced tardive dyskinesia and have found in rats that long-term neuroleptic treatment impairs Glu reuptake in the striatum (Price et al.,1981). Since neuro-leptics block dopamine receptors and dopamine inhibits Glu release from the cor-ticostriatal tract (Rowlands & Roberts, 1980), Glu release may be augmented (dis-inhibited) by neuroleptics. A combination of increased release and decreased re-uptake of Glu might cause a toxic accumulation of Glu at corticostriatal synapses with consequent degeneration of postsynaptic striatal neurons. Thus, we would entertain a combined Glu/dopamine hypothesis which might explain the irreversible symptoms of tardive dyskinesia better than the dopamine hypothesis alone.

Could ET play a role in senile dementia or the neuronal loss which occurs with aging? It is not difficult to conceive of homeostatic mechanisms wearing out with age to permit endogenous ET to accumulate in toxic concentrations at central synapses and destroy Glu-receptive neurons. Evidence presented by Bowen (this volume) that accumulation of Glu in K^+-stimulated human brain tissue increases as a function of age is consistent with this proposal. If an increased accumulation of synaptically released Glu were responsible for the diffuse loss of neurons that occurs during normal aging, this suggests a potentially promising prophylactic application for inhibitors of Glu release or antagonists of ET receptors. It is more difficult to relate ET mechanisms to the pattern of neuronal loss in senile dementia since a particular species of neuron, the cholinergic neuron, appears to be the victim of the senile dementia neurodegenerative process and no specific link is apparent between Glu or Asp systems and cholinergic neurons that would explain how an ET process might be responsible for the selective degeneration of these neurons.

As the emphasis of my own recent research suggests, I suspect that ET will even-tually be found to play a significant role in neurodegenerative phenomena asso-ciated with epilepsy. Whether ET mechanisms might be involved causally in the epileptic process itself remains unclear, i.e., no specific mechanism has been identified whereby ET activity in the presence of normal inhibitory containment mechanisms might result in either the initiation or maintenance of seizures. Given a defect in containment mechanisms, however, or any set of circumstances conducive to excessive firing of endogenous ET pathways, I propose that this can result in ET degeneration of structures innervated by those pathways.

Plaitakis et al. (1982) have shown that patients with a recessively inherited form of olivopontocerebellar degeneration (OPCD) have a deficiency of glutamic dehydrogenase (GDH) which impairs their ability to metabolize Glu. Intake of exogenous Glu in the diet results in abnormally high blood Glu levels. How this defect might give rise to degeneration of the OPC system remains to be elucidated but it is certainly a viable hypothesis that an ET mechanism might be involved.

SUMMARY

Here I have reviewed the foundations of the excitotoxin (ET) concept and, despite uncertainties regarding non-NMDA receptor subtypes,have emphasized that the evi-dence is quite strong for an NMDA receptor in the mammalian CNS which mediates both endogenous synaptic transmitter events and the excitatory and toxic actions of exogenous NMDA-type ET. By toxicological criteria, we have been able to iden-tify only two types of ET agonists, an NMA type and KA type. Both induce dendro-somatotoxic/axon-sparing local lesions when injected into brain and, in addition, KA-type ET induce seizures and a disseminated pattern of seizure-related brain damage (SRBD). Evidence is presented that the SRBD component of KA neurotoxicity can be reproduced by various methods which have sustained discharge activity as a common denominator. Because each SRBD syndrome, regardless of method of produc-tion, consists of typical ET cytopathology (dendrosomatotoxic/axon-sparing lesions) and sustained discharge activity may involve the release of endogenous

ET (Glu or Asp) at many of the tissue sites incurring damage, we hypothesize that SRBD is both a seizure-mediated and ET-mediated form of brain damage, i.e., it may represent the toxic consequence of seizure-induced release and intrasynaptic accumulation of endogenous ET (Glu or Asp). If this interpretation is correct, the most important implication is that an endogenous ET process may play a role in the brain damage that occurs in human epilepsy. A variety of challenging issues confronting the ET researcher are discussed and the possible role of ET in human neurodegenerative disorders is explored.

ACKNOWLEDGMENTS

This work was supported in part by USPHS Grants NS-09156, DA-00259, NIMH Research Career Scientist Award MH-38894 and a grant from the Epilepsy Foundation of America.

REFERENCES

Ben-Ari Y, Tremblay E, Ottersen OP and Naquet R (1979). Brain Res 165, 632-635.
Biscoe TJ, Davies J, Dray A, Evans RH, Martin MR and Watkins JC (1977). Eur J Pharmac 45,315-316.
Collins RC and Olney JW (1982). Science, in Press.
Colonnier M, Steriade M and Landry P (1979). Brain Res 172, 552-556.
Coyle JT and Schwarcz R (1976). Nature 263, 244-246.
Coyle JT, McGeer EG, McGeer PL and Schwarcz R (1978). In: Kainic Acid as a Tool in Neurobiology, McGeer EG, Olney JW, McGeer PL (Eds), Raven Press, New York.
Curtis DR and Watkins JC (1960). J Neurochem 6, 117-141.
DeMontigny C and Lund JP (1980. Neuroscience 5, 1621-1628.
Di Chiara G, Morelli M, Imperato A, Faa G, Fussarello M and Porceddu ML (1981). In: Glutamate as a Neurotransmitter, Di Chiara G and Gessa GL (Eds), Raven Press, New York.
Evans RH (1980). J Physiol 298, 25-35.
Evans RH, Francis AA, Hunt K, Oakes DJ and Watkins JC (1979). Br J Pharmacol 67, 591-603.
Fuller TA and Olney JW (1981). Neurobehav Toxicol Teratol 3, 355-361.
Fuller TA, Olney JW and Conboy VT (1981). Neurosci Abst 7, 811, 1981.
Hall JG, Hicks TP and McLennan H (1977). Neurosci Lett 8, 171-175.
Hattori T and McGeer EG (1977). Brain Res 129, 174-180.
Heggli DE, Aamodt A, Malthe-Sorenssen D (1981). Brain Res 230, 253-262.
Honchar MP, Olney JW and Sherman WR (1982). Neurosci Abst 8.
Hosli L, Andres P and Hosli E (1979). J Physiol (Paris) 75, 655-659.
Krespan B, Berl S and Nicklas WJ (1982). J Neurochem 38, 509-517.
Labruyere J, Olney JW and Collins RC (1982). Neurosci Abst 8.
London ED and Coyle JT (1979). Eur J Pharmacol 56, 287-290.
London ED, Klemm N and Coyle JT (1980). Brain Res 192, 463-476.
McLennan H (1981). In: Glutamate as a Neurotransmitter, Di Chiara G, Gessa GL (Eds), Raven Press, New York.
McLennan H and Hall JG (1978). Brain Res 149, 541-545.
Olney JW (1971). J Neuropathol Exp Neurol 30, 75-90.
Olney JW (1978). In: Kainic Acid as a Tool in Neurobiology, McGeer EG, Olney JW, McGeer PL (Eds), Raven Press, New York.
Olney JW (1979). In: Huntington's Disease, Chase TN, Wexler NS, Barbeau A (Eds), Raven Press, New York.
Olney JW (1981). In: Glutamate as a Neurotransmitter, Di Chiara G, Gessa GL (Eds) Raven Press, New York.
Olney JW and deGubareff T (1978a). Brain Res 140, 340-343.
Olney JW and deGubareff T (1978b). In: Kainic Acid as a Tool in Neurobiology, McGeer EG, Olney JW, McGeer PL (Eds), Raven Press, New York.
Olney JW and Price MT (1980). Brain Res Bull 5, Suppl 2, 361-368.

Olney JW and Sloviter RS (1981). J Neuropath Exp Neurol 40, 340.
Olney JW, Ho OL and Rhee V (1971). Exp Brain Res 14, 61-76.
Olney JW, Sharpe LG and deGubareff T (1975). Neurosci Abst 1, 371.
Olney JW, deGubareff T and Labruyere J (1979a). Life Sci 25, 537-540.
Olney JW, Fuller T and deGubareff T (1979b). Brain Res 176, 91-100.
Olney JW, deGubareff T and Collins JF (1980a). Neurosci Lett 19, 277-282.
Olney JW, Fuller TA, Collins RC and deGubareff T (1980b). Brain Res 200, 231-235.
Olney JW, Fuller TA and deGubareff T (1981a). Nature 292, 165-167.
Olney JW, Fuller TA, deGubareff T and Labruyere J (1981b). Neurosci Lett 25,
    185-191.
Olney JW, Labruyere J, Collins JF and Curry K (1981c). Brain Res 221, 207-210.
Olney JW, Collins JF and deGubareff T (1982a). Brain Res in press.
Olney JW, deGubareff T and Labruyere J (1982b). Neurosci Abst 8.
Plaitakis A, Berl S and Yahr MD (1982). Science 216, 193.
Price MT, Haft R and Olney JW (1981). Neurosci Abst 7, 714.
Price MT, Olney JW and Cicero TJ (1978). Neuroendocrinology 26, 352-358.
Rowlands GJ and Roberts PJ (1980). Europ J Pharmacol 62, 241.
Ruck A, Kramer S, Metz J and Brennan MJW (1980). Nature 287, 852-853.
Schwarcz R, Scholz D and Coyle TJ (1978). Neuropharmacology 17, 145-151.
Schwarcz R, Hokfelt T, Fuxe K, Johnson G, Goldstein M, Terenius L (1979). Exp
    Brain Res 37, 199-216
Simon JR, Contrera JF and Kuhar MJ (1976). J Neurochem 26, 141-147.
Sloviter RS and Damiano BP (1981). Neurosci Lett 24, 279-284.
Stone TW and Perkins MN (1981). Eur J Pharmacol 72, 411-412.
Stone TW, Perkins MN, Collins JF and Curry K (1981). Neuroscience 6, 2249-2252.
Watkins JC (1978). In: Kainic Acid as a Tool in Neurobiology, McGeer EG, Olney
    JW, McGeer PL (Eds), Raven Press, New York.
Watkins JC, Davies J, Evans RH, Francis AA and Jones AW (1981). In: Glutamate
    as a Neurotransmitter, Di Chiara G, Gessa GL (Eds), Raven Press, New York.

MECHANISMS OF EXCITOTOXICITY

Chairman: J. W. Olney

NEURONAL DEGENERATION AFTER INTRACEREBRAL INJECTIONS OF EXCITOTOXINS. A HISTOLOGICAL ANALYSIS OF KAINIC ACID, IBOTENIC ACID AND QUINOLINIC ACID LESIONS IN THE RAT BRAIN

CHRISTER KÖHLER

Department of Pharmacology, Astra Läkemedel AB, Södertälje, Sweden

KEYWORDS

Neurotoxicity; kainic acid; ibotenic acid; quinolinic acid; neuronal degeneration; mechanisms; immunocytochemistry.

INTRODUCTION

It is now well established that systemic and intracerebral injections of kainic acid (KA), a potent excitatory analogue of the endogenous amino acid glutamic acid (21), cause degeneration of neuronal cell bodies while leaving axons and nerve-terminals in the lesion area intact. (3,20,21,23,25,26,27,30)

With the discovery that KA causes axon-sparing lesions of central neurons, a novel lesioning tool was introduced in neurobiology and the KA lesions of the neostriatum and hippocampus have provided animal models for studies of neurode-generative disease (e.g. Huntingtons disease) (20,30) and the pathophysiology of status epilepticus (1,23,35,2), respectively. The subsequent extensive use of KA has revealed, however, certain features of its toxic properties that may partly limit the usefulness of this toxin as a selective lesioning tool. Thus, several studies have demonstrated that neurons differ with regard to their vulnerability to KA (3,4,10,11,14,17,24) and that injections of the relatively large quantities of KA required to degenerate resistant cells may result in neuronal degeneration in brain areas located distant from the site of KA infusion. (1,3,16,19,27,35,37)

Recently, several different acidic amino acids with potent neuroexcitatory properties have been reported to cause neuronal degeneration when injected into the brain. (see 24) Intracerebral injections of ibotenic acid (IBO), an isoxazole isolated from the mushroom amanita muscaria (5,6) have been shown to produce axon sparing lesions of neurons in the hippocampus (14,15), striatum (15,32) and sub-stantia nigra (32) of the rat. Although the mechanism(s) by which IBO induces neuronal degeneration is not known at present, experimental studies (14) have suggested that it may differ from that of KA.

The validity of KA and IBO lesions as animal models for human neurodegenerative disease is limited by the fact that neither KA nor IBO are endogenously present in mammals and, thus, the neuronal degeneration caused by either of these compounds does not relate directly to the aetiology of the disease processes in humans that are triggered by endogenous factors. Quinolinic acid (QUIN), a metabolite of tryptophan which is endogenously present in mammals have been

recently shown to cause neuronal degeneration when injected into the hippocampus
and the striatum of rats (34). Biochemical studies have suggested that the extrinsic afferents to the lesion area remain intact (34) after QUIN infusion
(See also Schwacz et al, this volume). This selective, axon-sparing type of lesion
caused by intracerebral injections of QUIN makes it an interesting candidate as an
endogenous factor involved in neurodegenerative disease.

While numerous previous studies have been devoted to the study of KA lesions (23)
little is known about the morphology of IBO and QUIN induced neuronal degeneration after intracerebral injections. In the present study KA, IBO and QUIN lesions
have been analyzed and compared at the light microscopic level after intracerebroventricular, hippocampal and cerebellar injections of either toxin into the rat's
brain.

METHODS

Subjects.   Adult male Sprague Dawley albino rats (175 g, Anticimex, Stockholm)
have been used throughout the study.

Surgery and histology.   Under pentobarbital anaesthesia (Mebumal, 60 mg/kg) the
rat was positioned in a Kopf$^{(R)}$ stereotaxic instrument and different concentrations of KA, IBO and QUIN (dissolved in phosphate buffer, ph 7.4) was injected
into the lateral ventricle, hippocampus, piriform cortex, or cerebellum. After
survival periods ranging from 3 hrs to 7 days, the rats were killed through trans-
cardial perfusion with saline followed by paraformaldehyde and glutaraldehyde as
previously described (14). In some experiments rats were injected intracerebro-
ventricularly with an inhibitor of axonal transport (colchicine, SIGMA, 60 μg/10 μl)
24 hours before sacrifice. The colchicine injections were made 2 to 3 days after
injection of the excitotoxins. A majority of the fixed brains were cut at 30 um
in a cryostat (Dittes, Heidelberg) and the sections stained with thionin to
visualize normal cell bodies, or processed according to the Fink-Heimer method
(procedure II) for the visualization of degenerated neurons and nerve-terminals.
Some brains from each group was embedded in araldite and cut at 1 um and stained
with toloudine blue.

One series of brains injected with KA, IBO or QUIN was processed according to the
copper-thiocholine method of Koelle (13) for the demonstration of acetylcholinesterase (AChE) as described by Geneser-Jensen and Blackstad (9). Unspecific
cholinesterase was inhibited by adding ethopropazine to the incubation medium.

Immunohistochemistry.   Pieces of fixed brain-tissue containing the lesion area
were cut on a Vibratom$^{(R)}$ (Oxford) and the sections (50 - 100 um thick) were incubated free-floating for 2 days with antibody to 5-hydroxytryptamine;(5HT
serotonin: diluted 1:1200 in PBS containing 0.3 % Triton x-100), somatostatin
(SOM; diluted 1:500), vasoactive intestinal polypeptide (VIP; diluted 1:500) or
glutamic acid decarboxylase (GAD; diluted 1:500). The antigen-antibody complex
was visualized using the biotin-avidin complex method of Hsu (12). The reacted
sections were stained with thionin, defatted and coverslipped with Permount.

RESULTS

The hippocampus

Kainic Acid.   Several previous studies have provided detailed descriptions of the
morphology of KA induced lesions of the hippocampus after systemic and intracerebral injections in the rat. (21,23) Thus, the present discussion will focus
primarily on aspects of KA toxicity relevant to comparisons with IBO and QUIN
toxicity in the hippocampal formation.

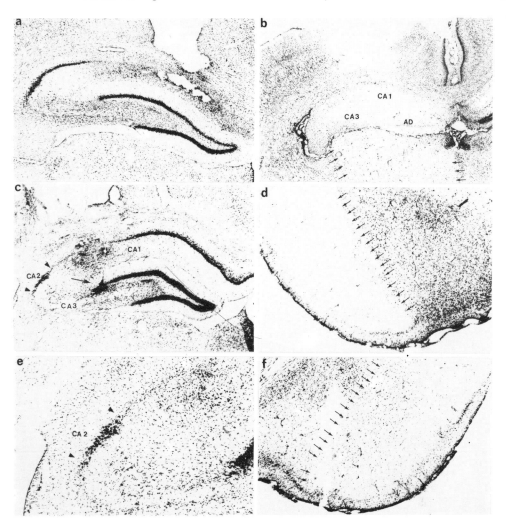

Figure 1 (a-f) Photomicrographs of local and distal cell loss one
week after the injection of KA into the dorsal hippocampus of the rat.
Micrographs in (a)and(b)demonstrate the selective resistance of granule
and CA2 pyramidal cells to KA. In(a) KA (0.5 µg/0.5 µl) was infused
into the medial aspect of the hippocampus and in(b)the same amount was
injected at its most lateral part (arrow). As can be seen in both(a)
and (b) the pyramidal cells of CA3 a-c have undergone degeneration while
pyramidal cells of CA2 (arrow heads in c and e) remain intact. Injections of a higher dose (1 µg/0.5 µl) result in total cell loss in the
dorsal hippocampus (b), in the dorsal and medial thalamic nuclei
(arrows in b) and in the ipsi (d) and contra (f)-lateral piriform
cortex. Thionine stain. Abbreviations: AD = area dentata, CA1, CA2,
CA3 = hippocampal subfields. Magn. x 20 (a,b,c) x 85 (d,e,f)

Although the lesions produced by KA are of a so-called axon sparing type in all brain regions examined so far, two factors may partly limit its usefulness as a selective lesioning tool. First, certain classes of neurons appear to be more vulnerable to the toxin than others. This selective toxicity of KA towards certain neurons is well illustrated in the hippocampal formation (Fig. 1).

After intracerebroventricular or intrahippocampal injections of KA (0.5 µg/0.5 µl) the pyramidal cells in subfield CA3 a-c are preferentially degenerated. On the basis of dose-response studies the different hippocampal cell types have been found to express the following relative vulnerability to KA: CA3 > CA1 > granule cells > CA2. The degeneration of CA3 and CA1 pyramidal cells proceed relatively rapidly and signs of neuronal degeneration are observed at the light microscopic level already after 4 hrs. At this time the pyramidal cells appear basophilic with displacement of Nissl substance into distal parts of the dendrites. In silver stained sections a majority of the cells are clearly argyrophilic and extensive dendritic degeneration is observed. Importantly, however, is the observation that the granule cells show few signs of degeneration at this time after KA infusion. At eight hours after KA injection, however, a large number of degenerated granule cells are present, thus suggesting that these two neuronal populations (granule and pyramidal cells) undergo degeneration with different time course and could indicate that different mechanisms are responsible for the degeneration by KA of these two hippocampal cell-types.

The different vulnerability of nerve-cells to KA creates a problem when complete degeneration of a structure is required. This problem can be overcome by increasing the dose of KA ($\geqslant$ 1 ug for the hippocampus). However, this maneuver introduces a second major disadvantage of KA: cell death in brain regions located distant from the site of KA infusion (Fig.1 d,f). Such distant degeneration is most frequently observed in the piriform cortex, the antero- and medidorsal thalamic nuclei, the claustrum and the medial prefrontal cortex (see 35).

The mechanism by which KA induces such distant cell loss is not known at present but since all damaged brain areas receive afferents from the hippocampal region (including the entorhinal area) it is possible that the seizures triggered by KA within the hippocampal region play an important role for this type of pathology (for a discussion of this topic, see refs. 1, 35).

Interesting in this regard is the observation that the piriform cortex, which is an area extremely vulnerable to KA when injected into the hippocampus is not particularly sensitive to direct intracortical application of a small amounts of KA. Thus, relatively little damage to neurons in the piriform cortex is seen after injection of 0.3 - 0.5 µg/0.5 µl of the toxin directly into the anterior parts of the piriform cortex. However, injections of the same amounts at more posterior sites, close to the ventral hippocampus, resulted in extensive degeneration of cells in layers II and III throughout a major part of the piriform cortex. (16)

Ibotenic Acid Intrahippocampal injections of IBO cause a dose-dependent degeneration of pyramidal, granule and a large number of other multipolar and bipolar cells (see below). The area of neuronal degeneration is dependent on the dose and volume of IBO injected and a dose of 5 µg/0.5 ml of IBO results in hippocampal cell death in a radius extending approximately 1.5 mm from the center of the injection. Within the hippocampal formation, IBO is about 5 - 10 times less potent than KA towards the pyramidal cells. In contrast to KA, however, a complete degeneration of the entire hippocampus can be accomplished by successive injections of IBO without any detectable damage to neurons in distant brain areas.

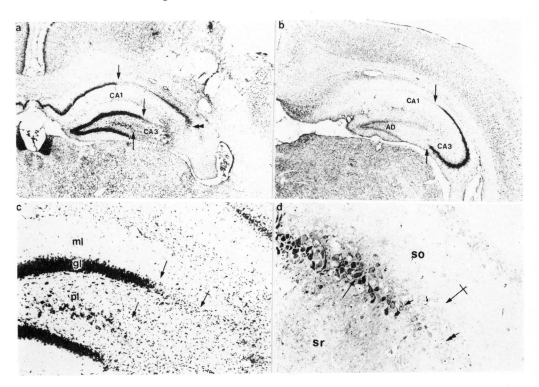

Figure 2 (a-d) Photomicrographs of local cell loss one week after the injection of IBO into the dorsal hippocampal formation (a,c) and lateral ventricle (b) of the rat. After both intrahippocampal (5 ug/0.5 µl) and intraventricular (10 µg/1 ul) injections there is a sharp border between intact and degenerated neurons. (Arrows in a, b and c.) Photomicrograph in(c)is a high-power micrograph of area dentata and part of subfield CA3. The sharp border between intact and degenerated neurons is clearly seen. The crossed arrow points at the lateral tip of the granule cell layer. Thionine stain Photomicrograph in (d)show a semithin (1 µm) section through the border between the CA1/CA2 and CA3 regions three hours after an intrahippocampal IBO (5 µg/0.5 µl) injection. Arrows point at neurons in different stages of degeneration. Double arrow-head show normal looking cell. Crossed arrow indicates the sharp border between neurons undergoing degeneration and intact neurons. Toluidine stain. Abbreviations: gl = granule cell layer, ml = molecular layer, pl = plexiform cell layer. Magn. x 20 (a,b); x 85 (d,c).

Signs of neuronal degeneration in the hippocampus can be observed at the light microscopic level as early as 3 - 4 hrs after intraventricular or intrahippocampal injections of IBO (Fig 2d). At this time pyramidal cells in CA1 and CA3 show dilatation of their dendrites and displacement of Nissl substance into distal parts of the dendrites as well as clear signs of disintegration of the soma membrane. In silver stained preparations the cells are argyrophilic with intense staining of soma and dendrites after 3 hrs. After 12 hrs the hippocampal neurons are shrunken and pyknotic and after 2 weeks a majority of the degenerated cells have been completely removed. Comparative studies of the early reaction of neurons to IBO and KA in the hippocampus clearly indicate a more rapid degeneration of

granule cells after IBO than after KA infusions. Thus, 3-4 hours after IBO injections (5 µg/0.5 µl) the granule cells are in an advanced stage of degeneration as
seen both in Nissl and silver stained sections. At the same time after KA
(1.0 µg/0.5 µl) infusions, however, only some of the granule cells are argyrophilic (see above).

It has been shown previously (33) using biochemical markers for presynaptic elements in the hippocampus (e.g. 5HT and noradrenalin uptake) that intrahippocampal
IBO does not degenerate hippocampal afferents or fibers passing through this
structure. An important question in this context, which is not answered using biochemical methods, is to what extent the afferents to the lesion area retain their
original position(s) and morphology after IBO injections. Studies of the cholinergic input to the hippocampus from the medial septum (22) using AChE-histochemistry (13) show a normal pattern of AChE staining within the area of neuronal
degeneration (Fig. 3). With the exception of the area in close vincinity of the
needle track no clear distortion of these cholinergic afferents is present.

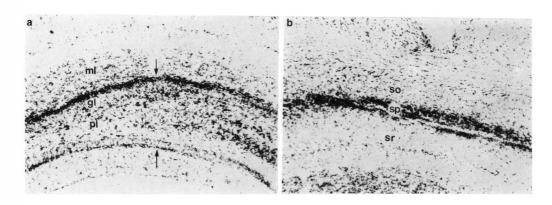

Figure 3 (a,b) Photomicrographs of the area dentata (a) and regio
superior (b) stained for the demonstration for AChE activity to mark
cholinergic nerve-terminals after an intrahippocampal injection of IBO
(5 µg/0.5 µl). Complete neuronal cell loss is found throughout the
dorsal hippocampal formation. Normal distribution of AChE reaction
product is found adjacent to degenerated granule cells (arrows in a)
and degenerated pyramidal neurons in (b) Abbreviations: so = stratum
oriens, sp = stratum pyramidale, sr = stratum radiatum. Magn. x 85

In fact, a closer examination revealed that in most cases the band of AChE staining in the inner molecular layer is more intense on the lesion as compared to the
non-lesion side. This increased staining of AChE positive fibers adjacent to degenerated cell bodies could be secondary to a shrinkage of the hippocampus due to
the lesion or could reflect processes such as sprouting or increased turn-over
within the cholinergic terminals in the lesioned hippocampus.

The axon sparing properties of IBO is not restricted to the cholinergic septohippocampal pathway.
Incubation of IBO - lesion hippocampi with antibody to serotonin in order to
visualize the serotonin innervation of the hippocampal formation from the raphe
nuclei shows a rich plexus of normal looking 5HT fibers adjacent to degenerated
granule and pyramidal cells. It should be pointed out, however, that although a
majority of the fibers appear normal a small number of individual serotonin con-

taining axons show morphological distortions within the lesion area, that suggest degeneration of at least some 5HT-fibers.

The neurotoxicity of IBO differs from that of KA in two major ways. First, intra-hippocampal injections of IBO cause degeneration of pyramidal and granule cells to about the same extent. This apparent lack of differential vulnerability of hippocampal neurons to IBO is illustrated in Figs.1 and 2. In this experiment KA (0.5 μg) and IBO (5 μg) was injected into the lateral part of the CA1 subfield. As can be seen (Fig. 1) KA degenerates pyramidal cells of CA1 and CA3 a-c while CA2 pyramidal and granule cells remain intact. In contrast, IBO injections cause degeneration of pyramidal cells in CA1 and CA3 subfields to approximately the same extent. As can be seen in Fig. 2 a-c there is a sharp border between intact and degenerated cells that cuts right through the hippocampal formation. The same pic-ture is seen when the toxin is injected into the ventricle close to the hippo-campus (Fig. 2b) which suggest that after IBO infusion the extent of neuronal de-generation is restricted primarily by the diffusion of the active compound with-in the hippocampal formation, and not by differential vulnerability of granule and pyramidal cells to the toxin.

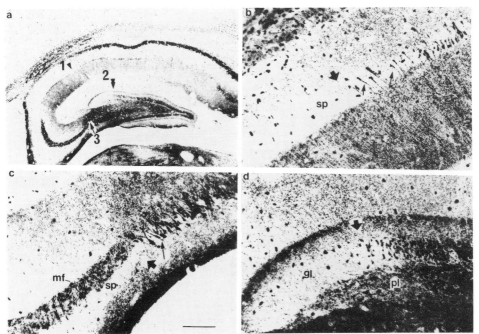

Figure 4 (a-d) Photomicrographs of the hippocampus two days after in-jection of QUIN (40 μg/1 μl) into the lateral ventricle. Fink-Heimer silverstain. (a) Neuronal cell loss is found from the midline to the level of the arrows (1, 2 and 3) in regio superior, area dentata and regio inferior, respectively. High power photomicrographs of the borders between intact and degenerated cells (large arrows) in regio superior (b; 1 in fig. a), regio inferior (c, 3 in fig. a) and area dentata (d; 2 in fig. a). Magn x 85 (a); x 85 (b-d)

Quinolinic acid. Intrahippocampal or intracerebroventricular injections of QUIN result in a dose-dependent degeneration of pyramidal and granule cells (Fig. 4). Within the hippocampal formation, QUIN is approximately 3 - 4 times less potent than IBO. The threshold dose for degeneration of the pyramidal cells is around

5 µg for QUIN while doses between 10 - 20 µg is required for degeneration of a
major portion of the dorsal hippocampal formation, including the granule cells.
No evidence for cell loss in distant brain regions has been found after intrahippocampal injections of large doses (40 µg) of QUIN. In studies where small
(5 µg) doses of QUIN was injected into the hippocampal formation only pyramidal
cells of CA4 and CA1 are found to undergo degeneration. In this respect, QUIN
toxicity seems to resemble that of KA. If the dose is increased ($>$10 µg),
however, degeneration of both pyramidal and granule cells is found. Similar to
IBO, but unlike KA, after QUIN injections into the ventricle a sharp border is
found between intact and degenerated pyramidal as well as granule cells (Fig. 4).

The degeneration of pyramidal and granule cells proceeds rapidly and at the light
microscopic level hippocampal cells are found to be argyrophilic in silverstained
sections after 3 to 4 hrs. In Nissl stained material the CA3/CA4 pyramidal cells
are pyknotic with signs of extensive reactive gliosis throughout the lesioned
hippocampus. After one week the damaged cells are fully degenerated and removed
by phagocytosis.

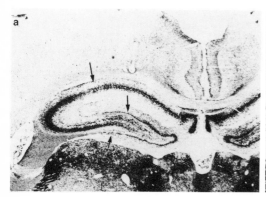 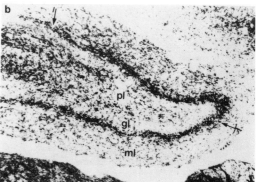

Figure 5 (a-b)
Photomicrographs of an AChE stained section through the hippocampal
formation after an intrahippocampal injection of QUIN (20 ug/0.5 µl).
Arrows in (a) mark the borders between areas of intact (left) and degenerated (right) neurons. As can be seen the AChE containing terminals remain at their normal position both in regio superior and area
dentata (b) adjacent to degenerated neuronal cell bodies. Magn. X.
20 (a) 85 (b)

The effects of intrahippocampal or intraventricular injections of QUIN on the
cholinergic nerve-terminals in the pyramidal and granule cell layers was evaluated
using AChE-histochemistry and serotonin immunohistochemistry of QUIN lesioned
hippocampi. Analysis of this material contrastained with thionin reveal a normal
or slightly intensified band of AChE reaction products adjacent to degenerated
neurons (Fig. 5) which is similar to that observed after IBO injections. Furthermore, the 5HT innervation of the lesioned hippocampus remain essentially intact
after QUIN injections. Taken together these findings support biochemical evidence
(34 and Schwacz et al, this volume) that QUIN, like IBO and KA cause neuronal
degeneration of an axon-sparing type.

Hippocampal neurons resistent to excitotoxins

Inspection of the hippocampal formation after IBO injections show numerous intact
neurons of non-pyramidal shape that are located within and outside the pyramidal
cell layer. Recently, immunohistochemical studies have shown that the hippocampal

non-pyramidal neurons contain cholecystokinin octapeptide (CCK-8), somatostatin (SOM) (7), vasoactive intestinal polypeptide (VIP) (18), enkephalin (ENK) (8) or GAD (29)-like immunoreactivity. In order to determine if the surviving cells belong to one particular class of chemically identified neurons, IBO-lesioned hippocampi were incubated with antibodies to SOM, VIP,ENK, CCK-8 and GAD. These studies clearly show that a majority of all IBO-resistant neurons are GAD positive (Fig. 7), while no VIP or SOM-L immunoreactive cells are present within the lesion area. The reason for this resistance of GAD cells to IBO toxicity is not known but may not necessarily be related to their neurochemical identity but rather to the possible existence of certain types of surface receptors that (a) either do not recognize IBO or (b) are coupled to a different effector in the plasma membrane of the cell thus, protecting the cell from degeneration. An interesting observation in this regard is the strong cholinoceptive nature of surviving neurons whithin the hilus of the area dentata. It remains to be shown if these cholinoceptic cells that survive the IBO injection also are GAD positive. Similar studies with KA show that this toxin, too, does not degenerate all non-pyramidal cells in the hippocampal formation. However, an analysis of the histochemical identity of these resistant cells shows that many different GAD and peptide containing neurons survive. Taken together, these findings further emphasize the different toxic action of IBO and KA which may reflect basic differences in their mechanism(s) of action. Hippocampal "interneurons" are not the only cell group showing selective resistance to high concentration of excitotoxins, but cells in a large number of brain areas have been shown to exhibit this feature (4). It is possible that a more intensive study of the factors contributing to the selective resistance of certain neurons to KA and IBO may be a fruitful approach in trying to understand the mechanism(s) behind neuronal degeneration.

Cerebellum

Kainic Acid   Intracerebellar injections of KA result in a dose dependent degeneration of cerebellar granule, Purkinje and stellate cells at the center of the injection as described in previous light and electron-microscopic studies (10,11). Three days after an injection of KA (0.5 μg/0.5 μl) pyknotic granule cells are found in an area extending approximately 1 mm from the center of the infusion. In most cases, a relatively irregular pattern of degeneration is seen in different folia, probably due to diffusion of the toxin and the special morphology of the cerebellum. At higher doses of KA (1 μg/1 μl) a major part of the vermis contained degenerated neurons. In addition, extensive degeneration of cells is seen in the deep cerebellar nuclei, in spite of the fact that they are situated relatively far from the injection site and that they are separated from the center of the injection by numerous intact cerebellar neurons. Analysis of serial sections through the lesion area revealed, however, complete degeneration of granule cells at locations where the adjacent Purkinje cells remain intact. This observation is at variance with earlier observations on the hamster cerebellum (10) and studies on the effects on cerebellar cultures in vitro (36) but is in good agreement with the observations by Lovell and Jones (19) which have shown intact Purkinje cells adjacent to degenerated granule cells after intra-cerebellar injections in the mouse. The reason(s) for these discrepancies is unclear at present. However, the fact that the Purkinje cells remain intact in rat and mouse cerebellum after KA infusion represents another example of differences in vulnerability of various neuronal cell types to KA and challenges the original hypothesis (20) that KA toxicity is directly related to its binding to cell-surface glutamate receptors.

Ibotenic acid   Similar to KA, intracerebellar injections of IBO cause a dose dependent degeneration of all cerebellar neurons. At the center of infusion, all neuronal cell types undergo degeneration if sufficiently high doses are injected. ($\geqslant$ 10 μg/0.5 μl). The area of complete degeneration of all cellbodies is very small and analysis of folia located 50 - 100 um away from the needle track show a remarkable selectivity with regard to damage to certain neurons: although granule and stellate cells undergo degeneration the Purkinje cells are intact as shown by Nissl, silver and immunohistochemical staining method. Although, selective sparing of Purkinje cells is related to the dose given as measured at the center of infusion, intact Purkinje cells are always present close to degenerated granule cells at more distantly located folia. The fact that intact Purkinje cells contain GAD-like immunoreactivity indicates that these cell retain their ability to synthetize GAD when the cell is situated in close vicinity of the injection site and thus must have been exposed to large quantities of toxin (Fig. 6).

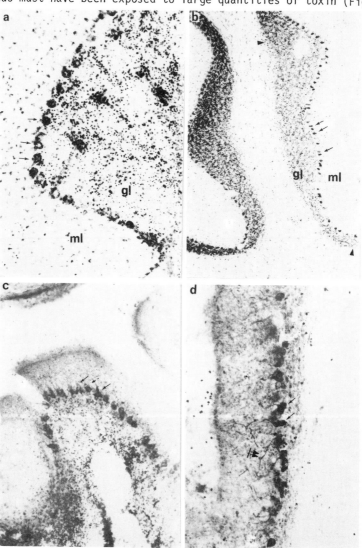

Figure 6 (a-d) Photomicrographs of one cerebellar folia after injection of IBO (5 μg/0.5 μl) (a,c) and QUIN (40 μg/1 ul) (b,d) in two individual rats. Photomicrographs in (a) and (b) show degenerated granule cells and intact Purkinje cells (arrows) in close vicinity of the injections. Arrow heads in (b) delimits the area containing degenerated granule cells after QUIN infusion. In (c) and (d) intact GAD-immunoreactive

Purkinje cells are shown adjacent to degenerated granule cells in
close proximity to the injection site. Double arrow-heads in d indicate Purkinje cell dendrites.
Abbreviations: gl = granule cell layer, ml = molecular cell layer,
Magn: X 210 (a); 20 (b) 210 (c,d)

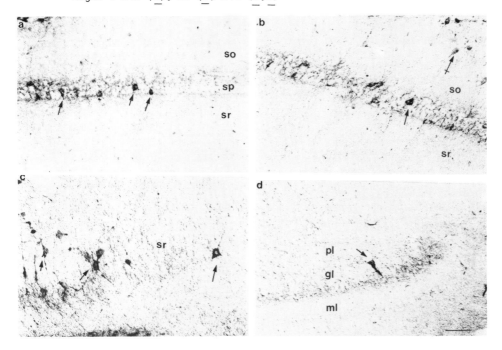

Figure 7 (a-d)   Photomicrographs showing intact GAD-immunoreactive
                  neuronal cell-bodies one week after the injection
                  of IBO (5 ug/0.5 ul) into the dorsal hippocampus
                  of the rat. The immunoreactive cells (arrows) are
                  surrounded by degenerated perikarya. Photomicro-
                  graphs are from the regio superior (a, b) regio
                  inferior (c) and area dentata (d). Crossed arrow
                  in b shows intact GAD positive neuron in stratum
                  oriens of the regio superior. Abbreviations as in
                  Figs. 2 and 3. Nomarski optics. Magn. x 210.

Quinolinic acid Both KA and IBO have been shown previously to be relatively
toxic towards cells of the cerebellar cortex and deep cerebellar nuclei. In
order to examine the toxicity of QUIN in other structures than the hippocampus
different doses of QUIN were injected into the vermis of the cerebellum at
positions similar to those for KA and IBO injections. Intra cerebellar injections of QUIN resulted in a dose-dependent degeneration of granule, stellate
and Purkinje cells. Compared to the area of degeneration observed in the hippocampus after equipotent doses the region of cerebellar tissue containing degenerated cells around the site of QUIN-infusion is relatively small. Even after
high doses (40 µg) of QUIN the area of degeneration does not extend more than
0.5-1.0 mm from the injection site. Systematic comparisons of the total area
containing nerve cell loss after injections into the cerebellum with that
observed after injections into the hippocampus, striatum or substantia nigra

suggests a remarkable variation in the vulnerability of cells in different brain regions to QUIN as compared to both KA and IBO (see also Schwarcz, this volume).

Since QUIN is endogenously present in mammalian tissue, and thus, potentially also present in the brain, this regional variation in neurotoxic potency of QUIN may relate to the regional variations in tissue concentrations of QUIN or its receptor in different brain regions.

Neurons of the hippocampus and the striatum have been shown to undergo degeneration in chronic epilepsy (see Meldrum, this volume) and Huntingtons disease, respectively. The fact that the hippocampus and the striatum are particularly sensitive to QUIN, an endogenous excitatory aminoacid, may suggest a role of this or some related compound in these neurological diseases.

SUMMARY

The morphology of the neuronal degeneration caused by two exogenous (KA; IBO) and one endogenous (QUIN) excitotoxic aminoacids have been studied in the rat brain. All three excitotoxins cause neuronal degeneration of an axon sparing type but the pattern of neuronal degeneration is sufficiently different between the three excitotoxins to suggest basic differences in their mechanisms of action. Certain neurons within the hippocampus are resistant to IBO, KA and QUIN. Immunohistochemical studies showed a selective resistance of GAD-containing neurons to IBO toxicity while many GAD, VIP and SOM-containing cells survive KA infusions. It is possible that a further characterization of those neurons in the hippocampus (and other brain areas) that survive infusions of high doses of excitotoxic aminoacids will contribute to our understanding of the mechanism(s) underlying their neurotoxicity.

ACKNOWLEDGEMENT

The excellent technical assistance of L.G. Eriksson is gratefully acknowledged. The 5-HT antiserum was kindly provided by Dr. H. Steinbusch, Free University, Amsterdam, The Netherlands and the GAD-antiserum by Dr. J.Y. Wu, Baylor College of Medicine, Houston, Texas, USA.

REFERENCES

1. Ben-Ari, Y., I. Lagowska, E. Tremblay and G. LeGal la Salle (1979). Brain Res. 163, 176-180.
2. Collonier, M., M. Steriade and P. Landry (1979). Brain Res. 172, 552-556.
3. Coyle, I.T., S.J. Bird, R.H. Evans, R.L. Gulley, I.V. Nadler, W.I. Nicklas and I.W. Olney (Eds.) (1981). Neurosci. Res. Prog. Bull. 19.
4. De Montigny, C. and J.P. Lund (1980). Neurosci. 5, 1621-1628.
5. Eugster, C.H. (1967). In: Ethnopharmacological Search for Psychoactive Drugs. Efron, D.H., Holmstedt, B. and N.S. Kline (Eds.) p. 416. MS Public Health Service.
6. Eugster, C.H. (1968). Natur Wiss. 55, 305-313.
7. Finley, J.C.W., I.L. Maderdrut, L.J. Roger and P. Petrusz (1981). Neurosci. 6, 2173-2192.
8. Gall, C., N. Brecha, H.I. Karten and K.I. Chang (1981). J. Comp. Neurol. 198. 335-350.
9. Geneser-Jensen, F.H. and T.W. Blackstad (1971). 2. Zellforschmikrosk. Anat. 114, 460-481.
10. Herndon, R.M. and J.T. Coyle (1977). Science N.Y. 198, 71-72.
11. Herndon, R.M., J.T. Coyle and E. Addicks (1980). Neurosci. 5, 1015-1027.
12. Hsu, S.M., L. Raine and H. Fanger (1981). J. Histochem. Cytochem. 29, 577-580.
13. Koelle, G.B. (1954). J. Comp. Neurol. 100, 211-228.

14. Köhler, Ch., R. Schwarcz and K. Fuxe (1979). Brain Res. 175, 366-371.
15. Köhler, Ch. and R. Schwarcz (1981). Meeting Int. Soc. Neurochem. (Abstract 272).
16. Köhler, Ch. and R. Schwarcz (1982). (Submitted).
17. Krammer, E.G., M.F. Lischka, M. Karobath and G. Schönbeck (1979). Brain Res. 177, 577-582.
18. Lorén, I., P.C. Emson, I. Fahrenkrug, A. Björklund and F. Sundler (1979). Neurosci. 4, 1953-1976.
19. Lovell, K.L. and M.Z. Jones (1980). Brain Res. 186, 245-249.
20. McGeer, P.L., E.G. McGeer and T. Hattori (1978). In: Kainic acid as a tool in neurobiology. McGeer, E.G., J.W. Olney and P.L. McGeer (Eds.) p. 123, Raven Press N.Y.
21. McGeer, E.G., J.W. Olney and P.L. McGeer (Eds.) (1978). Kainic acid as a tool in neurobiology. Raven Press N.Y.
22. Mellgren, S.I. and B. Srebro (1973). Brain Res. 52, 19-36.
23. Nadler, J.V. (1979). Life Sci. 24, 289-300.
24. Nadler, J.V., D.A. Evenson and G.J. Cuthbertson (1981). Neurosci. 12, 2505-2517.
25. Olney, J.W., V. Rhee and O.L. Ho (1974). Brain Res. 77, 507-512.
26. Olney, J.W. and T. DeGubareff (1978). Brain Res. 140, 340-343.
27. Olney, J.W. (1978). In: McGeer, E.G., J.W. Olney and P.L. McGeer (Eds.) Raven Press N.Y.
28. Olney, J.W., T. Fuller and T. DeGubareff (1976). Brain Res. 176, 91-100.
29. Ribak, C.E., J.E. Vaughn and K. Saito (1978). Brain Res. 140, 315-332.
30. Schwarcz, R. and J.T. Coyle (1977). Life Sci. 20, 431-436.
31. Schwarcz, R., D. Scholtz and J.T. Coyle (1978). Neuropharmacol. 17, 145-151.
32. Schwarcz, R., T. Hökfelt, K. Fuxe, G. Jonsson, M. Goldstein and L. Terenius (1979). Exp. Brain Res. 37, 199-216.
33. Schwarcz, R., Ch. Köhler, K. Fuxe, T. Hökfelt and M. Goldstein (1979). In: Advances in neurology, vol 23, Chase, T.N., N. Wexler and A. Barbeau (Eds.) p. 655-667, New York.
34. Schwarcz, R., Ch. Köhler and R. Mangano (1982). Neurosci. (Abstract).
35. Schwob, J.E., T. Fuller, J.L. Price and J.W. Olney (1980). Neurosci. 5, 991-1014.
36. Seil, F., N.K. Blank and A.L. Leiman (1979). Brain Res. 161, 253-265.
37. Wuerthele, S.M., K.M. Lovell, M.Z. Jones and Moore K.E. (1978). Brain Res. 149, 489-497.

KAINIC ACID: INSIGHTS INTO ITS RECEPTOR-MEDIATED NEUROTOXIC MECHANISMS

J. T. COYLE, J. FERKANY, R. ZACZEK, J. SLEVIN and K. RETZ

Division of Child Psychiatry, Departments of Psychiatry, Neuroscience Pharmacology and Pædiatrics, Johns Hopkins University, School of Medicine, Baltimore, Maryland 21205

INTRODUCTION

Historically, kainic acid (KA) was selected as a potential exitotoxin because the evidence at the time was consistent with the notion that, as a conformationally restricted analogue of L-glutamate, it was a potent agonist at glutamate receptors (Olney et al., 1974; Coyle and Schwarcz, 1976). Since the first reports of the perikaryal-specific neurotoxic action of intracerebrally injected KA, it has become increasingly apparent that the mechanism of its neurotoxic effects is complex. Consequently, it has been our strategy for clarifying the mechanism of neurotoxicity of KA to focus on receptor specific interactions of the drug. We have felt that this approach might lead to a better understanding of the proximate physiologic events that result in perikaryal-specific neuronal degeneration. Furthermore, the effects of KA might be distinguished from other receptor-specific excitatory amino acid analogues (Watkins and Evans, 1981) such as N-methyl-D-aspartic acid (NMDA) and quisqualic acid as well as more generalized consequences of excessive stimulation of the broad class of the acidic amino acid receptors. These studies have provided evidence of the unique physiologic, pharmacologic and toxicologic properties associated with activation of receptors for KA.

RESULTS

Ligand binding of [3H]-kainic acid. Simon et al. (1976) first described the specific, saturable and high affinity binding of [3H]-KA to brain membranes. Their study provided evidence that [3H]-KA bound to a site that was enriched in synaptic membranes and that had the pharmacologic characteristics of an acidic excitatory amino acid receptor. In subsequent studies, we have focused on the specific binding of [3H]-KA in order to characterize the receptor mediating its neurotoxic effects. Saturation isotherms as well as competitive displacement studies indicated the existence of at least two binding sites in the rat brain: the higher affinty site with a K_D of 5 nM was found in forebrain regions whereas the lower affinty site with a K_D of 50 nM was found in all major brain regions examined (London and Coyle, 1979a). The regional distribution of the binding sites for [3H]-KA was markedly uneven; the highest density of sites was found in the striatum followed by the frontal cortex and hippocampus with the cerebellum having intermediate levels and the medulla pons having the lowest density of binding sites. Specific binding of [3H]-KA could not be demonstrated in peripheral tissue such as the liver, lung, kidney or intestine.

Although L-glutamate exhibits a uM affinity for the [^{3}H]-KA labeled site, D-glutamate has a 60-fold lower affinty than the L-isomer whereas these stereo-isomers are nearly equipotent as neuroexcitants. Furthermore, the neurophysio-logically weak analogue of KA, dihydrokainic acid, in which the isopropylene side-chain is reduced, exhibited a several hundred fold lower affinity for the receptor than KA although the glutamate portion of the KA molecule is unaffected by side-chain reduction. Subsequent detailed displacement studies indicated that both L-glutamate and dihydrokainate exhibited shallow displacement curves with Hill coefficients significantly less than one, which was not consistent with isographic binding of these two compounds to the [^{3}H]-KA labeled site (London and Coyle, 1979b). These findings have called into question the origi-nal assumption that [^{3}H]-KA was labeling a "glutamate" receptor.

Structural Activity Relations. With the recent availability of several structural analogues of KA, it has been possible to better delineate the topography of the [^{3}H]-KA recognition site. It should be emphasized that the physiologic relevance of ligand-binding sites must be defined in terms of the correlation between receptor affinity and physiologic potency of related ligands. In this regard, affinity of the KA analogues for the receptor have been correlated with neurotoxic potency and neurophysiologic activity (Biscoe et al., 1976) where known (Table I). However, it must be kept in mind that

TABLE 1

Neurotoxic and Electrophysiologic Potency of Kainate Analogues
in the Striatum Versus [^{3}H]-Kainate Receptor Affinity

Compound	K$_I$ at KA Receptor (nM)	Physiologic Potency [X]/[Glu]	Toxic Potency [X]/[KA]
Domoic Acid	13*	36-109	1
α-Kainic Acid	21	18- 54	1
α-Keto Kainic Acid	430	10	40
α-Kainic Acid Diethylester	1,040	< 1	>>50
Dihydrokainic Acid	7,400*	0.06-0.8	>>50
α-Allo Kainic Acid	>10,000	0.5-2	50
L-Glutamic Acid	722*	1	>>100
Quisqualic Acid	610	22-90	>50 (est)
Ibotenic Acid	9,400	2-7	40
N-Methyl-D-Aspartic Acid	>10,000	4-12	120

Specific binding of [^{3}H]-kainic acid was performed in the rat cerebellum with displacement curves consisting of 10 or more concentrations of drug. Neurotoxicity was based upon the reductions in the presynaptic markers for cho-linergic and GABAergic neurons following stereotaxic injection into the rat cor-pus striatum (Schwarcz et al., 1978; Zaczek and Coyle, 1982). Physiologic potency are based upon the values for mammalian neurons of Biscoe et al. (1976). *Hill coefficient significantly less than one.

alterations in molecular structure that may radically reduce affinity for the [^{3}H]-KA binding site could enhance affinity for other excitatory receptors so that an exact correlation between receptor affinity and neurophysiologic potency might not be expected. Finally, in order to avoid the interpretational problems associated with kinetics of displacement at two receptors, we have used rat cerebellar membranes, which possess only the low affinity 50 nM site to which [^{3}H]-KA acid binds with a Hill coefficient of 1.0 (London and Coyle, 1979b). Domoic acid, an analogue of kainic acid with a more extended side-chain, is two-to three-fold more potent than kainic acid in neurophysiologic studies and exhibits a three-fold higher affinity for the receptor; it is at least as potent as kainic acid as a neurotoxin. Alpha-keto-kainic acid has a ketone substituted for the methylene group on the side-chain; this analogue has approximately 10-fold lower potency in terms of excitatory activity and a 20-fold lower affinity for the KA receptor, which is approximately equivalent to its neurotoxic efficacy. As noted above, dihydrokainate, in which the double-bond in the isopropylene side-chain has been reduced, has a 200-fold lower affinity for the receptor and is devoid of neurotoxic action at doses 100-fold above the threshold dose of KA. Alpha-allo-kainate is a stereoisomer, in which the isopropylene side-chain has a trans configuration; this compound has weak excitatory effects and exhibits greater than a 500-fold lower affinity for the KA receptor. Curiously, this stereoisomer exhibits significant neurotoxic effects, albeit at 50-times the effective dose of KA. Thus, these studies indicate a relatively close correspondence between receptor affinity, neurophysiologic potency and neurotoxicologic effects among a series of analogues for KA. Furthermore, these results point to the critical role played by the isopropylene side-chain in binding to the kainate receptor.

Recently, Ruck et al. (1980) suggested that folates, naturally occurring cofactors ubiquitously distributed in brain albeit in low concentrations, have high affinity for KA receptors and therefore may serve as endogenous ligands for these receptors. In contrast, we found that N-5-methyltetrahydrofolic acid, tetrahydrofolic acid and dihydrofolic acid had affinities less than 2,000-fold of that of KA for the receptor (e.g., K_I's >> 50 uM). Furthermore, these folate derivaties were virtually devoid of local neurotoxic effects when injected into the rat corpus striatum in saturating solutions (1 ul of 250 mM). Finally, none of the folate derivatives stimulated the formation of cyclic GMP in cerebellar slices incubated in vitro at 1 mM concentration, in contrast to KA, which has significant effects at 20-fold lower concentrations. Thus, we could find no evidence to support the hypothesis that folates serve as endogenous agonists at the KA receptor (Ferkany et al., in press).

Kainate Receptor Distribution. In a phylogenetic study, the specific binding of [^{3}H]-KA was examined in the nervous tissue from fourteen species ranging from invertebrates to man (London et al., 1980). In all species except the sea anemone, significant specific binding of [^{3}H]-KA was observed. Notably, at intermediate levels of the phylogenetic tree including the spiny dog fish, the goldfish, the frog and the chicken, the density of binding sites in brain were more than 10-fold greater than found in the brains of mammals including rat and man. An intriguing feature of these results is that receptor density of sites in the cerebella of the dog fish, goldfish, frog and chick were several magnitudes greater than in the mammalian cerebellum, a brain region with a relatively low density of binding sites. Curiously, displacement of the bound [^{3}H]-KA by unlabeled KA in chick cerebellum resulted in complex curves (Malouf and Coyle, unpublished).

Aside from the convincing correlation between neurotoxic potency and affinity for KA receptors observed with KA analogues, additional evidence for the role of these receptors in neurotoxicity comes from the demonstration of a high degree of localization of KA receptor binding sites on neurons vulnerable to the excitotoxin. Thus, prior KA lesion of the rat corpus striatum (London and Coyle, 1979a) or the chick neural retina (Biziere and Coyle, 1979a) resulted in a dramatic loss of KA binding sites. Evidence that these receptors are required for the neurotoxic effects of KA is supported by the results of a developmental study in which vulnerability to the neurotoxic effects was shown to increase postnatally in the rat in association with the accrual of KA receptor binding sites (Campochiaro and Coyle, 1978). In the rat cerebellum, the development of

KA receptors occurs contemporaneously with the elaboration of the granule cell parallel fiber synapses (Slevin and Coyle, 1981). Notably, the developmental profile for the KA receptor differs from that of the [^{3}H]-L-glutamate binding site (Slevin et al., in press), which reaches adult levels more rapidly and has a 20-fold greater density.

Marked reductions in the density of KA binding sites after KA lesion of the striatum have led to the suggestion that the bulk of these receptors are located on vulnerable neuronal perikarya within the striatum; however, nearly 40% of the binding sites persisted after the KA lesion and decortication resulted in a 25% reduction in total specific binding at 7 and 15 days after the surgery (Biziere and Coyle, 1979b). This result suggests a partial presynaptic localization of the KA receptors. To assess better the localization of these receptor sites, we examined the effects of drug induced or inherited lesions of the cerebellar neurons on the binding sites for [^{3}H]-KA and [^{3}H]-L-glutamate (Table 2). Neonatal treatment of the mouse with the potent alkylating agent

TABLE 2

Excitatory Receptor Binding to Membranes Prepared from Lesioned
Mouse Cerebellum

	Density	Total per Cerebellum
	Percent of Control	
[^{3}H]-Kainic Acid (50 nM)		
Granule cell deficient	93 + 8	57 + 5*
Purkinje cell deficient	96 + 12	56 + 6*
[^{3}H]-L-Glutamic Acid (600 nM)		
Granule cell deficient	165 + 8*	95 + 5
Purkinje cell deficient	139 + 10*	76 + 11*

The specific binding of [^{3}H]-kainic acid and [^{3}H]-L-glutamic acid to washed cerebellar membranes was determined in mice deficient in granule cells induced by neonatal treatment with methylazoxymethanol acetate or deficient in Purkinje cells due to the nervous mutation. The results are the mean of 7 or more preparations, which were compared to litter mate controls assayed at the same time (Slevin et al, 1982; Slevin and Coyle, unpublished).

methylazoxymethanol acetate (MAM) causes a selective and marked hypoplasia of the granule cells while sparing the Purkinje cells (Slevin et al., 1982). This lesion was associated with an enrichment in the binding sites for [^{3}H]-L-glutamate but not those for [^{3}H]-KA. In other words, loss of granule cells did not significantly affect the total number of glutamate receptors in the cerebellum but did result in a 43% decrease in the KA receptors; this finding suggests that the latter receptors are located on the affected granule cell population. In the case of the nervous mutant, there is a selective degeneration of the Purkinje cells with sparing of the granule cells. In this somewhat hypoplastic cerebellum, the density of KA receptors was unchanged, resulting in a 44% decrement in the total number of KA receptor sites for the cerebellum. While the glutamate binding was increased by 39% in concentration, the total number of glutamate binding sites per cerebellum was significantly reduced by 24%. Thus, these results clearly indicate that the glutamate receptor and the KA receptor have different neuronal sites of distribution in the cerebellum and suggest that nearly half of the KA receptors have a "presynaptic" localization on the excitatory, presumably glutamatergic, parallel fiber system.

Kainate-induced release of endogenous acidic excitatory amino acids. It has been well established that the mechanism of neurotoxicity of KA in several brain regions is indirect and requires the integrity of excitatory afferents. For example, decortication, which causes degeneration of the cortico-striate glutamatergic projection, protects against the neurotoxic effects of KA injected into the striatum (Biziere and Coyle, 1978b). An interesting feature of the protective effects of these lesions is that the onset is delayed; thus, termination of impulse flow within the pathway appears to be insufficient for providing protection (Biziere and Coyle, 1979b). Recently, Krespan et al. (1982), using precursor prelabeling techniques, demonstrated that KA stimulates the release of radiolabeled glutamate from cerebellar slices incubated in vitro. In light of the evidence that nearly half of the KA receptors are located on the cerebellar granule cells, we wondered whether these receptors might account for the release of prelabeled glutamate from cerebellar slices incubated in vitro and, in a broader sense, might explain the apparent potentiation of glutamatergic neurotransmission in axotomized afferent systems such as the cortico-striate pathway.

To avoid the interpretational problems associated with prelabeling techniques, we have measured the release of endogenous amino acids from cerebellar slices incubated in vitro by the precolumn derivitization technique of Hill et al (1979). Elevated potassium stimulated a significant release of aspartate, glutamate and GABA from the slices but did not alter the spontaneous efflux of glutamine (Table 3). Although 0.5 mM KA significantly enhanced the release of aspartate and glutamate, it did not affect the release of glutamine, alanine, taurine or GABA (Ferkany et al., 1982). The potassium-induced release of glutamate and aspartate was blocked by 1 uM tetrodotoxin whereas tetrodotoxin was ineffective in inhibiting the release of the excitatory amino acids induced by KA. This finding effectively rules out the possibility that the KA-induced release resulted from elevated extracellular concentrations of potassium, a known effect of kainate. Nevertheless, the KA-induced release appeared to be occurring by an exocytotic process since calcium-free media containing EGTA inhibited it. Furthermore, the response appeared to be mediated by receptor interaction of KA since dihydrokainate and alpha-allo-kainate, two inactive analogues, were ineffective in stimulating glutamate and aspartate release. Since dihydrokainate is a more potent inhibitor of the glutamate uptake process (Biziere and Coyle, 1978b), this finding also discounted the possibility that enhanced release simply reflected inhibition of the terminal uptake process. Finally, this response appeared to be specific for KA receptors because the excitatory amino acid analogue, N-methyl-D,L-aspartate, did not affect glutamate release.

To establish further that KA was acting on a neuronal pool of the acidic excitatory amino acids, we examined amino acid release in cerebellar slices deficient in granule cells as a result of postnatal treatment with MAM (Slevin et al., 1982). In the granulo-prival cerebellum, KA-induced release of glutamate was reduced by 67% whereas the release of aspartate was not significantly affected. Since aspartate is thought to be the excitatory neurotransmitter of a component of the climbing fiber system (Wikilund et al., 1982), which is spared by the MAM lesion, these findings are consistent with the KA acting on neuronal pools of the acidic excitatory amino acid. In further support of this interpretation, we have found that KA does not significantly

TABLE 3

Endogenous Amino Acid Release from Cerebellar Slices

Condition	Aspartate	Glutamate
	nmoles/mg protein/15 min	
Control	0.6 + 0.0	1.5 + 0.1
KCl (40 mM)	1.4 + 0.3*	2.6 + 0.2*
α-KA (0.5 mM)	1.4 + 0.1*	4.0 + 0.3*
TTX (5 uM)	0.4 + 0.1	1.0 + 0.1
KCl + TTX (5 uM)	0.4 + 0.1	1.1 + 0.2
α-KA + TTX (5 uM)	1.1 + 0.1**	3.0 + 0.3*
α-KA + 0 Ca^{++}	0.7 + 0.1	1.6 + 0.1
Dihydro-KA (5 mM)	0.9 + 0.3	2.1 + 0.4
Allo-KA (5 mM)	0.9 + 0.3	2.2 + 0.3
NMDA (10 mM)	ND	1.7 + 0.3
AMPA (1 mM)	0.6 + 0.1	1.5 + 0.4

Cerebellar slices prepared from adult mice were incubated in oxygenated Krebs buffer in the presence of the drugs. The results are expressed in terms of the net amount of the amino acids released into the medium in the presence of drug compared with control slices incubated in parallel. Values are the mean + S.E.M. of five or more preparations. Under no condition did the levels of glutamine differ significantly from control. Abbreviations: ND, not detectable (due to interference of NMDA); TTX, tetrodotoxin; KCl, potassium chloride; KA, kainic acid; NMDA, N-methyl-D-aspartic acid.
*p < 0.02 versus control.

enhance the release of glutamate from slices of ten day old rat cerebellum, in which the granule cell parallel system has yet to be established. The KA-induced stimulation of excitatory amino acid release is not restricted to the cerebellum; in fact, marked and selective KA stimulation of aspartate and glutamate release, that occurs predominantly by a calcium-dependent process, has also been demonstrated in perfused hippocampal and striatal slices (Ferkany et al., 1982). Thus, these studies have demonstrated a second, important site of action of KA aside from its direct excitatory effects on neurons.

Acute metabolic effects of excitotoxins. The proximate cause of for excitotoxin-induced neuronal degeneration has not been directly assessed although neurophysiologic results indicate that depolarization block and profound swelling of the affected neuronal dendrites are early concomitants of the neurodegenerative process (Coyle et al., 1978). It has been hypothesized that the profound depolarization induced by excitotoxins overwhelms the energy capability of the neurons to extrude the intracellularly accumulated sodium and water (Olney et al., 1971). Consistent with this hypothesis, [^{14}C]-2-deoxyglucose autoradiographic studies have demonstrated a profound, acute increase in glucose turnover in brain areas affected by neuronal degeneration after intracerebral administration of KA (Wooten and Collins, 1980). However, interpretation of [^{14}C]-2-deoxyglucose studies is confounded by problems of distinguishing the contribution of increased impulse flow of afferent systems from activity of intrinsic neurons, both of which may be affected by a locally injected excitotoxin. Accordingly, we have examined the effects of intrastriatally injected excitotoxins on the disposition of high energy phosphates and glucose, which would provide a better insight into the metabolic status of the brain region.

Studies were performed in the striatum of the mouse because this species was most amenable to nearly instantaneous termination of metabolic activity by focused microwave irradiation. High energy phosphate levels and metabolite profiles obtained in the striatum of the mouse after focused microwave irradiation closely approximated those occurring in whole brain after freeze-blowing techniques or cerebral cortex after freeze clamping with liquid nitrogen (Retz and Coyle, 1982). As shown in Table 4, intrastriatal injection of KA caused rapid and significant decreases in the levels of phosphocreatine, ATP, energy charge and glucose. Intrastriatal injection of ibotenic acid, an

TABLE 4

Effects of Intrastriatal Kainic Acid and Ibotenic Acid on
Metabolic Parameters

Treatment	PCr	ATP	Ad-P Total	Energy Charge	Lactate	Glucose
			Percent of Control			
Kainic Acid	75 + 5*	68 + 4*	80 + 3*	91 + 2*	144 + 6*	44 + 11*
Ibotenic Acid	62 + 10*	88 + 4*	93 + 2*	93 + 4*	214 + 6*	75 + 11
Decortication	106 + 8	91 + 6	90 + 5	99 + 2	161 + 10*	110 + 6
Decortication plus Kainic Acid	99 + 8	95 + 5	96 + 4	101 + 1	312 + 9*	85 + 5

Mice received unilateral injections of either kainic acid (0.35 ug) or ibotenic acid (7 ug) two hours prior to sacrifice by focused microwave irradiation (0.95 sec; 1.25 KW). Decortication was performed seven days prior to the kainate injection. Results are the mean + S.E.M. of 10-16 preparations assayed in parallel with controls (Retz and Coyle, 1982). Abbreviations: PCr, phosphocreatine; Ad-P, total adenosine phosphates. *p < 0.05 versus control by ANOVA.

excitotoxin with a mechanism of action different than KA, produced comparable but less severe alterations in cellular energy parameters at 2 hours after injection. Although the fall in energy charge appears relatively modest, the severity of the decrement is minimized due to the significant loss of total adenosine phosphates. If one takes into account the loss of adenosine phosphates in calculating the energy charge, the corrected energy charge would have fallen to 0.66, a level associated with inhibition of macromolecular synthesis (Svedes et al., 1975).

With KA, it is essential to distinguish those effects related to its direct excitatory action from those responsible for its neurotoxic effects. Prior decortication, which prevents the neurotoxic action of KA in the mouse striatum, completely prevented the alterations in high energy phosphates, glucose levels, and energy charge. However, KA injection into the decorticate striatum was associated with a dramatic increase in the concentration of lactate, considerably greater than that found after KA injection in the intact striatum. This finding is consistent with the maintenance of the excitatory effects of KA shown neurophysiologically in the absence of neurotoxicity in the decorticate striatum (McLennan, 1980).

DISCUSSION

Kainic acid has proved to be the most potent excitotoxin available, being 20- to 100-fold more active on intracerebral injection than ibotenate, quisqualate and N-methyl-D-aspartate, excitatory amino acid analogues that act at different receptor sites (Schwarcz et al., 1978; Zaczek and Coyle, 1982). This unusual neurotoxic potency is discrepant from the excitatory efficacy of kainic acid, which is equivalent to quisqualate and only 2- to 3-fold greater than ibotenate and N-methyl-D-aspartic acid (Biscoe et al., 1976). This disparity may be related to the indirect mechanism of neurotoxicity of KA, which differs from the apparent uniform and presumably direct effects of ibotenate, N-methyl-D-aspartate and quisqualate. Neurophysiologic and ligand binding studies now indicate the existence of a distinct receptor that responds to KA (Watkins and Evans, 1981). The molecular determinants for activation of the receptor not only include the glutamate aspect of the molecule with the amino and two carboxyl groups but also the appropriate orientation of the Pi electron containing isopropylene side-chain.

While it is clear from ligand binding and neurophysiologic studies that KA receptors are concentrated on neuronal perikarya or their dendritic extensions, it is now apparent that they are also localized on excitatory amino acid terminals such as the cortico-striatal projection and the cerebellar parallel fiber system. It should be emphasized that the kinetics of binding of $[^3H]$-KA in the cerebellum reveal only a single population of recognition sites; thus, pre- and post-synaptic receptors cannot be distinguished on the basis of agonist affinity for the recognition site. Results obtained thus far suggest a selective localization of these presynaptic KA receptors on aspartergic and glutamatergic terminals in the cerebellum, striatum and hippocampus, in which KA-induced release is calcium dependent but insensitive to tetrodotoxin (Ferkany et al., 1982). Notably, KA does not induce the release of endogenous GABA or prelabeled norepinephrine by a comparable mechanism.

As indicate in Figure 1, the combined interaction of KA with pre-synaptic receptors, which enhance the release of excitatory amino acid neurotransmitters, and at post-synaptic excitatory receptors undoubtedly plays a reinforcing role contributing to the potent neurotoxic action of this agent. Since the neurotoxic effects of KA require the integrity of excitatory afferents in most regions, stimulation of post-synaptic KA receptors on neurons is insufficient for neurotoxicity although these receptors appear to be required for neurotoxic effects. On the other hand, while the direct excitatory amino acid receptor agonists such as quisqualate and N-methyl-D-aspartate, are clearly neurotoxic, they produce lesions comparable to KA at molar ratios 40- to 100-fold greater than KA. The combined pre- and post-synaptic actions of KA are also consistent with the uneven pattern of neuronal vulnerability to KA which may reflect both the density of KA receptors on vulnerable neurons as well as on the excitatory afferents (Coyle et al., 1978). In addition, since KA appears to be rather metabolically inert and to diffuse widely in the brain after intracerebral injection (Zaczek et al., 1980), the presynaptic effects of KA in promoting excitatory neurotransmission, especially in the hippocampal formation, may contribute to its potent convulsant effects within the limbic system.

The proximate cause of neuronal cell death, which occurs undoubtedly quite rapidly after intracerebral injection of excitotoxins, remains to be precisely defined. While the effects of KA and ibotenic acid on the disposition of high energy phosphates and glucose metabolism is consistent with the excitotoxin hypothesis, it should be noted that the total adenosine pool falls contemporaneously with the decrease of phosphocreatine and ATP. This profile differs

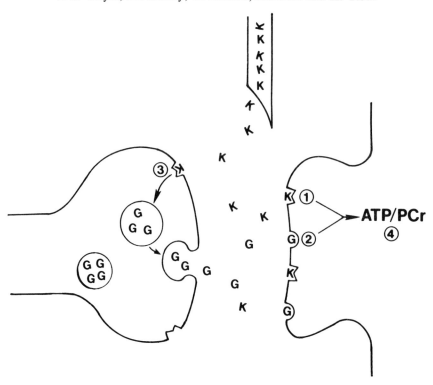

Figure 1. Schematic representation of the sequence of events involved in kainate-induced neuronal degeneration. Kainate (K) acts at post-synaptic excitatory receptors (1) and at pre-synaptic receptors (2) that release endogenous excitatory amino acids (G). The cooperative interaction between the activation of kainate receptors and excitatory amino acid receptors on vulnerable neurons precipitates a sequence of events resulting in neuronal cell energy depletion, dendritic and perikaryal endomosis and neuronal cell death.

from that seen with anoxia or seizures (Sacktor et al., 1966; Duffy et al., 1972), in which there is a quantitative shift of high energy metabolites to the lower energy form. The disparity between metabolic effects of seizures and excitotoxins suggests that energy depletion may be an epiphenomenon of excitotoxin-induced neuronal degeneration and not the proximate event. Prolonged stimulation of nicotinic receptors at the neuromuscular junction produces acute ultrastructural pathology of the muscle fibers similar to the acute dendridic alteration caused by excitotoxins (Salpeter et al., 1979). Notably, the myotoxic effects of profound nicotinic receptor stimulation is dependent upon extracellular calcium and appears to involve activation of intracellular calcium dependent proteases. This observation raises the question whether disruption of the intracellular disposition of calcium may be the proximate cause of neuronal degeneration caused by excitotoxins. Consistent with this hypothesis, glutamate has been shown to enhance the influx of calcium in brain homogenates (Retz et al., 1982). The search for the initial event responsible for neuronal degeneration produced by excitotoxins remains a critical issue since it may provide an important link between excitatory amino acid transmitter mechanisms and dysfunctional processes responsible for selective neuronal loss in hereditary and acquired neurodegenerative disorders in man.

ACKNOWLEDGEMENT

We thank Carol Kenyon and Dorothea Stieff for excellent secretarial assistance and appreciate the support of USPHS grants RSDA MH-00125, NS-13584 and the Surdna Foundation.

REFERENCES

Biscoe, T.J., Evans, R.H., Headley, P.M., Martin, M.R. and Watkins, J.C. (1976). Br. J. Pharmacol., 58, 373-382.
Biziere, K. and Coyle, J.T. (1978a). J. Neurochem., 31, 513-520.
Biziere, K. and Coyle, J.T. (1978b). Neurosci. Lett.,8, 303-310.
Biziere, K. and Coyle, J.T. (1979a). Neuropharmacology, 18, 409-413.
Biziere, K. and Coyle, J.T. (1979b). J. Neurosci. Res., 4, 383-398.
Campochiaro, P. and Coyle, J.T. (1978). Proc. Natl. Acad. Sci. USA, 75, 2025-2029.
Coyle, J.T. and Schwarcz, R. (1976). Nature, 263, 244-246.
Coyle, J.T., Molliver, M.E. and Kuhar, M.J. (1978). J. Comp. Neurol., 180, 301-324.
Curtis, D. and Johnston, G.A.R. (1974). Eben Physiol. 69, 97-188.
Duffy, T.E., Nelson, S.R. and Lowry, O.H. (1972) J. Neurochem., 19, 959-977.
Ferkany, J.W., Slevin, J.T., Zaczek, R. and Coyle, J.T. Neurobehavioral Toxicology, in press.
Ferkany, J.W., Zaczek, R. and Coyle, J.T. (1982) Nature, 298, 757-759.
Hill, D.W., Walters, F.H., Wilson, T.D. and Stuart, J.D. (1979). Anal. Chem., 51, 1338-1341.
Krespan, B., Berl, S. and Nicklas, W.J. (1982). J. Neurochem., 38, 509-518.
London, E.D. and Coyle, J.T. (1979a). Mol. Pharmacol., 15, 492-505.
London, E.D. and Coyle, J.T. (1979b). Eur. J. Pharmacol., 56, 287-290.
London, E.D., Klemm, N. and Coyle, J.T. (1980). Brain Res., 192, 463-476.
McGeer, E.G., McGeer, P.H. and Singh, K. (1978). Brain Res., 139, 381-383.
McLennan, H. (1980) Neurosci. Letts., 18, 313-316.
Olney, J.W., Ho, O.L. and Rhee, V. (1971) Exp. Brain Res., 14, 61-70.
Olney, J.W., Rhee, V. and Ho., O.L. (1974) Brain Res., 77, 507-512.
Retz, K.C. and Coyle, J.T. (1982) J. Neurochem., 38, 196-203.
Retz, K.C., Young, A.C. and Coyle, J.T. (1982). European Journal of Pharmacology, 79, 319-322.
Ruck, A., Kramer, S., Metz, J. and Brennan, M.J.W. (1980). Nature, 287, 852-853.
Sacktor, B., Wilson, J.E. and Tiekert, C.G. (1966) J. Biol. Chem., 241, 5071-5075.
Salpeter, M.M., Kasprzak, H., Fong, H. and Fertuck, H. (1979) J. Neurocytol., 8, 95-115.
Schwarcz, R. and Coyle, J.T. (1977). Brain Res., 127, 235-247.
Schwarcz, R., Scholz , D. and Coyle, J.T. (1978). Neuropharmacology, 17, 145-151.
Simon, J.R., Contrera, J.F. and Kuhar, M.J. (1976). J. Neurochem., 26, 141-147
Slevin, J., Collins, J., Lindsley, K. and Coyle, J.T. Brain Res., in press.
Slevin, J.T. and Coyle, J.T. (1981). J. Neurochem., 37, 531-533.
Slevin, J.T., Johnston, M.V., Biziere, K. and Coyle, J.T. (1982). Developmental Neuroscience, 5, 3-12.
Svedes, J.S., Sedo, R.J. and Atkinson, D.E. (1975) J. Biol. Chem., 250, 6930-6938.
Watkins, J.C. and Evans, R.H. (1981). Ann. Rev. Pharmacol., 21, 165-204.
Wikilund, L., Toggenburgen, G. and Cuenod, M. (1982). Science, 216, 78-80.
Wooten, G.F. and Collins, R. (1980) Brain Res., 201, 173-184.
Zaczek, R. and Coyle, J.T. (1982). Neuropharmacology, 21, 15-26.
Zaczek, R., Simonton, S. and Coyle, J.T. (1980) J. Neuropathol. Exp. Neurol., 39, 245-264.

THE NEURODEGENERATIVE PROPERTIES OF INTRACEREBRAL QUINOLINIC ACID AND ITS STRUCTURAL ANALOG CIS–2,3–PIPERIDINE DICARBOXYLIC ACID

ROBERT SCHWARCZ*, WILLIAM O. WHETSELL Jr.** and ALAN C. FOSTER*

*Maryland Psychiatric Research Center, University of Maryland School of Medicine, Baltimore, Maryland, USA

**Division of Neuropathology, University of Tennessee Center of the Health Sciences, Memphis, Tennessee, USA

INTRODUCTION

Experiments using intracerebral injections in rodents of kainic (KA) or ibotenic (IBO) acid, two amino acids of plant and fungal origin, respectively, have led to the hypothesis that human neurodegenerative diseases, e.g. Huntington's disease (HD) and temporal lobe epilepsy, may be related to a pathological overproduction of endogenous neuroexcitatory amino acids (Coyle et al., 1977; Divac, 1977; Olney and de Gubareff, 1978; French et al., 1982). Of these, glutamate, aspartate and cysteine sulfinate, all putative neurotransmitters in the central nervous system (Roberts et al., 1981; Recasens et al., 1982), do not appear to posses pronounced neurotoxicity, even when introduced into the brain at very high concentrations (Olney and de Gubareff, 1978; Mangano and Schwarcz, 1983). Also, examinations of acidic amino acids in tissues and body fluids of patients suffering from HD or epilepsy have merely yielded equivocal results (Perry et al., 1975; Gray et al., 1980; Perry and Hansen, 1981; Mangano and Schwarcz, 1981, 1982). Their dysfunction in neuro-psychiatric disorders has as yet not been established.

Recently, our attention was drawn to the tryptophan metabolite quinolinic acid (QUIN; 2,3-pyridine dicarboxylic acid) because of its convulsive and neuroexcitatory potency (Lapin, 1978; Stone and Perkins, 1981; cf. also Herrling, this volume). These qualities as well as its chemical structure, which resembles that of established excitotoxins (Figure 1) appeared to justify a thorough evaluation of QUIN's possible neurotoxic properties (Schwarcz et al., 1982a). In this report, we present data on QUIN-induced neuronal degeneration after intracerebral application as assessed by morphological and neurochemical techniques. Its neurotoxic effects were compared with those of cis-2,3-piperidine dicarboxylic acid (cis-2,3-PDA; Figure 1), an excitant of spinal neurons (Watkins, 1981), and the blocking action of (-) 2-amino-7-phosphonoheptanoic acid (-APH), a selective antagonist of IBO-neurotoxicity (Schwarcz et al., 1982b), vis-a-vis QUIN and cis-2,3-PDA was investigated. Finally, we examined possible interactions of QUIN and cis-2,3-PDA with glutamate uptake sites and receptors for glutamate and KA in vitro.

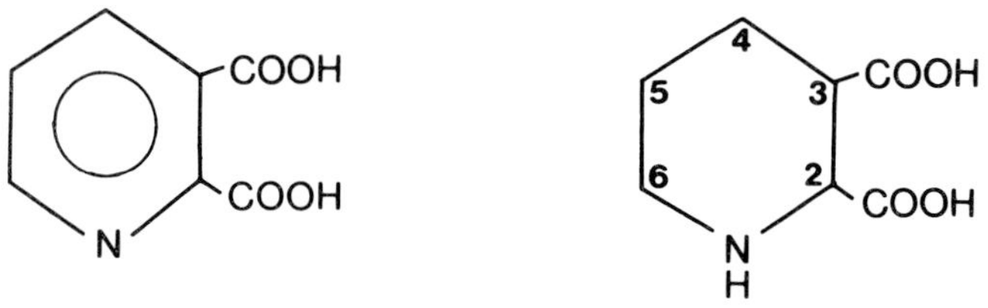

Quinolinic acid   2,3-Piperidine dicarboxylic acid

FIGURE 1: Chemical structures of QUIN and 2,3-PDA

MATERIALS AND METHODS

Male Sprague-Dawley rats (170-250g) or 7-day old Sprague-Dawley pups were used
for all experiments described here. For intracerebral injections, adult animal.
were anesthetized with nembutal (50 mg/kg, i.p.) and placed in a David Kopf
stereotaxic apparatus. Coordinates for striatal (A: 7.9, L: 2.6, V: 4.8) and hippocampal (A: 4.5, L: 2.6, V: 3.0) injections were chosen according to König and
Klippel (1963). All test compounds were dissolved in 1N NaOH or distilled water,
the solutions titrated to pH 7.4 and injected in a volume of 1 µl over 2 minutes.
Following surgery, the scalp was apposed with would clips.

For intrastriatal injections into 7-day old rats (coordinates: A: 0.7 mm anterior
to the bregma, L: 2.2 mm from the midline, V: 4.2 mm from the dura), pups were
anesthetized with ether and placed in the stereotaxic frame. Compounds were injected (1 µl) with a 30 gauge Hamilton needle via a hole carefully pierced
through the skull. After the injection, the skin was closed with Permabond-glue,
the pups were allowed to recover from anesthesia and then returned to their
mother.

Injected animals were sacrificed 3-4 days later and their brains processed for
measurement of choline acetyltransferase (CAT; Bull and Oderfeld-Novak, 1971) and
tyrosine hydroxylase (TH; Waymire et al., 1971) activities or for light or electron microscopic analysis. For experiments in which the blocking capacity of
-APH was assessed, the drug was co-injected with QUIN or cis-2,3-PDA, respectively. Its effects were determined by examining thionin-stained sections of injected tissue at the light microscopic level. Antagonism of neurotoxicity was
defined by the absence of neuronal degeneration beyond a sphere of 100 µm in
diameter around the injection site. The number of separate animals examined was
3-5 for every set of morphological analyses (dose, brain region) reported in this
communication.

L-^{3}H-glutamate binding to striatal and hippocampal P_2 membranes was determined by
a modification of the method of Foster and Roberts (1978). Briefly, aliquots of
washed membrane suspensions (corresponding to approximately 4 mg original tissue
weight) were brought to a volume of 1 ml with either 50 mM Tris-HCl (pH 7.4) or
50 mM Tris-acetate (pH 7.4). After a 6 minute preincubation at 30°C, assay tubes

were incubated for 28 minutes at 30°C with L-^{3}H-glutamate (20 nM final concentration). Two pharmacologically distinct populations of binding sites for L-glutamate were assayed in the same membrane preparation by using different buffer systems: in 50 mM Tris HCl buffer, L-glutamate binds predominantly to a Cl$^-$-stimulated population of sites, whereas binding measured in 50 mM Tris-citrate is predominantly to a Cl$^-$-insensitive population of sites (Fagg et al., 1982; Mena et al., 1982). ^{3}H-kainic acid binding was assessed simultaneously in the same striatal or hippocampal membranes using a modification (Schwarcz and Fuxe, 1979) of the method of Simon et al. (1976). For both glutamate and KA-binding assays, test drugs were included at a final concentration of 1 mM prior to commencement of the assay. Specific binding was determined as the binding which is displaced by a 1 mM concentration of the respective unlabelled ligand. Drug effects were expressed as the percentage of control specific binding.

Compounds (1 mM) were also tested for inhibition of the high-affinity uptake of L-^{3}H-glutamate into striatal and hippocampal P$_2$ preparations, assayed by the method of Storm-Mathisen (1977).

Cis-2,3-PDA and -APH were generously supplied by Dr. J.F. Collins, London. QUIN and nicotinic acid were purchased from Sigma (St. Louis, MO). L-^{3}H-glutamate (44 Ci/mmol) and ^{3}H-kainate (4 Ci/mmol) were obtained from New England Nuclear (Boston, MA).

RESULTS

Characteristics of intracerebral QUIN injections: Unilateral intrastriatal injection of >120 nmoles QUIN resulted in tonic-clonic movements of the contralateral forelimb lasting approximately 4-6 hours after awakening from anesthesia. This behavior was virtually indistinguishable from that observed after identical treatments with KA or IBO (Coyle and Schwarcz, 1976; Schwarcz et al., 1979). No abnormal behaviors could be observed on the days following QUIN-application.

Upon histological examination, nerve cell loss at the site of injection could be noticed at doses as low as 12 nmoles. Glial cells did not seem to be reduced in number, and myelinated internal capsule fibers appeared unchanged. The typical appearance of a QUIN-treated rat striatum is depicted in Figures 2A and C and contrasted to that of a striatum injected with 800 nmoles nicotinic acid (Figures 2B and D), a decarboxylation product of QUIN devoid of neurotoxic effects. Lesions induced by QUIN extended spherically from the tip of the injected cannula. Neuronal loss distant from the injection site, such as that known from striatal KA-application (Wuerthele et al., 1978; Zaczek et al., 1980; Schwob et al., 1980), was never detected, even when large doses (600 nmoles) of QUIN were applied.

Electron microscopic analysis of striatal tissue four days after injection of 60 nmoles of QUIN showed a pronounced disturbance of neuropil and nerve cells (Figures 3A and C). Clearly, the number of synaptic complexes was markedly reduced as compared to the contralateral uninjected striatum (Figures 3B and D) or to tissue treated with 800 nmoles nicotinic acid (micrographs not shown). Prominent swelling of dendritic processes was common. Postsynaptic densities could often be seen on dilated dendrites in apposition to seemingly unaffected presynaptic elements. Myelinated axons appeared to be well-preserved.

Once the axon-sparing properties of QUIN were established on the ultrastructural level, we proceeded to measure striatal enzyme activities after QUIN lesions. CAT-activity decreased in a dose-dependent fashion, with 600 nmol QUIN causing an 84% loss of the cholinergic marker enzyme, while TH-activity did not change significantly in the same tissue homogenates (Table 1). Control injection of 800 nmoles nicotinic acid did not cause any detectable changes in CAT or TH (data not shown).

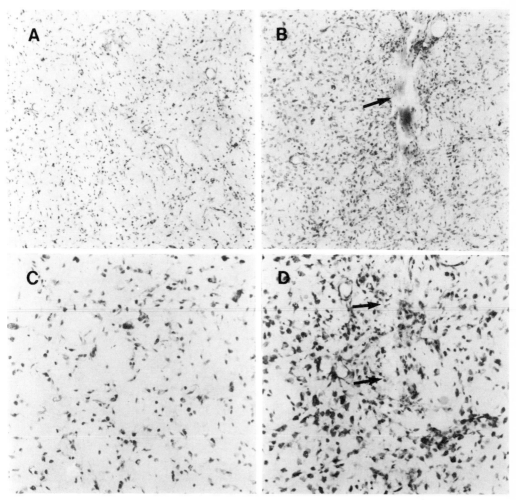

FIGURE 2: Light microscopic appearance of striata four days after local injection of 60 nmoles QUIN (A, C) or 800 nmoles nicotinic acid (B, D). Arrows
in B and D indicate track of the injection cannula. C and D are higher mag-
nifications (50X) of micrographs A and B (25X).

Intrahippocampal injections of <500 nmoles QUIN produced no obvious behavioral abnormalities. Doses in excess of 500 nmoles reliably resulted in generalized convulsions characterized by intermittent jumping, running fits, ipsilateral turning
and pronounced exophthalmos, lasting for 2-4 hours. Histological analysis showed
that a low dose of QUIN (30 nmoles) led to a selective degeneration of the pyramidal cell population (Figure 4A), while 60 nmoles or more caused the degeneration
of all neuronal types in the hippocampus (Figure 4B). Nerve cell loss was always
limited to the site of injection (as in the case of striatal lesions) and never
extended beyond the dorsal thalamic nuclei. Control injections of nicotinic acid
(800 nmoles) failed to produce neuronal damage in the hippocampal formation (micrograph not shown).

Preliminary experiments were performed to assess QUIN-toxicity in two other brain
regions. As depicted in Figure 5A, neurons in the pars compacta of the substantia
nigra were quite resistant to 60 nmoles QUIN. Intracerebellar infusions of 120

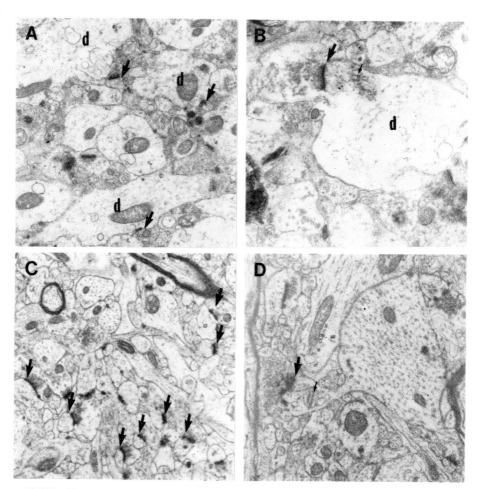

FIGURE 3: A. Appearance of neuropil of striatum of adult rat three days
after intrastriatal injection of QUIN (30 nmoles). Arrows show three synapses associated with swollen dendrites (d). 8,900X.   B. Detail of neuropil of striatum of rat three days after injection of QUIN (30 nmoles). Larger arrow points to probable axospinous synapse. Small arrow indicates
swollen vesicular structure within dendritic process (d) suggestive of disturbed spine apparatus.   14,600X.   C. Neuropil of striatum on uninjected
side. Arrows indicate numerous normal asymmetrical synapse.   8,900X.
D. Detail of neuropil of striatum on uninjected side showing axospinous
synapse (larger arrow). Spine apparatus in dendritic spine is denoted by
small arrow.   14,600X.

nmoles of QUIN, while toxic to all neuronal cell types in close vicinity of the
needle track, revealed a higher vulnerability of granule as compared to Purkinje
cells with increasing distance from the injection site (Figure 5B). Thus, it
appeared that hippocampal and striatal neurons in general were more susceptible to
the neurodegenerative effects of QUIN than those in the substantia nigra and in
the cerebellum (cf. also Köhler, this volume).

	CAT	% of contra-lateral striatum	TH	% of contra-lateral striatum
QUIN				
300 nmoles	424 ± 56*	50	3.0 ± 0.1	112
600 nmoles	116 ± 31*	14	2.9 ± 0.1	86
cis-2,3-PDA				
600 nmoles	484 ± 108*	47	3.9 ± 0.7	101

TABLE 1: Striatal enzyme activities after intrastriatal injection of QUIN and cis-2,3-PDA. Amino acids were administered as described in the text four days before killing the rats. Enzyme activities are expressed as pmoles/mg tissue/min and represent the mean ± S.E.M. of 5 individual animals each. *P < 0.01 by paired t-test as compared to the uninjected contralateral striatum.

No local or distant neuronal degeneration was detected by our light microscopic analysis after intrastriatal injection of up to 120 nmoles QUIN in 7-day old rats (Figure 6).

Intracerebral application of cis-2,3-PDA: Injections of cis-2,3-PDA into the striatum (Figure 7A) or hippocampus (Figures 7B and C) of adult rats resulted in circumscribed local neuronal lesions. Unilateral intrastriatal infusion of >250 nmoles cis-2,3-PDA also caused the characteristic short-lasting tonic-clonic behavioral syndrome observed after instrastriatal application of KA, IBO and QUIN. Its axon-sparing properties (Table 1), the lack of "distant" cell death, preferential vulnerability of hippocampal pyramidal cells at lower doses (Figure 7B), necrosis of the entire hippocampal formation at higher doses (Figure 7C) and lack of neurotoxicity in the developing striatum (micrograph not shown) indicated a close resemblance between the neurotoxic characteristics of cis-2,3-PDA and QUIN. In quantitative terms, as judged from the extent and quality of cis-2,3-PDA induced hippocampal damage (cf. Figures 4 and 7) and the decrease of CAT-activity after intrastriatal application (Table 1), the piperidine derivative was approximately half as potent as QUIN.

Antagonism of neurotoxicity by -APH: Co-administration of equimolor quantities of -APH with either QUIN (Figure 8A and B) or cis-2,3-PDA (micrographs not shown) in both striatum and hippocampus resulted in a total blockade of the neurotoxic effects of both compounds. Notably, in the striatum -APH also antagonized the acute behavioral syndrome characteristic for excitotoxins (see above).

In vitro assays: QUIN and cis-2,3-PDA were tested for activity in glutamate and kainate binding and glutamate uptake assays. Both compounds were poor inhibitors of L-^{3}H-glutamate binding to striatal or hippocampal membranes measured in Tris-HCl or Tris-citrate buffer. At a concentration of 1 mM, cis-2,3-PDA was slightly more potent than QUIN and both compounds appeared to be more active at Cl$^-$-independent glutamate binding sites (Table 2). At the same concentration, cis-2,3-PDA was a weak inhibitor of ^{3}H-kainate binding to striatal or hippocampal membranes while QUIN was devoid of any activity. At a concentration of 1 mM, neither compound caused significant inhibition of L-^{3}H-glutamate uptake into hippocampal or striatal P_2 preparations (data not shown).

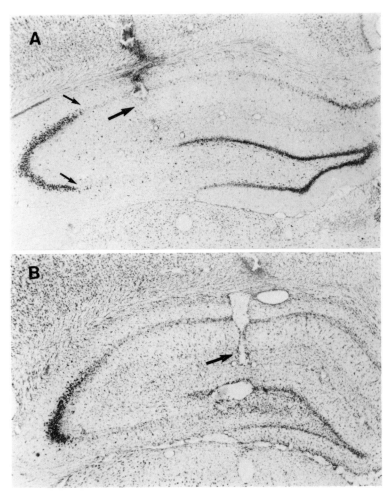

FIGURE 4: Effects of intrahippocampal injection of 30 nmoles (A) and 60 nmoles (B) QUIN. Large arrows point to the needle tracks. Small arrows in A indicate the sharp border between degenerated and intact pyramidal cells. Mag. 10X.

DISCUSSION

The excitotoxic hypothesis, based on electrophysiological data accumulated in the 1960s and experimental neuropathological studies performed in the early 1970s, causally links the neuroexcitatory and selective neurodegenerative properties of some acidic amino acids (for review see Olney, 1980). While the cellular and molecular mechanisms underlying excitotoxicity are not understood in detail, it seems clear that for a compound to exert excitotoxic actions it must have certain structural features. Two acidic groups in sterical proximity to each other and to an amino group appear essential, as exemplified in glutamate, aspartate, N-methyl-D-aspartate, KA, IBO and related molecules (Watkins, 1981). On theoretical grounds, both QUIN and cis-2,3-PDA therefore fit the structural pattern expected

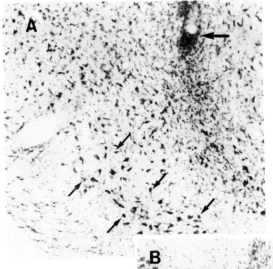

FIGURE 5: Micrographs illustrating the effects of 60 nmoles QUIN into the substantia nigra (A) and 120 nmoles QUIN into the cerebellum (B). Large arrow in A indicates needle track. Small arrows in A point to surviving zona compacta cells. Arrows in B delineate intact Purkinje cells next to degenerated granule cells. Mag.: 25X.

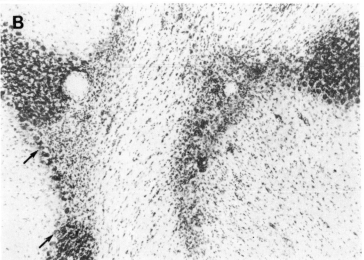

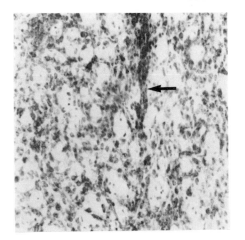

FIGURE 6: Micrograph showing lack of neurotoxicity of QUIN (120 nmoles) in the developing striatum. Note the abundance of healthy neurons in the immediate vicinity of the needle track (arrow). Mag. 50X.

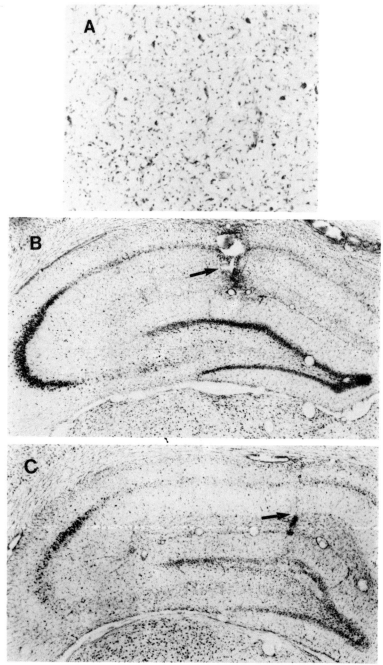

FIGURE 7: Neuronal loss after intrastriatal injection of 120 nmoles (A) and intrahippocampal administration of 60 (B) and 120 nmoles (C) cis-2,3-PDA. Arrows in B and C point to needle tracks. Mag. 25X (A), 10X (B, C).

	QUIN (1 mM)	cis-2,3-PDA (1 mM)
^{3}H-Glutamate (Tris-HCl)		
Striatum	99.2 ± 7.9	67.6 ± 11.4
Hippocampus	116.4 ± 8.1	58.8 ± 7.3
^{3}H-Glutamate (Tris-citrate)		
Striatum	70.0 ± 9.1	38.8 ± 8.2
Hippocampus	91.0 ± 4.9	42.6 ± 2.6
^{3}H-Kainate		
Striatum	93.6 ± 9.3	76.6 ± 9.6
Hippocampus	76.6 ± 9.6	60.8 ± 9.3

TABLE 2: Effects of QUIN and cis-2,3-PDA on the binding of ^{3}H-glutamate and ^{3}H-kainate. Data are expressed as percent of specific binding and represent the mean ± S.E.M. of 3-10 separate experiments.

from excitotoxin candidates (cf. Figure 1). Indeed both compounds have been shown to possess neuroexcitatory activity at striatal and hippocampal neurons (Herrling, McLennan, this meeting).

Stereotaxic unilateral microinjections of nmol amounts QUIN into the striatum of the adult rat resulted in an acute excitatory response as judged by the short-lasting tonic-clonic movements of the contralateral forelimb. This behavior, which is possibly linked to rapid activation of the ipsilateral nigrostriatal dopaminergic system (Andersson et. al., 1980), had previously also been described after intrastriatal application of KA (Coyle and Schwarcz, 1976; Di Chiara et al., 1977) and IBO (Schwarcz et al., 1979) and thus appears to be a characteristic excitotoxic phenomenon. Notably, cis-2,3-PPA caused identical spontaneous movements at somewhat larger doses than QUIN, thus meeting the excitotoxic criterion as judged by a behavioral paradigm.

Probably the best established quality of excitotoxic lesions is their axon-sparing nature (Olney, 1980). In the present series of experiments, the resistance of striatal axons of extrinsic origin to QUIN was examined both ultrastructurally and neurochemically. These analyses revealed the survival of fibers of passage and termination as well as glial elements in the immediate vicinity of degenerated dendro-somatic structures. Electron micrographs taken four days after intrastriatal QUIN were indistinguishable from those obtained after KA (Hattori and McGeer, 1977; Olney, 1978). Tyrosine hydroxylase activity, marking the nigro-striatal dopaminergic neurons, was unchanged after intrastriatal QUIN or cis-2,3-PDA in the same tissue where CAT-activity was significantly reduced. This bio-chemical picture, too, is qualitatively identical to that observed after KA or IBO (Coyle and Schwarcz, 1976; McGeer and McGeer, 1976; Schwarcz et al., 1979). Thus, both the pyridine derivative QUIN and its saturated analog cis-2,3-PDA apparently fulfil essential excitotoxic criteria.

As reported earlier by us and others (Köhler et al., 1979 a, b; Nadler et al., 1981), there exist pronounced differences between various excitotoxins beyond the common features described above. One of the major dissimilarities between KA and IBO is the presence of neuronal lesions distant from the site of injection after intracerebral KA (Wuerthele et al., 1978; Zazcek et al., 1980; Schwob et al., 1980) but not IBO (Schwarcz et al., 1979). This distant damage has been suggest-ed to be causally related to the powerful convulsant properties of KA (Ben-Ari et al., 1980). IBO, on the other hand, precipitates only mild seizures upon intra-cerebral injection (Aldinio et al., submitted). In vivo, other major differences between KA and IBO, summarized in Table 3, are: the selectivity of toxic effects

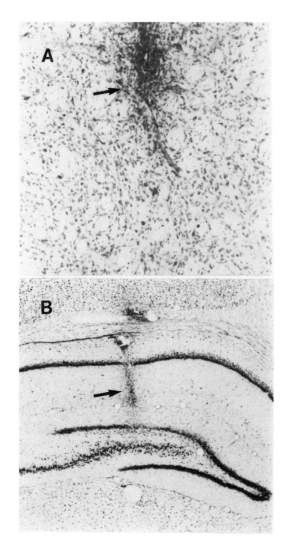

FIGURE 8: Blockade of the neurotoxic effects of 300 nmoles (intrastriatal; A) and 120 nmoles (intrahippocampal; B) QUIN by co-administration of equimolar -APH. Arrows
point to cannula tracks.   Mags.
25X (A) and 10X (B).

for certain nerve cell groups or brain regions (pronounced for KA, marginal for
IBO; Köhler et al., 1979a), the antagonism of IBO- but not of KA-neurotoxicity by
-APH (Schwarcz et al., 1982b), the exclusive antagonism of KA-toxicity by prior
deafferentation of the targeted brain area (McGeer et al., 1978; Biziere and
Coyle, 1978; Köhler et al., 1979b) and the resistance of brain tissue early during
ontogeny to KA (Campochiaro and Coyle, 1978) but not to IBO (Köhler and Schwarcz,
1981).   Additionally, as judged from in vitro experiments performed in a number
of laboratories and test systems (for review see Watkins and Evans, 1981), it is
clear that KA and IBO do not interact with the same membrane components when
exerting their neuroexcitatory (and hence, according to the excitotoxic theory,
neurotoxic) effects.

As demonstrated here (cf. also Table 3), intracerebral QUIN shares some of the
qualities of both KA and IBO. Although QUIN lesions remain localized at the site

of injection similar to those caused by IBO, the individual susceptibility of neurons vis-a-vis QUIN differs markedly. In particular, the lesser vulnerability to QUIN of hippocampal granule cells and cell bodies in the substantia nigra is reminiscent of KA (Schwarcz and Coyle, 1977; Nadler et al., 1978). In contrast, most neurons in the brain, including the dentate granule cells and neurons of the substantia nigra, appear to be equally affected by IBO (Köhler and Schwarcz, submitted), i.e. there exists no pronounced neurodegenerative selectivity of IBO. Unlike KA, QUIN is a mild convulsant, as judged by preliminary intrahippocampal depth recordings after local injections in unanesthetized rats (unpublished observation). Moreover, both QUIN-induced seizures and neurodegenerative effects, like those of IBO, can be powerfully antagonized by pretreatment or, as shown here, coadministration of equimolar quantities of -APH. Both KA-induced convulsions and neurotoxicity remain virtually unaffected by -APH (Schwarcz et al., 1982b). Finally, intrastriatal QUIN or KA treatment does not cause nerve cell loss in seven-day old rat pups, an age at which IBO is neurotoxic. The onset of QUIN-neurotoxicity during development is currently being studied in our laboratories. It will be interesting to examine if the ontogenetic appearance of neuronal susceptibility parallels that of KA-toxicity (Campochiaro and Coyle, 1978).

While we have not performed the respective deafferentation experiments in vivo, studies in tissue culture indicate that, at least in the cortico-striatal system, QUIN-toxicity may be critically dependent on intact and fully developed afferent fibers (see Whetsell and Schwarcz, this volume).

Using a number of different in vivo and in vitro paradigms, we were unable to identify significant qualitative differences between the excitotoxic properties of QUIN and cis-2,3-PDA. In vitro, neither of the two amino acids appears to act via one of the well-characterized membrane sites functionally related to other excitatory amino acids. In particular, kainate and glutamate binding sites (see Roberts, 1981 for review), which are implicated in the actions of KA and IBO (Foster and Roberts, 1978; Coyle et al., 1981), are very little affected by QUIN and cis-2,3-PDA. Similarly, QUIN and cis-2,3-PDA do not inhibit synaptosomal glutamate uptake and therefore do not appear to exert their action by increasing the synaptic concentration of glutamate (McGeer et al., 1978). The data presented here, combined with the assessment of detailed structure-activity relationships of numerous pyridine- and piperidine derivatives (Foster et al., submitted), suggest the specific cellular sites mediating the actions of QUIN and cis-2,3-PDA to be very similar or identical. Structural considerations indicate that these sites may be closely related to the receptor for N-methyl-D-aspartate, one of the pharmacologically best characterized amino acid agonists (Watkins, 1981).

While the presence of cis-2,3-PDA in biological material has not been investigated to date, QUIN and its metabolic machinery has been known for many decades to exist in plant and animal tissues (see e.g. Henderson and Ramasarma, 1949). While most of the published literature on QUIN deals with its role in hepatic tissue (Gholson et al., 1964; Maxwell and Ray, 1980), its presence in mammalian brain has recently also been demonstrated (Wolfensberger et al., in preparation). In the liver, QUIN constitutes a metabolic intermediate of the kynurenine pathway, which is responsible for the conversion of tryptophan to nicotinamide adenine dinucleotide (NAD), the ubiquitous oxido-reductive coenzyme. While the first steps of the kynurenine pathway - from tryptophan to 3-hydroxyanthranilic acid - have been described to occur in brain tissue (Gal, 1974; Gal and Sherman, 1978), it is currently not clear if the biosynthesis of NAD in brain also involves the formation of QUIN as a necessary intermediate. At any rate, production and metabolic breakdown of QUIN can be reasonably assumed to take place in the brain and ought to be carefully investigated in light of our present data.

	Kainic acid	Ibotenic acid	Quinolinic acid
in vivo			
Lesion	local + distant	local, discrete	local, discrete
Bleedings	yes	no	no
Neurotoxic range	0.5 - 2 µg	2 - 20 µg	5 - 50 µg
Selectivity of toxicity	pronounced	marginal	pronounced
Seizure threshold	5 - 10 ng	1 - 2 µg	2 - 5 µg
Antagonism by -APH	no	yes	yes
Antagonism by deafferentation	yes	no	N.T.
Developing brain	resistant	vulnerable	resistant
in vitro			
Kainate binding	IC_{50} = 40 nM	no affinity at 1 mM	no affinity at 1 mM
Glutamate binding	no affinity at 1 mM	IC_{50} = 10 µM	no affinity at 1 mM
Glutamate uptake	IC_{50} = 500 µM	no affinity at 1 mM	no affinity at 1 mM

TABLE 3: In vivo and in vivo properties of kainic, ibotenic and quinolinic acid. N.T. = not tested.

The idea that an endogenous neuroexcitatory acidic amino acid may be involved in the pathogenesis of HD arises directly from earlier animal work with exogenous drugs such as KA and IBO (Coyle and Schwarcz, 1976; McGeer and McGeer, 1976; Schwarcz et al., 1979). A series of putative neurotransmitters, which seemed to meet both structural and functional criteria for such an endogenous excitotoxin - glutamate, aspartate, homocysteate, cysteine sulfinate - have now been scrutinized in experimental neurotoxic paradigms and shown to have only weak neurodegenerative properties, particularly in the adult animal (Olney and de Gubareff, 1978; Schwarcz et al., 1978a; Mangano and Schwarcz, 1983). Their more prominent toxicity on the developing nervous system (Olney et al., 1971) also argues against their participation in HD, which usually does not manifest itself before early adulthood (Bruyn, 1968).

While it is premature at this point to even speculate upon a possible role of QUIN as a neurotransmitter, its excitotoxic properties make it an attractive candidate which should be considered as an etiological factor in HD. Although a detailed ontogenetic study has yet to be completed in the animal model, its lack of effect early during development coincides with the temporal sequence of the human disorder (see above). The apparent high vulnerability to QUIN of striatal neurons as compared to, e.g., nigral or cerebellar nerve cells, parallels the neuropathological picture of HD, which preferentially afflicts the caudate/putamen complex (Bruyn, 1968). Finally, our preliminary experiments (Wolfensberger et al., in preparation) indicate that there exists a relatively narrow margin between the brain tissue levels of QUIN and the threshold dose for its excitotoxicity ($< 10 \mu M$ as judged by tissue culture experiments; cf. Whetsell and Schwarcz, this volume). Thus, it appears conceivable that an increased accumulation of QUIN, due to any of a number of genetically determined defects, could preferentially destroy adult striatal cells in HD. Fortunately, such a QUIN-hypothesis of HD is testable and an answer about an involvement of QUIN in HD should be forthcoming in the not too distant future.

From our experiments, it is more difficult at present to make a link between QUIN and temporal lobe epilepsy. As for the HD-model, the idea of a participation of excitotoxins in seizure phenomena originated from work with KA (Nadler et al., 1978; Schwarcz et al., 1978b; Ben-Ari et al., 1979). As outlined in Table 3 and discussed above, QUIN and KA do share, inter alia, one particular property which may be of relevance for epilepsy research, namely a preferential neurotoxicity for hippocampal CA_3/CA_4 pyramidal cells. This selective hippocampal neurotoxicity of KA has repeatedly been associated with the epileptogenic nature of these particular cells (see e.g. Menini et al., 1980), an idea which is supported by neuropathological findings in epileptic brain tissue (Falconer, 1974). Compared to KA, QUIN is a relatively mild convulsant (this report),though it is by far the most convulsive of all tryptophan catabolites (Lapin, 1978). Careful electroencephalographic analysis, similar to that performed with intrahippocampal KA (French et al., 1982) and IBO (Aldinio et al., submitted), will have to become available before a possible involvement of QUIN in seizure phenomena can be realistically evaluated.

Finally, should a causal link between QUIN and human neurodegenerative phenomena be established, our present data on the remarkable blocking ability of -APH vis-a-vis QUIN-neurotoxicity could be viewed from a potential therapeutic angle. -APH has recently been shown to possess pronounced anticonvulsant properties in two experimental seizure models (Croucher et al., 1982), a finding which would be compatible with a role of QUIN or a QUIN-like agent (possibly cis-2,3-PDA?) as an endogenous epileptogenic factor. Thus, in addition to its obvious usefulness as a research tool for unraveling QUIN-related excitotoxic mechanisms (cf. also Whetsell and Schwarcz, this volume), -APH may represent a class of compounds with considerable clinical potential for the treatment of HD, epilepsy and possibly other degenerative disorders of the nervous system. Studies are currently in progress to further investigate the respective therapeutic value of -APH and some of its congeners.

ACKNOWLEDGEMENTS

This work was supported by USPHS grants NS-16941 and NS-16102. We gratefully appreciate the expert technical assistance of Deborah Parks and William Zinkand and the secretarial help of Beverly Rheubottom.

REFERENCES

Andersson, K., R. Schwarcz and K. Fuxe (1980): Nature, 283:94-96.
Ben-Ari, Y., J. Lagowska, E. Tremblay and G. Le Gal La Salle (1979): Brain Res., 163:176-180.
Ben-Ari, Y., E. Tremblay and O.P. Ottersen (1980): Neuroscience, 5:515-528.
Biziere, K. and J.T. Coyle (1978): Neurosci. Lett., 8:303-310.
Bruyn, G. (1968); In: Handbook of Clinical Neurology, Vol. 6 (P.J. Vinken and G. W. Bruyn, eds.), pp. 298-378, North-Holland, Amsterdam.
Bull, G. and B. Oderfeld-Novak (1971): J. Neurochem., 19:935-947.
Campochiaro, P. and J.T. Coyle (1978); Proc. Natl. Acad. Sci. (USA), 75:2025-2029.
Coyle, J.T. and R. Schwarcz (1976): Nature, 263:244-246.
Coyle, J.T., R. Schwarcz, J.P. Bennett and P. Campochiaro (1977): Progr. Neuro-Psychopharmac., 1:13-30.
Coyle, J.T., R. Zaczek, J. Slevin and J. Collins (1981): In: Glutamate as a Neurotransmitter (G. Di Chiara and G.L. Gessa, eds.), pp. 337-346, Raven, New York.
Croucher, M.J., J.F. Collins and B.S. Meldrum (1982): Science, 216:899-901.
Di Chiara, G., M.L. Porceddu, W. Fratta and G.L. Gessa (1977): Nature, 267:270-272.
Divac, I. (1977): Acta Neurol. Scand., 56:357-360.
Fagg, E.G., A.C. Foster, E.E. Mena and C.W. Cotman (1982): J. Neurosci., 2:958-965.
Falconer, M.A. (1974): Lancet, 2:767-770.
Foster, A.C. and P.J. Roberts (1978): J. Neurochem., 31:1476-1477.
French, E.D., C. Aldinio and R. Schwarcz (1982): Neuroscience, in press.
Gal, E.M. (1974): J. Neurochem., 22:861-863.
Gal, E.M. and A.D. Sherman (1978): J. Neurochem., 30:607-613.
Gholson, R.K., I. Ueda, N. Ogasawa and L.M. Henderson (1964): J. Biol. Chem., 239:1208-1214.
Gray, P.N., P.C. May, L. Mundy and J. Elkins (1980): Biochem. Biophys. Res. Comm., 95:707-714.
Hattori, T. and E.G. McGeer (1977): Brain Res., 129:174-180.
Henderson, L.M. and G.B. Ramasarma (1949): J. Biol. Chem., 181:687-692.
Köhler, C. and R. Schwarcz (1981): Int. Soc. Neurochem. Abstr., p. 272.
Köhler, C., R. Schwarcz and K. Fuxe (1979a): Neurosci. Lett., 15:223-228.
Köhler, C., R. Schwarcz and K. Fuxe (1979b): Brain Res., 175:366-371.
König, J.F.R. and R.A. Klippel (1963): The Rat Brain. A Stereotaxic Atlas of the Forebrain and Lower Parts of the Brainstem, Williams and Wilkins, Baltimore.
Lapin, I.P. (1978): J. Neural Transm., 42:37-43.
Mangano, R.M. and R. Schwarcz (1981): J. Neurochem., 37:1072-1074.
Mangano, R.M. and R. Schwarcz (1982): J. Neurol. Sci., 53:489-500.
Mangano, R.M. and R. Schwarcz (1983): Brain Res. Bull., in press.
Maxwell, J.R. and P.D. Ray (1980): Biochim. Biophys. Acta, 614:163-172.
McGeer, E.G. and P.L. McGeer (1976): Nature, 263:517-519.
McGeer, E.G., P.L. McGeer and K. Singh (1978): Brain Res., 139:381-383.
Mena, E.E., G.E. Fagg and C.W. Cotman (1982): Brain Res., 243:378-381.
Menini, C., B.S. Meldrum, D. Riche, C. Silva-Comte and J.M. Stutzmann (1980): Ann. Neurol., 8:501-509.

Nadler, J.V., D.A. Evenson and G.L. Cuthbertson (1981): Neuroscience, 6:2505-2517.
Nadler, J.V., B.W. Perry and C.W. Cotman (1978): Nature, 271:676-677.
Olney, J.W. (1978): In: Kainic Acid as a Tool in Neurobiology (E.G. McGeer, J.W. Olney and P.L. McGeer, eds.), pp. 95-121, Raven, New York.
Olney, J.W. (1980): In: Experimental and Clinical Neurotoxicity (P.S. Spencer and H.H. Schaumburg, eds.), pp. 272-294, Williams and Wilkins, Baltimore.
Olney, J.W. and T. de Gubareff (1978): Nature, 271:557-559.
Olney, J.W., O.H. Ho and V. Rhee (1971): Exp. Brain Res., 14:61-76.
Perry, T.L. and S. Hansen (1981): Neurobiology, 31:872-876.
Perry, T.L., S. Hansen, J. Kennedy, J.A. Wada and G.B. Thompson (1975): Arch. Neurol., 32:752-754.
Recasens, M., T.V. Varga, D. Nanopoulos, F. Saadoun, G. Vincendon and J. Benavides (1982): Brain Res., 239:153-173.
Roberts, P.J., J. Storm-Mathisen and G.A.R. Johnston (1981): Glutamate: Transmitter in the Central Nervous System, Wiley, New York.
Schwarcz, R., J.F. Collins and D.A. Parks (1982b): Neurosci. Lett., in press.
Schwarcz, R. and J.T. Coyle (1977): Life Sci., 20:431-436.
Schwarcz, R. and K. Fuxe (1979): Life Sci., 24:1471-1480.
Schwarcz, R., T. Hökfelt, K. Fuxe, G. Jonsson, M. Goldstein and L. Terenius (1979): Exp. Brain Res., 37:199-216.
Schwarcz, R., D. Scholz and J.T. Coyle (1978a): Neuropharmac., 17:145-151.
Schwarcz, R., W.O. Whetsell, Jr. and R.M. Mangano (1982a): Science, in press.
Schwarcz, R., R. Zaczek and J.T. Coyle (1978b): Europ. J. Pharmac., 50:209-220.
Schwob, J.E., T. Fuller, J.L. Price and J.W. Olney (1980): Neuroscience, 5:991-1014.
Simon, J.R., J.F. Contrera and M.J. Kuhar (1976): J. Neurochem., 26:141-147.
Stone, T.W. and M.N. Perkins (1981): Europ. J. Pharmac., 72:411-412.
Storm-Mathisen, J. (1977): Brain Res., 120:376-386.
Watkins, J.C. (1981): In: Glutamate: Transmitter in the Central Nervous System (P.J. Roberts, J. Storm-Mathisen and G.A.R. Johnston, eds.), pp. 1-25, Wiley, New York.
Watkins, J.C. and R.H. Evans (1981): Ann. Rev. Pharmac. Toxic., 21:165-204.
Waymire, J.C., R. Bjur and N. Weiner (1971): Anal. Biochem., 43:588-600.
Wuerthele, S.M., K.L. Lovell, M.Z. Jones and K.E. Moore (1978): Brain Res., 149:489-497.

STUDIES ON EXCITATORY AMINO ACID RECEPTORS AND THEIR INTERACTIONS AND REGULATION OF PRE- AND POSTSYNAPTIC DOPAMINERGIC MECHANISM IN THE RAT TELENCEPHALON

K. FUXE*, L. F. AGNATI**, M. F. CELANI*, F. BENFANATI**,
K. ANDERSSON*, and J. COLLINS***

*Department of Histology, Karolinska Institute, Stockholm, Sweden
**Departments of Human Physiology and Endocrinology, University of Modena, Modena, Italy
***Department of Chem., City of London Polytechnic, 32 Jewry Street, London, England

KEYWORDS

Dopamine receptors; dopamine turnover; striatum; limbic system; N-methyl-D-aspartate; kainic acid; glutamate; ibotenic acid; excitatory amino acid antagonists.

ABSTRACT

Evidence has been obtained for the existence of receptor – receptor interactions between ^{3}H-glutamate and ^{3}H-kainic acid binding sites in rat striatal membranes. Kainic acid (10^{-6} M) in vitro rapidly reduces the number (11 %) and increases the affinity (12%) in the striatal ^{3}H-glutamate binding sites, while glutamate (10^{-8} M) in vitro increases the number of striatal ^{3}H-kainic acid binding sites (18 %) and reduces their affinity (46%). The specificity of this interaction is indicated from the fact that N-methyl-D-aspartate (10^{-6} M) did not modulate the binding characteristics of ^{3}H-glutamate and ^{3}H-kainic acid striatal binding sites. Ibotenic acid (10^{-6} M) which has a substantial affinity for the ^{3}H-glutamate binding site, mimicked the effects of glutamate on the ^{3}H-kainic acid binding sites. These results may help to explain the important role glutamate seems to play for the neurotoxic action of kainic acid, at least in the striatum where the present experiments indicate that activation of glutamate receptors increases the number of ^{3}H-kainic acid binding sites, so that they may reach a certain critical number required for neurotoxicity. Furthermore, kainic acid by increasing the affinity of the ^{3}H-glutamate binding sites may set the excitatory glutamate synapses into operation at lower concentrations of glutamate, in this way increasing the vulnerability of the striatal nerve cells to kainic acid neurotoxicity. The small percent changes in the ^{3}H-glutamate and ^{3}H-kainic acid binding sites are probably amplified considerably as the signal pass via the membrane to its final biological effector.

It is also reported that N-methyl-D- aspartate (NMDA) given intraventricularly (0.1 μg) into male conscious rats can selectively reduce dopamine (DA) turnover in the diffuse cholecystokinin (CCK) negative systems of the nuc. accumbens and tuberculum olfactorium without changing the DA levels in these DA terminal systems. This action could not be antagonized by simultaneous intraventricular injections of the selective NMDA antagonist (-)-2-amino-7-phosphonoheptanoate (1 µg), which unexpectedly by itself had the same action as NMDA on limbic DA turn-over. These results indicate the existence of a special type of NMDA receptor, reducing DA turnover and release in a subpopulation of mesolimbic DA neurons and probably belonging to cortico limbic glutamate-aspartate systems. Selective NMDA agonists for this receptor may represent new potential drugs for the treatment of schizophrenia.

We also report that l-glutamate (10^{-6} M), but not NMDA (10^{-6} M) and quisqualate (10^{-6} M), can significantly reduce the affinity (27 %) of the high affinity ago-nist binding sites of striatal DA receptors and produce a small increase (8 %) in the number of these receptors. Instead these excitatory amino acids (l-gluta-mate, NMDA; 10^{-6} M) have no significant action on the neuroleptic binding sites of the DA receptors. These results give evidence for a differential regulation of the neuroleptic and DA agonist striatal binding sites by l-glutamate. Thus, the results indicate the existence of receptor - receptor interactions between glutamate receptors and a subpopulation of DA receptors in the striatum, which may represent an important integrative mechanism in the processing of sensory motor information in the local circuits of the striatum. It may be stated that under the influence of high activity in the striatal glutamate receptors high affinity types of DA receptors (D_2-D_3 type) may require higher concentrations of released DA to operate, but when in operation the maximal DA transmission may be increased in view of the weakly increased density of these types of DA receptors caused by l-glutamate.

The results furthermore demonstrated that the neuropeptide CCK-8 (10^{-8} M) can exert a most powerful downregulation of striatal ^{3}H-glutamate binding sites by producing a 63% reduction of their affinity and a 26% reduction of their densi-ty. These results open up new ideas about treatment of Huntington's Chorea assu-ming that the degeneration of striatal nerve cells is enhanced by activation of glutamate receptors. Thus, by developing drugs which activate receptors for CCK peptides a marked downregulation of striatal glutamte receptor mechanisms may be obtained.

INTRODUCTION

A large number of neurophysiological and biochemical studies have demonstrated the existence of multiple excitatory amino acid receptors in the mammallian brain (see McLennan et al., 1981, Roberts et al., 1981, Coyle et al., 1981, Watkins et al., 1981). These investigations have led to the description of at least three types of excitatory amino acid receptors, the N-methyl-D-aspartate (NMDA) receptor, the quisqualate receptor and the kainic acid receptor. Recently amino acid antagonists have been developed for the NMDA receptor, such as 2-amino-7-phosphonoheptanoate (APH) (McLennan, 1982, Evens and Watkins 1981, Purkins et al., 1981). It has been shown by Schwarcz et al., (1982a,b) that the neurotoxic and convulsant effects of ibotenic acid are antagonized by (-)-2-amino-7-phosphonoheptanoate. Previous studies by Coyle and colleagues (1981) have indicated that activity at glutamate receptors in the striatum is essential for the neurotoxic activity of kainic acid. In the present paper we have there-fore investigated possible interactions between striatal ^{3}H-glutamate and ^{3}H-kainic acid binding sites. Glutamate is an excitatory amino acid receptor ago-nist, which may act at several types of excitatory amino acid receptors. The ability of striatal CCK-8 positive afferents to modulate striatal ^{3}H-glutamate binding sites have also been evaluated.

It is presently unknown to which extent excitatory amino acid receptors regulate DA turnover and release in striatum, nuc. accumbens and tuberculum olfactorium

as well as the characteristics of several types of DA receptors by way of receptor - receptor interactions (Fuxe et al., 1981, 1982b, Agnati et al., 1982a,b).
In the present paper the in vitro effects of l-glutamate, NMDA and quisqualate
have been evaluated on the binding characteristics of ^{3}H-spiperone (DA receptor
antagonist) and ^{3}H-N-propylnorapomorphine (^{3}H-NPA; DA receptor agonist) binding
sites, which label D_2 and D_2 - D_3 receptors respectively (see Seeman, 1980).
Furthermore, the effects of NMDA on regional DA levels and turnover have been
evaluated in vivo by intraventricular injections into male awake rats with or
without a prior intraventricular injection of the NMDA antagonists (-) or (+)
2-amino-7-phosphonoheptanoate ((-)-APH (most active form) or (+)-APH). The results show that certain types of excitatory amino acid receptors are important
modulators of pre- and postsynaptic dopaminergic properties in limbic and striatal areas of the rat brain, respectively.

MATERIAL AND METHODS

Male specific pathogen free Sprague-Dawley rats (150 g, b.wt) have been used.
The rats were given food pellets and water ad libitum and kept under standarized
light and dark conditions (lights on at 6.00 a.m. and off at 8.00 p.m.). The
following types of experiments have been performed:

1. Effects of NMDA and NMDA antagonists on DA levels and turnover in various
   areas of the forebrain.

The rats were implanted with an intraventricular cannula in the lateral ventricle two days before the experiments by means of a stereotaxic procedure. The
following drugs were administered into the lateral ventricle dissolved in 30 μl
of physiological saline during a period of 3 minutes. NMDA was administered in a
dose of 0.1 μg. The (-) and (+) form of APH was each administered in a dose of 1
μg per rat. In the combined experiment (+) or (-) APH was administered 5 min
prior to the NMDA injection (0.1 μg). In the DA turnover experiment the tyrosine
hydroxylase inhibitor, α-methyl tyrosine methyl ester (H 44/68, 250 mg/kg, i.p.)
was administered immediately before the intraventricular injections of the drugs
mentioned above. All rats were rapidly decapitated 1 h following the injection
of H 44/68 or in the experiments on DA levels alone 1 h after the injection of
NMDA. Immediately after decapitation the telencephalon was dissected out and
taken to amine fluorescence histochemistry in combination with quantitative
microfluorimetry (Löfström et al., 1976, Agnati et al., 1979). It must be under-
lined that NMDA in the dose used did not change the gross behaviour of the animals.

2. Effects of NMDA, glutamate and ibotenic acid on striatal ^{3}H-kainic acid binding sites and of kainic acid, NMDA and CCK-8 on ^{3}H-glutamate binding sites..

The ^{3}H-kainic acid (2 Ci/mmol; Amersham, U.K.) binding procedure was principally
based on that of Schwarcz and Fuxe (1979). Tris (50 mM)-citrate (1mM) buffer was
used at pH 7.1. Unspecific binding was defined as the binding in the presence of
10^{-4} M of kainic acid. The striatal homogenate contained 5 mg tissue/ml. The
freshly prepared and washed membranes were preincubated for 30 min at +37°C
followed by further washing to remove a possible endogenous inhibitor. The influence of NMDA (10^{-6} M), ibotenic acid (10^{-6} M) and l-glutamate (10^{-8} M) on
^{3}H-kainic acid binding in striatum was tested by preincubating the striatal
membranes with the respective drug for 10 min at +4°C. The ^{3}H-kainic acid binding assay was performed at +4°C for 20 min.

The ^{3}H-glutamate (44 Ci/mmol, Boston, Mass. U.S.A.) binding procedure was principally performed as described by Baundry and Lynch (1980). The buffer used was
Tris-HCl 50 mM containing 1 mM of calcium chloride, which is known to induce a

two fold increase in specific sodium independent ^{3}H-glutamate binding (pH 7.4).
Unspecific binding was defined as the binding in the presence of l-glutamate
(10^{-4} M). The striatal homogenate contained 2.5 mg tissue/ml. To remove a possible endogenous inhibitor of l-glutamate binding (Roberts, 1981) the striatal
membranes were preincubated at +37° C for 30 min. The striatal membranes were
preincubated for 10 min at room temperature with NMDA (10^{-6} M), kainic acid
(10^{-6} M) and CCK-8 (10^{-8} M) in order to study their influence on the characteristics of ^{3}H-glutamate binding. The assay was performed at room temperature
during a period of 15 min.

3. The effects of glutamate, NMDA and quisqualate on the characteristics of striatal ^{3}H-spiperone and ^{3}H-NPA binding sites

The ^{3}H-spiperone (25-35 Ci/mmol, NEN, Boston, Massachussetts, U.S.A.) binding
procedure was performed according to Creese et al., (1977). Unspecific binding
was defined as the binding in the presence of (+)butaclamol (10^{-6} M) and the
majority of the ^{3}H-spiperone binding sites are linked to D_2 receptors (see Seeman, 1980). The tissue concentration was 2.5 mg/ml. The striatal membranes were
preincubated for 10 min at +37° C to remove endogenous DA. After resuspension of
the final pellet the influence of the excitatory amino acids l-glutamate and
NMDA was evaluated by preincubating the striatal membranes with the drugs in a
concentration of 10^{-6} M at +4°C during a period of 10 min followed by incubation
at 37°C for 10 min.

The ^{3}H-NPA binding procedure was principally performed as described by Leysen
and Gommersen (1981) for ^{3}H-apomorphine binding. Unspecific binding was defined
as the binding in the presence of 10^{-6} M of (+)butaclamol. The tissue concentration was 3.3 mg/ml. The buffer used (for the homogenization washing and assay)
was Tris-HCl 15 mM, pH 7.6 containing ascorbic acid 0.01% and EDTA 1 mM. The
striatal membranes were preincubated for 10 minutes at +37°C to remove endogenous DA, and preincubation with the drugs was also performed for 10 minutes but
at +4°C. The assay took place at room temperature for 30 minutes.

In all the binding experiments the influence of the various excitatory amino
acids and CCK-8 was analyzed by studying their influence on the binding characteristics of the respective radioligand as evaluated by saturation analysis
using 8-10 concentrations. 5-9 replications were made, and a possible significant modulation of the K_D and B_{max} values was tested by the use of Student's
paired t-test.

RESULTS AND DISCUSSION

1. Effects of intraventricular injections of NMDA and a NMDA receptor antagonist on regional telencephalic DA levels and turnover

NMDA did not produce any significant effects on DA levels in striatum, nuc.
accumbens and tuberculum olfactorium. Instead, NMDA markedly reduced DA turnover
in the diffuse types of DA nerve terminals in the tuberculum olfactorium and the
nuc. accumbens leaving the dotted type of CCK positive DA terminals in these
areas unaffected (Table 1) (figs. 1-2). With the present dose used of NMDA no
effects were observed in the various DA nerve terminal networks analyzed in the
striatum. All the measurements were made at the rostro-caudal level A 8500 according to König and Klippel (1963), except the analysis in the nuc. accumbens (A
9500 for diffuse types of DA terminals). Unexpectedly, it found that the NMDA
antagonist (-)APH in a dose of 1 µg had the same action as NMDA and selectively
reduced DA turnover in the diffuse types of CCK negative DA nerve terminal systems of nuc. accumbens and tuberculum olfactorium. When NMDA and (-)APH were
given intraventricularly together, no additive effects were observed, indicating

TABLE 1

The effects of an intraventricular injection of NMDA on DA levels in various forebrain areas

NMDA was given in a dose of 0.1 µg (in 30 µl saline) 1 h before decapitation. Means±s.e.m. are shown in per cent of saline treated group mean value. Sample size: 4-6. Mann-Whitney U-test. NS Absolute amounts of DA in nmol/g are shown in parenthesis.

Treatment	Dose µg/rat	Cma	Cme	Cce	Adif	Adot	Tdot	Tdif
Saline	–	100 ± 10	100 ± 7	100 ± 7	100 ± 9	100 ± 6	100 ± 6	100 ± 12
		(80 ± 7)	(114 ± 7)	(77 ± 5)	(75 ± 7)	(200 ± 12)	(190 ± 12)	(80 ± 10)
NMDA	0.1	111 ± 5	101 ± 3	106 ± 5	111 ± 3	116 ± 7	113 ± 9	120 ± 4

Abbreviations used: Cma= marginal zone of the caudate nucleus; Cme= medial part of the caudate nucleus; Cce= central part of the caudate nucleus; Adif= diffuse type of DA fluorescence of the anterior part of the nuc. accumbens; Adot= dotted type of DA fluorescence of the posterior part of the nuc. accumbens; Tdot= dotted type of DA fluorescence of the medial-posterior part of the tuberculum olfactorium; Tdif= diffuse type of DA fluorescence of the lateral part of the tuberculum olfactorium.

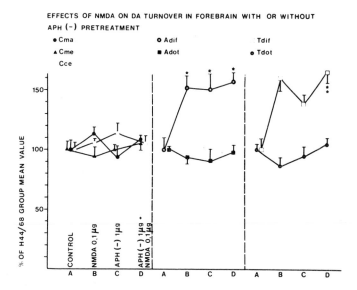

Fig. 1. The effects of an intraventricular injection of NMDA
(0.1 μg) on the H 44/68 induced DA fluorescence disappearance
in various forebrain areas of the male awake rat with or without prior treatment with (-)APH (1 μg). (-)APH was injected 5
min prior to the NMDA injection and H 44/68 (250 mg/kg) was administered immediately before the i.v.t. injection. The rats were
decapitated 1 h following the H 44/68 injection. Means $\pm$ s.e.m.
are shown in per cent of H 44/68 group mean value. n= 5. The
statistical analysis has been performed by way of Wilcoxon test,
comparing all possible pairs of treatment. The significances
indicated in the figure refer to the H 44/68 alone group treated
with saline alone. *= p< 0.05; **= p< 0.01.

that these two drugs act at the same receptor to reduce DA turnover. The less
active form of APH, the (+) form, could in part counteract the ability of NMDA
to reduce DA turnover in the diffuse types of DA nerve terminal systems, in the
subcortical limbic areas (figs. 1-2).

These results imply that there exists a special type of NMDA receptor within
nuc. accumbens and tuberculum olfactorium, which cannot be blocked by known NMDA
antagonists and which can markedly reduce DA turnover in the diffuse types of DA

nerve terminals (CCK negative) in these two areas. At this type of NMDA receptor the known NMDA antagonist (–)APH seems to act as an agonist, since it also produced a marked reduction of DA turnover in these systems. Instead, the less active form of the NMDA antagonist (+)APH in part counteracted the action of NMDA on DA turnover in the tuberculum olfactorium (fig. 2). Herrling (this symposium) has also described the existence in the striatum of a NMDA receptor, which is not blocked by the selective NMDA antagonist d-α-aminoadipic acid. He suggests that

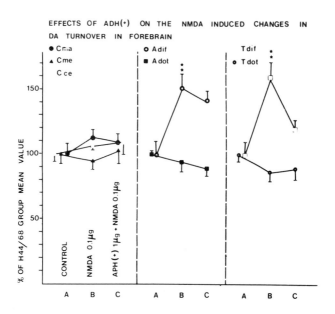

Fig. 2. The effects of (+)APH on the NMDA (0.1 µg, i.v.t.) induced reduction of the H 44/68 induced DA fluorescence disappearance in certain limbic areas of the awake male rat. (+)APH was administered 5 min prior to the NMDA injection in a dose of 1 µg. H 44/68 was administered i.p. immediately before the (+)APH injection in a dose of 250 mg/kg. All animals were killed 1 h after the H 44/68 injection by decapitation. Means ± s.e.m. are shown in per cent of H 44/68 group mean value. n= 5. Wilcoxon test has been performed comparing all possible pairs of treatments. The significances indicated in the figure refer to the control group mean value treated with saline alone. **= p< 0.01.

this receptor may be of the kainic acid type. The present results upen up the possibility of developing new treatments of schizophrenia, since by activating special types of NMDA receptors it seems possible to selectively reduce DA activity within subcortical limbic areas. Furthermore, the present results indicate that NMDA receptors are not involved in the regulation of DA turnover in various areas of the striatum. In line with these results Herrling (this symposium) has in electrophysiological studies obtained evidence that receptors of the NMDA type do not mediate cortically evoked excitations in the cat caudate nucleus. Fonnum et al., (1981) have described that cortical ablations especially of the medio-frontal cortex lead to a considerable disappearance of D-aspartate uptake in the olfactory tubercle, and transection of the fimbria-fornix system leads to a 50 % reduction of glutamate uptake in the nuc. accumbens. Thus, the special type of NMDA receptor present in these areas may belong to cortico-limbic systems operating with aspartate-glutamate as neurotransmitters.

2. The effects of excitatory amino acids and CCK-8 on ^{3}H-glutamate and ^{3}H-kainic acid binding in striatal membranes.

The results on ^{3}H-kainic acid binding are summarized in fig. 3.1-Glutamate (10^{-8} M) significantly increased the K_D values by 46 % and increased the B_{max} values of the ^{3}H-kainic acid binding sites by 18% (fig. 4), while NMDA 10^{-6} M) had no significant action on ^{3}H-kainic acid binding (fig. 5). Ibotenic acid (10^{-6} M) did not have any significant action on the density of ^{3}H-kainic acid binding sites, but significantly increased the K_D values by 52% in this way mimicking the action of 1-glutamate (fig. 5).

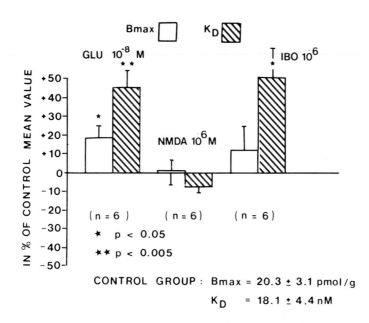

Fig. 3. Summary of the results obtained on striatal ^{3}H-kainic acid binding sites after modulation in vitro with 1-glutamate (10^{-8} M), NMDA (10^{-6} M) and ibotenic acid (10^{-6} M). The mean per cent change ($\pm$ s.e.m.) is shown. Student's paired t-test.

The results on ^{3}H-glutamate binding are summarized in fig. 6. Kainic acid (10^{-6} M) produced a significant reduction of the K_D value by 11% and of the B_{max} value by 12% (fig. 7). NMDA (10^{-6} M) had no effect on the binding characteristics of the ^{3}H-glutamate binding sites. Instead CCK-8 (10^{-8} M) produced a marked (63%)

reduction the affinity of the striatal glutamate binding sites and a 26% reduction in the B_{max} values of these sites (fig. 8). Thus, CCK-8 may be a powerful
downregulator of transmission at the striatal ^{3}H-glutamate binding sites. In
this way the CCK-peptides may have the possibility to counteract the neurotoxicity of kainic acid and of ibotenic acid. If so, CCK-peptides may have a role in
the treatment of Huntington's Chorea by protecting the striatal nerve cells from
degeneration.

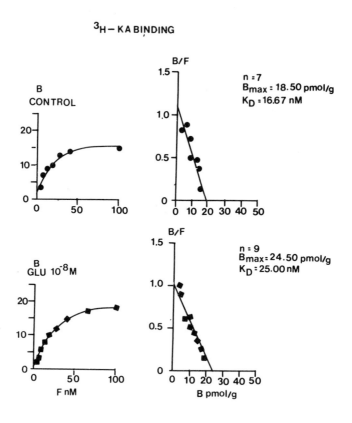

^{3}H – KA BINDING

Fig. 4. The effects of l-glutamate (10^{-8} M) on the binding
characteristics of striatal ^{3}H-kainic acid binding sites.
The saturation analysis is shown to the left in the figure
and the corresponding Scatchard plots are shown to the
right. 6 to 7 concentrations of ^{3}H-kainic acid have been
used. In the Scatchard plot the best fit to the experimental points was shown to be a straight line calculated by
standard parametrical procedures. In this way the K_D and
B_{max} values were obtained.

These results give evidence that in the striatum there exist receptor – receptor
interactions between glutamate and kainic acid receptors. Thus, when high affinity glutamate receptors are activated a larger number of kainic acid receptors
may become operational, but higher amounts of the possible endogenous ligand are
now required in view of the reduced affinity. It is known that glutamate is

required in the striatum in order for the neurotoxic effect of kainic acid to develop (Biziere and Coyle, 1979). In view of the present findings it seems possible that the role of glutamate in kainate neurotoxicity may in part be related to its ability to increase the number of ^{3}H-kainic acid binding sites. A lowering of affinity of these receptors is of no consequence for neurotoxic activity in view of the high concentrations of kainic acid present in the injected area. It might also be that glutamate may enhance the coupling of the kainic acid binding sites to its ion channel. Furthermore, in view of the discovery in the present paper that kainic acid can increase the affinity in the ^{3}H-glutamate binding sites, it must be considered that the glutamate receptors are now operational in synaptic transmission at lower concentrations of glutamate in the synaptic cleft compared with untreated rats. These changes in the glutamate

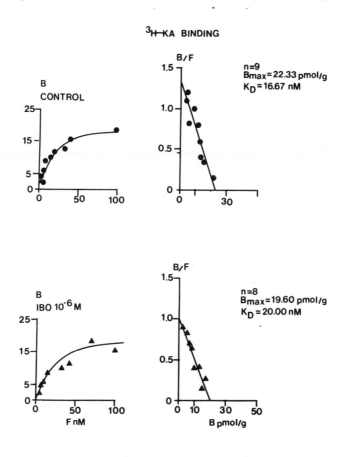

Fig. 5. The effects of ibotenic acid (10^{-6} M) on the binding characteristics of striatal ^{3}H-kainic acid binding sites. The saturation analysis is shown to the left in the figure and the corresponding Scatchard plot is shown to the right. For further details, see text to fig. 4.

receptors may lead to increases in excitability and firing of the striatal nerve cells under resting conditions, which also may be an important factor in determining the vulnerability of the striatal nerve cells to the neurotoxic effects of kainic acid receptor activation. Finally, the maximal transmission over ^{3}H-glutamate binding sites may, however, be reduced in view of the small reduction in the density of these sites induced by kainic acid. Although the per cent changes in the binding characteristics of ^{3}H-kainic acid and ^{3}H-glutamate binding sites may be small the amplifier gain of the receptor system is probably at least 1:30 (see Seeman, 1980, Fuxe et al., 1982a,b). In this way a 10 % change can lead to a 300 % change of synaptic transmission.

The present paper also reports the discovery of CCK-glutamate receptor interactions in striatal membranes. Under the influence of CCK-8 receptor activation, the glutamate binding sites undergo a marked reduction of affinity and are in addition reduced in number. These receptor changes probably reflect the development of receptor subsensitivity, since they may now operate only at higher concentrations of l-glutamate and with a reduced maximal capacity. It is therefore possible that CCK-peptides may reduce the neurotoxicity of excitotoxins provided they act over excitatory amino acid receptors, especially the ^{3}H-glutamate binding site. This type of receptor-receptor interaction may represent an allosteric interaction in a macromolecule containing both CCK-8 and glutamate binding sites in view of the ability of CCK-8 to displace ^{3}H-glutamate from its binding site.

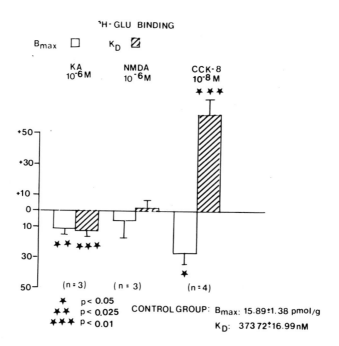

Fig. 6. Summary of results obtained on striatal ^{3}H-glutamate binding sites after modulation in vitro with kainic acid (10^{-6} M), NMDA (10^{-6} M) and CCK-8 (10^{-8} M). The mean per cent change ($\pm$ s.e.m.) is shown. Student's paired t-test.

3. Excitatory amino acid receptors and their modulation of striatal ^{3}H-spiperone and ^{3}H-NPA binding sites

The results are summarized in figs. 9 and 10. Glutamate (10^{-6} M), but not NMDA (10^{-6} M) are shown to significantly increase the K_D value of the ^{3}H-NPA binding sites in the striatum by 26% (fig. 11). In addition, glutamate produces a 8% increase in the number of ^{3}H-NPA binding sites. Furthermore, quisqualate (10^{-6} M) did not produce any significant change in the characteristics of the ^{3}H-NPA binding sites. Also the influence of glutamate (10^{-6} M) and NMDA (10^{-6} M) on ^{3}H-spiperone binding sites in striatal membranes was evaluated. None of these excitatory amino acids produced significant changes in the binding characteristics of the striatal ^{3}H-spiperone binding sites (fig. 12). In one experiment it was shown that cis-2,3-piperidine dicarboxylic acid (10^{-6} M), which seems to block the action of both NMDA and quisqualate could counteract the modulatory effects of glutamate (10^{-6} M) on the ^{3}H-NPA binding sites (see Davis et al., 1981).

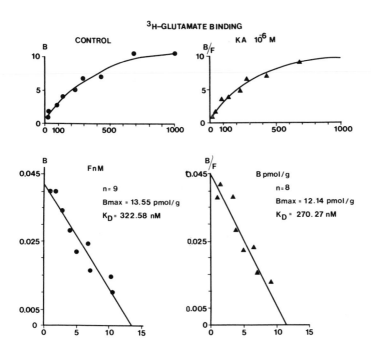

Fig. 7. The effects of kainic acid (10^{-6} M) on the binding characteristics of striatal ^{3}H-glutamate binding sites. The saturation curves are shown to the left in the figure and the corresponding Scatchard plot is shown to the right. The number of concentrations ranged from 7 to 10. For further details, see text to fig. 4.

[3]H-NPA probably labels DA receptors of the D_2 and D_3 type and ^{3}H-spiperone labels the DA receptors of the D_2 type (see Seeman, 1980). Thus, glutamate receptors, which do not appear to be of the NMDA or the quisqualate type and high affinity agonist binding sites of the D_2 and D_3 receptors may interact with each other. At the D_2 type of DA receptor glutamate receptors exclusively regulate the agonist binding sites, since the neuroleptic receptors do not seem to be modulated by glutamate. These results give evidence that receptor - receptor interactions exist in the central nervous system (CNS) of the mammallian brain at the local circuit level.

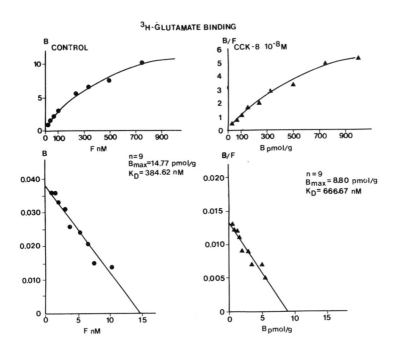

Fig. 8. The effects of CCK-8 (10^{-8} M) on the binding characteristics of striatal ^{3}H-glutamate binding sits. The saturation analysis is shown to the left in the figure and the corresponding Scatchard plot is shown to the right. 6 to 7 concentrations of ^{3}H-glutamate were used. In this analysis the binding was formed in the presence of 10^{-6} M of basitracin and 0.05% bovine serum albumin. For further details, see text to fig. 4.

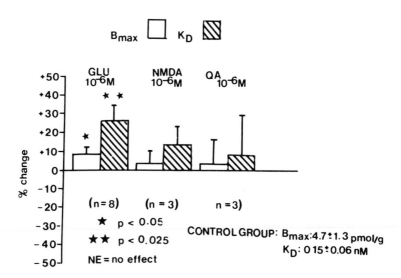

Fig. 9. Summary of results obtained on striatal ^{3}H–NPA
binding sites after modulation <u>in vitro</u> with 1-glutamate,
NMDA and quisqualate (QA). The mean per cent change
(<u>+</u> s.e.m.) is shown. Student's paired t-test.

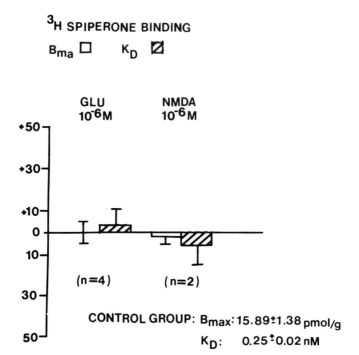

Fig. 10. Summary of results obtained on striatal ^{3}H-spi-perone binding sites after modulation in vitro with 1-glutamate (10^{-6} M) and NMDA (10^{-6} M). The mean per cent change ($\pm$ s.e.m.) is shown. Student's paired t-test.

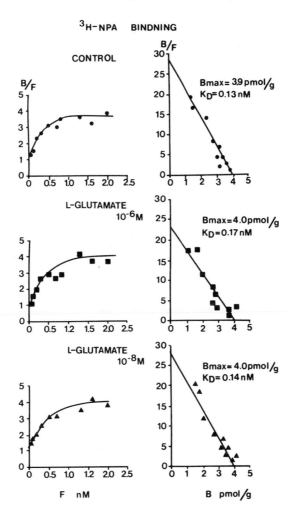

Fig. 11. The effects of l-glutamate (10^{-6} M and 10^{-8} M) on the binding characteristics of ^{3}H-NPA binding sites in the striatum of rats. Saturation analysis is shown to the left in the figure and the corresponding Scatchard plot to the right. For further details, see text to fig. 4. 9 to 10 concentrations of ^{3}H-NPA have been used.

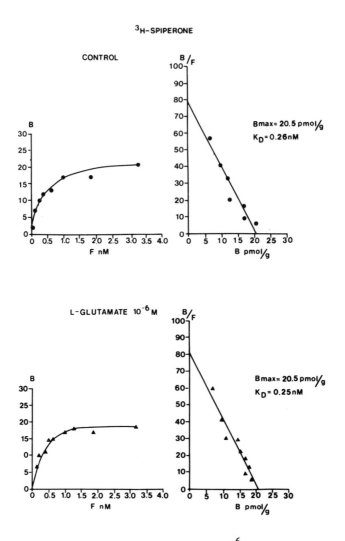

Fig. 12. The effects of l-glutamate (10^{-6} M) on the binding characteristics of ^{3}H-spiperone binding sites in striatum of rats. The saturation analysis is shown to the left in the figure and the corresponding Scatchard plot to the right. 9 to 10 concentrations have been used. For further details, see text to fig. 4.

Most of the glutamate receptors in the striatum probably belong to the cortico-striatal glutamate pathways, and most of the DA receptors belong to the nigro-striatal DA systems. Thus, these two powerful afferent systems to the striatum can interact with each other via a receptor - receptor interaction, which may be of importance for the integrative function of the striatum. Thus, when the cortical message via the corticostriatal glutamate pathway is increased, the high affinity DA receptors require higher amounts of DA in the synaptic cleft to become operational. However, the number seems to be increased, so that when the amounts released are sufficiently high to activate all the DA receptors, DA transmission at these receptor sites may be increased. It may be speculated that cortical pathways in this way take command in the regulation of striatal nerve cell activity so that the dopaminergic nigral control plays a more dominant role in states in which glutamate is released in reduced amounts in the local circuits of the striatum. This may e.g. take place when the glutamate synapses of the striatum are markedly downregulated by the striatal CCK afferents, which via release of CCK-8 markedly reduces the affinity and density of striatal glutamate receptors. At the same time CCK-8 (10^{-8} M) can produce a 9% increase in the density and a 17% increase in the K_D values of the striatal ^{3}H-NPA binding sites and a 10% reduction of the striatal spiperone binding sites (Fuxe et al., 1981, Fuxe, Agnati and Celani, 1982a). These results illustrate the chemical integrative processes occuring in the striatal local circuits via receptor-receptor interactions. These processes are probably of fundamental importance for sensory motor integration in the striatum and may also determine the sensitivity of the striatal nerve cells to the excitotoxins.

ACKNOWLEDGEMENT

This work has been supported by a grant (04X-715) from the Swedish Medical Research Council, by a grant from Magnus Bergvall's Stiftelse, by a grant (MH 25504) from the National Institute of Health, Bethesda, Maryland, U.S.A., and by a grant from Knut & Alice Wallenberg's Foundation. We are grateful for the excellent technical assistance of mrs. Ulla Altamimi, miss Birgitta Johansson, miss Siv Nilsson and miss Barbro Tinner and for the excellent secreterial assistance of miss Elisabeth Sandqvist.

REFERENCES

Agnati, L.F., Andersson, K., Wiesel, F. and Fuxe, K (1979). J. Neurosci. Meth., 1, 365-373.

Agnati, L.F., Fuxe, K., Benfenati, F., Calza, L., Battistini, N. and Ögren, S.-O (1982). In: Frontiers in Neuropsychiatric Research, CINP Satellite symposium, MacMillan Press, Corfu, Greece, June 28-30.

Agnati, L.F., Fuxe, K., Benfenati, F., Zini, I. and Hökfelt, T (1982b). Acta Physiol. Scand., in press.

Baudry, M. and Lynch, G (1979). Nature, Lond., 282, 748-750.

Biziere, K. and Coyle, J.T. (1979). J. Neurosci. Res., 4, 383-398.

Coyle, J.T., Zaczek, R., Slevin, J. and Collins, J (1981). In: Glutamate as a Neurotransmitter, (eds. G. Di Chiara and G.L. Gessa), pp. 337-346, Raven Press, New York.

Creese, I., Schneider, R. and Snyder, S.H (1977). Eur. J. Pharmacol., 46, 377-381.

Davies, J. and Watkins, J.C (1981). In: Glutamate as a Neurotransmitter, (eds. G. Di Chiara and G.L. Gessa), pp. 275-283, Raven Press, New York.

Evans, R.H. and Watkins, J.C (1981). Life Sci., 1303-1308.

Fonnum, F., Söreide, A., Kvale, I., Walker, J. and Wallas, I (1981). In: Glutamate as a Neurotransmitter, (eds. G. Di Chiara and G.L. Gessa), pp. 29-41, Raven Press, New York.

Fuxe, K., Agnati, L.F., Benfenati, F., Cimmino, M., Algeri, S., Hökfelt, T. and Mutt, V (1981). Acta Physiol. Scand., 113, 567-569.

Fuxe, K., Agnati, L.F. and Celani, M.F (1982a). Acta Physiol. Scand., in press.

Fuxe, K., Agnati, L.F., Benfenati, F., Celani, M.F., Zini, I., Zoli, M. and Mutt, V (1982b). In: Basic Aspects on Receptor Biochemistry, Symposium in Vienna, Austria, Sept. 10-12, J. Neural Trans., in press.

Herrling, P.L (1982). In: Excitotoxins, Wenner-Gren Center International Series, No. 39, (eds. K. Fuxe, P. Roberts and R. Scwarcz), Pergamon Press, in press.

Leysen, J. and Gommesen, W (1981). J. Neurochem., 36(1), 201–219.
Löfström, A., Jonsson, G., Wiesel, F.A. and Fuxe, K (1976). J. Histochem. Cytochem., 24, 430–442.
McLennan, H (1981). In: Glutamate as a Neurotransmitter, (eds. G. Di Chiara and G.L. Gessa), pp. 253–262, Raven Press, New York.
McLennan, H (1982). J. Physiol. Pharmacol., 60, 91–94.
Perkins, M.N., Stone, T.W., Collins, J.F. and Curry, K (1981). Neurosci. Lett., 23, 333–336.
Roberts, E (1981). In: Glutamate as a Neurotransmitter, (eds. G. Di Chiara and G.L. Gessa), pp. 91–102, Raven Press, New York.
Roberts, P.J. and Sharif, N.A (1981). In: Glutamate as a Neurotransmitter, (eds. G. Di Chiara and G.L. Gessa), pp. 295–305, Raven Press, New York.
Seeman, P (1980). Dopamine Receptors. Pharmacological Reviews, pp. 229–313, vol. 3, No. 3, William & Wilkins Comp., Baltimore.
Schwarcz, R., Aldinio, C., French, E.D. and Collins, J.F (1982a). Neurosci., 7, S 188.
Schwarcz, R., Collins, J. and Parks, D (1982b). Neurosci. Lett., in press.
Schwarcz, R. and Fuxe, K (1979). Life Sci., 24, 1471–1480.
Watkins, J.C (1981). In: Glutamate: Transmitter in the Central Nervous System, (eds. P.J. Roberts, J. Storm-Mathisen and G.A.R. Johnston), pp. 1–24, Wiley, New York.
Watkins, J.C., Davies, J., Evans, R.H., Francis, A.A. and Jones, A.W (1981). In: Glutamate as a Neurotransmitter, (eds. G. Di Chiara and G.L. Gessa), pp. 263–273, Raven Press, New York.

ELECTROPHYSIOLOGICAL AND PHARMACOLOGICAL STUDIES ON KAINIC ACID-INDUCED NEURONAL ACTIVATION

C. DE MONTIGNY, G. DE BONNEL AND D. TARDIF

Centre de Recherche en Sciences Neurologiques, Faculté de Médecine, Université de Montreal, P. O. Box 6128 Station "A", Montréal, Québec, Canada H3C 3J7

ABSTRACT

The excitotoxic hypothesis proposes that amino acids exert their neurotoxic action via an excessive neuronal excitation. In concordance with the extreme sensitivity of CA_3 pyramidal hippocampal neurons to the neurotoxic action of kaïnic acid (KA), these neurons were found to be exquisitely sensitive to the excitatory action of KA applied microiontophoretically. The excitatory action of KA on CA_1 but not on CA_3 neurons was selectively antagonized by low intravenous doses or low current microiontophoretic applications of benzodiazepines (BZD). This effect of BZD was not mimic by phenobarbital or chlorpromazine and was blocked by the specific BZD antogonist, RO 15-1788. The blockade of KA-induced activation of CA_1 pyramidal neurons is not due to an enhanced GABAergic activity since BZD, given at the same dose, failed to potentiate the effect of GABA; furthermore, direct microiontophoretic applications of GABA did not have any selective effect on KA-induced activation. It is proposed that the antagonism of an endogenous ligand for these "KA-sensitive" receptors might be related to their clinical anxiolytic effect.

KEYWORDS

Anxiety, benzodiazepines, epilepsy, hippocampus, Huntington's chorea, kainic acid, pyramidal neurons, RO 15-1788.

INTRODUCTION

The discovery of the neurotoxic action of certain amino acids has been initially perceived as a technical advance permitting axon-spearing neuronal lesions. However, it was quickly realized that they were potential keys to open new fields of investigations in neuroscience. For instance, the analogy between the kainate-induced neuronal degeneration and that found in Huntington's chorea and in temporal lobe epilepsy prompted many fruitful investigations (Coyle and Schwarcz, 1976; Mason et al., 1978; Nadler, 1981).

Besides this potential heuristic value for understanding the pathophysiology of certain neurological disorders, the mechanisms put into motion by these amino acids leading to neuronal death have attracted the attention of many investigators. Olney et al. (1971) and Johnston (1973) have formulated the excitotoxic hypothesis which proposes that amino acids exert their neurotoxic action via an excessive excitation of the target neurons. This was based on the similar ranking of the neurotoxic and neuroexcitatory potencies of amino acids. However, since there is an important regional variation of their neurotoxic effects, the validation of the hypothesis required assessing both neurotoxic and neuroexcitatory actions in the same neuronal populations. We have recently shown that rat mesencephalic trigeminal neurons are resistant to both neurotoxic and excitatory actions of kainic acid (KA) (de Montigny and Lund, 1980). Moving to the other extreme of the scale, we reported the exquisite sensitivity to KA excitatory action of CA3 hippocampal pyramidal neurons (de Montigny and Tardif, 1981) which extreme susceptibility to the neurotoxic action of this amino acid had been demonstrated by Nadler et al. (1978).

Diazepam (DZP) can block both convulsant and neurotoxic effects of KA (Ben-Ari et al., 1980; Fuller and Olney, 1979; Zaczek et al., 1978). The present studies were undertaken to determine if DZP and other benzodiazepines (BZD) can reduce the excitatory effect of KA.

MATERIAL AND METHODS

Male Sprague-Dawley rats (200-300 g) were anesthetized with urethane (1.25 g/kg, i.p.) and a catheter was inserted in the femoral vein. They were then mounted on a stereotoxic apparatus. Five-barrelled glass micropipettes were pulled in a conventional manner and their tips broken to 8-10 m under microscopic control. The central barrel, used for unitary recording, was filled with a 2 M NaCl solution saturated with Fast Green FCF. One side barrel, used for automatic current balancing, was filled with a 2 M NaCl solution. The remaining barrels were filled with three of the following solutions: KA 0.001 M in 0.4 NaCl, pH: 8 (Sigma); glutamate HCl (GLU) 0.05 M in 0.05 M NaCl, pH: 8 (Aldrich); acetylcholine chloride (ACh) 0.02 M in 0.2 M NaCl, pH: 4 (Sigma); GABA 0.01 M in .05 M NaCl, pH: 4 (Calbiochem); chlordiazepoxide HCl (CDP) 0.01 M in 0.02 M NaCl, pH: 3 (Hoffman-LaRoche); flurazepam 2HCl (FLU) 0.01 M, pH:3 (Hoffman-LaRoche).

Hippocampal pyramidal cells were identified by their long duration (0.8-1.5 ms) and large amplitude (0.5-2 mV) action potentials and by the presence of "complex spike" discharges alternating with simple spike activity (Kandel and Spencer, 1961). Spikes were amplified in a conventional manner and fed through a window discriminator generating signals counted for 10 s periods and recorded with a pen writer. At the end of the experiment, a Fast Green deposit was left at the last recording site with a -20 µA current for subsequent histological verification.

RESULTS

The differential action of KA on cortical, CA1 and CA3 dorsal hippocampus pyramidal neurons

The value of any scientific hypothesis can be measured by the accuracy of its predictions. Given the extreme sensitivity of CA3 pyramidal neurons to the neurotoxic action of KA (Nadler et al., 1978), the excitotoxic hypothesis (Johnston, 1973; Olney et al., 1971) would predict that these neurons should be exquisitely sensitive to the neuroexcitatory action of KA.

Fig. 1 illustrates the response of a cortical, a CA1 and a CA3 pyramidal neuron to microiontophoretic applications of KA. Whereas relatively high ejecting (negative) currents were necessary to activate cortical and CA1 hippocampal neurons with KA, a mere lowering of the retention (positive) current was often sufficient to bring an intense activation of CA3 pyramidal neurons. Interestingly, brief microiontophoretic applications of KA with out-going currents in the CA$_3$ region often resulted in a long-lasting activation of the neuron. This type of activation was never seen in the CA$_1$ region even when large ejecting currents (up to -100 nA) were used.

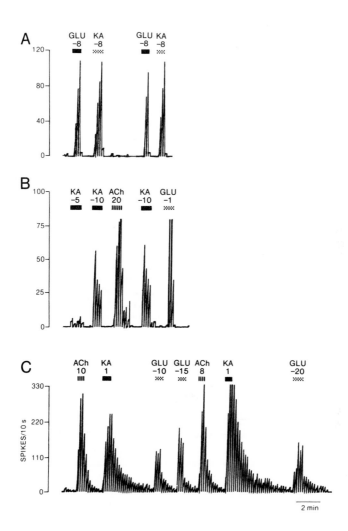

Fig. 1 Integrated firing rate histograms of a cortical neuron (A) and of pyramidal neurons recorded in the CA$_1$ (B) and CA$_3$ (C) hippocampal regions showing their response to KA, GLU and ACh. Note that a mere reduction of retention current suffices to induce an intense activation of the CA$_3$ neuron with KA, whereas negative out-going currents are required to activate the cortical and the CA$_1$ neurons. Currents indicated in nA in this and the following figures.

In order to evaluate the specificity of this differential effect of KA on these neuronal populations, GLU and ACh were tested on the same neurons. As illustrated in Fig. 1, CA$_3$ neurons did not display any greater responsiveness to both agents. From the responses evoked by GLU and KA, taking in account the ionic dilution of the solutions used and the currents applied, it could be estimated that KA was approximately 70 times more active than GLU in CA$_1$, whereas it was at least 3,000 times more active than GLU in CA$_3$. This clear regional dissociation between the effects of GLU and KA constitutes further evidence that they activate different receptors. Another electrophysiological observation which points to the same conclusion is the fact that most pyramidal neurons could be driven by KA to high rates of discharge (50-60 Hz) without any modification of the wave form whereas GLU induced a depolarization block at much lower rates of discharge.

It is noteworthy that the differential effect of KA on CA$_1$ and CA$_3$ neurons cannot be attributed to a non-specific susceptibility of CA$_3$ pyramidal neurons to neurotoxins since CA$_1$ and CA$_3$ pyramidal neurons are equally responsive to the excitatory action of ibotenic acid, another potent neurotoxin (Ouelette and de Montigny, unpublished observations).

The substratum for the differential sensitivity of CA$_1$ and CA$_3$ pyramidal neurons to KA is unknown. The simplest explanation would be that CA$_3$ pyramidal neurons have a greater number of receptors. This explanation is in keeping with the radioautographic demonstration by Foster et al. (1981) of a much denser labelling with ^{3}H-KA of the CA$_3$ region as compared to CA$_1$. However, the resolution of the photonic method used in that study does not allow differentiation of pre-vs postsynaptic localization of the labelling. It is impossible at present time to rule out the possibility that KA might act presynaptically to release an excitatory neurotransmitter from terminals of a fiber system projecting specifically to the CA$_3$ region. This possibility would be consistent with the findings of Nadler and Cuthbertson (1980) who described the protective effect against theneurotoxic effect of KA afforded by a lesion of the dentate - CA$_3$ mossy fiber projections. Finally, the presence of a calcium binding protein in the somata of CA$_1$ pyramidal neurons but not in the CA$_3$ neurons (Baimbridge and Miller, 1981) could also possibly account for the differential excitatory potency of KA in these two regions. Experiments adressed to verify each of these possibilities are currently in progress in our laboratory.

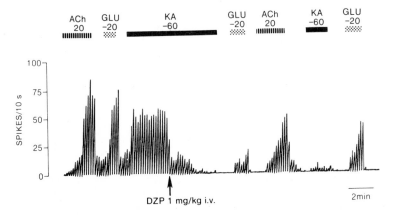

Fig. 2   Integrated firing rate histogram of a CA$_1$ pyramidal neuron illustrating the selective blockade of KA-induced activation by diazepam (DZP).

Blockade of the KA-induced activation of CA_1 pyramidal neurons by benzodiazepines

Intraventricular or systemic injections of KA in the rat induce seizures which can be abolished by DZP (Ben-Ari et al., 1980; Zaczec et al., 1978). Furthermore, Fuller and Olney (1979) reported that DZP could prevent the neurotoxic action of KA in CA_1 but not in CA_3. We thus thought it would be interesting to determine if DZP and other BZD could antagonize the neuroexcitatory action of KA.

We recently reported that the intravenous administration of low doses of BZD reverses the activation of CA_1 pyramidal neurons by KA applied microiontophoretically (de Bonnel and de Montigny, 1982). In Fig. 2, DZP almost completely blocked the activation of this CA_1 pyramidal cell by KA whereas the excitatory actions of ACh and GLU were much less affected. Similar results were obtained with lorazepam (LOR). The intravenous ED_{80} of DZP and LOR for reducing KA activation of CA_1 neurons were 0.4 and 1.5 mg/kg respectively.

In CA_3, however, BZD were found to be almost inactive at clinically relevant doses. The activation by KA of the CA_3 pyramidal neuron presented in Fig. 3 was hardly affected by a total intravenous dose of 3.5 mg/kg of DZP. Note that this CA_3 neuron, as mentioned in the previous section, is activated by a mere lowering (from +7 to +1 nA) of the retention current of KA, contrasting with the relatively high ejection current (-60 nA) used to activate CA_1 neuron presented in Fig. 2.

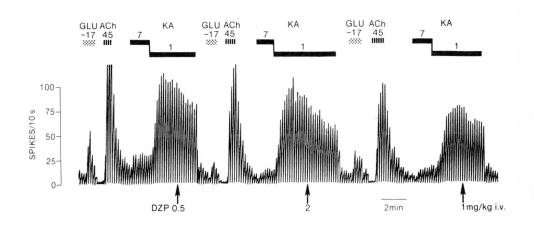

Fig. 3 Integrated firing rate histogram of a CA_3 pyramidal neuron showing that the administration of a cumulative dose of 3.5 mg/kg of DZP does not affect much the KA-induced activation.

To further investigate the regional selectivity of this effect of BZD, we studied the effect of LOR (0.5 mg/kg, i.v.) on parietal cortical neurons activated by microiontophoretic applications of KA, GLU and ACh. Contrasting with its long-lasting effect in CA_1, LOR exerted only a transient reduction of the KA-induced activation. Furthermore the selectivity for KA observed in the CA_1 region was not present in the cortex since GLU and ACh were affected to a similar degree (de Bonnel and de Montigny, 1982).

To determine if the blockade of the KA activation of CA_1 pyramidal neurons by intravenous BZD was attributable to their direct action on the membrane of the neurons recorded, we studied the effect of microiontophoretic applications of two water-soluble BZD, FLU and CDP. Fig. 4 illustrates the dose-related reduction of KA-induced activation during low current applications of FLU whereas the activation by ACh is not affected by identical applications of this BZD. Consistent with the weak effect of intravenous BZD, large currents of FLU and CDP were required to reduce the excitatory effect of KA in CA_3 (Fig. 5).

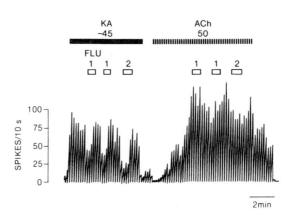

Fig. 4   Integrated firing rate histogram of a CA_1 pyramidal neuron showing the dose-related reduction of KA activation by microiontophoretic applications of flurazepam (FLU). Applications of FLU with the same currents did not modify the ACh-induced activation.

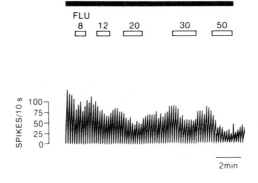

Fig. 5   Integrated firing rate histogram of a CA_3 pyramidal neuron which activation by KA is only slightly reduced by large current applications of FLU.

Pharmacological specificity of the suppression of KA-induced activation of CA₁ pyramidal cells by BZD

Specific binding sites for BZD have been identified in the rat CNS (Braestrup and Squires, 1978). Assuming that the suppressant action of BZD on KA activation was mediated through these sites, one could make two predictions: firstly, other non-BZD psychotropic drugs should not share this property since they do not displace BZD from their binding sites (Braestrup and Squires, 1978); secondly, the effect of BZD on the KA activation should be prevented by a BZD antagonist with a high affinity for these sites.

To verify the validity of the first prediction, we studied the effect of phenobarbital (10 mg/kg, i.v.), an anticonvulsant barbiturate, and of chlorpromazine (4 mg/kg, i.v.), a sedative neuroleptic, on the activation of CA₁ neurons by microiontophoretic applications of KA. Both psychotropic agents failed to alter consistently the excitatory action of KA on these neurons (de Bonnel and de Montigny, 1982).

The second prediction was put to the test using the BZD antagonist, RO 15-1788 (Darragh et al., 1981; Hunkeler et al., 1981; Möhler and Richard, 1981; Polc etal., 1981). As illustrated in Fig. 6, high doses of this antagonist markedly reduced the effect of LOR on KA activation of CA₁ pyramidal neurons. In another series of experiments, lower doses of RO 15-1788 (3.5 mg/kg, i.v.), produced a 60% reduction of the effect of LOR (0.35 mg/kg, i.v.) on CA₁ neurons activated with KA (de Bonnel and de Montigny, 1982).

Is the effect of BZD on KA activation mediated via an enhancement of GABAergic activity?

BZD have been shown to potentiate GABA-mediated inhibition in many CNS regions (see Tallman et al., 1980). Could an enhancement of the tonic action of GABA on CA₁ pyramidal neurons account for the effect of BZD on their activation by KA?

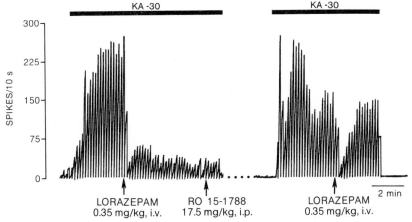

Fig. 6 Integrated firing rate histogram of a CA₁ pyramidal neuron showing the marked reduction of KA-induced activation by lorazepam. Following the administration of the benzodiazepine antagonist RO 15-1788, KA recovers its ability to activate the neuron and the same dose of lorazepam produces only a transient reduction of the firing rate. Note that traces are discontinuous.

As a first attempt to answer this question, we determined the effect of intravenous LOR on the depression of the ACh-induced firing of CA_1 pyramidal cells by repeated microiontophoretic applications of GABA. Results are presented in Table 1. No significant effect could be detected following the administration of 0.5 mg/kg of LOR, which dose is sufficient to produce a greater than 80% reduction of KA activation of these neurons. Higher cumulative doses (up to 2 mg/kg) also failed to potentiate the action of GABA (Table 1 and Fig. 7).

TABLE 1: Effect of intravenous lorazepam (LOR) on GABA-induced depression of CA_1 pyramidal neuron firing rate[+]

Cumulative doses of LOR (mg/kg)	Number of units tested	Effect of GABA (mean ± s.e.m.)
0	7	52.7 ± 3.6%
0.5	7	51.0 ± 7.6%
1.0	7	46.3 ± 6.4%
1.5	5	52.5 ± 9.3%
2.0	2	54.0 ± 3.0%

[+] Pyramidal neurons were activated with a small current of ACh to a discharge frequency of 10-15 Hz. The current of GABA (6.2 ± 0.7 nA) was adjusted for each neuron to obtain a depression of firing rate ranging from 40 to 60%. At least three applications of GABA with the same current were carried out before and following each dose of LOR (see Fig. 7). Only one cell per rat was tested. None of the values obtained after LOR were satistically different from the initial value.

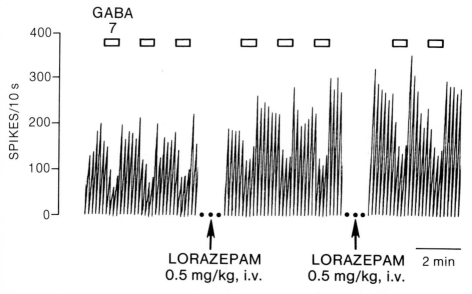

Fig. 7   Integrated firing rate histogram of a CA_1 pyramidal neuron activated with a low current fo ACh (3 nA) showing that its response to GABA is not modified by the intravenous injection of lorazepam.

In another series of experiments we used the same paradigm except that CDP was applied microiontophoretically using the same currents which were shown effective in reducing KA activation (see Fig. 4). Microiontophoretic applications of CDP failed to potentiate the depressant effect of GABA (Table 2 and Fig. 8).

TABLE 2: Effect of microiontophoretic applications of chlordiazepoxide (CDP) on GABA-induced depression of CA$_1$ pyramidal neuron firing rate[+]

Ranges of current (nA) of CDP	Number of neurons tested	Effect of GABA (mean ± s.e.m.) without CDP	Effect of GABA (mean ± s.e.m.) during CDP
1 - 5	19	55.4 ± 3.4%	50.2 ± 4.4%
6 - 10	22	54.8 ± 2.6%	61.6 ± 3.4%
11 - 15	9	52.6 ± 4.3%	56.6 ± 5.5%
16 - 30	8	56.8 ± 5.8%	61.5 ± 9.3%

[+] Pyramidal neurons were activated with a small current of ACh to a discharge frequency of 10 - 15 Hz. The current of GABA (5.8 ± 0.6 nA) was adjusted for each neuron before CDP application to obtain a depression of the firing rate ranging from 40 to 60% and the same current of GABA was reapplied during CDP (see Fig. 8).

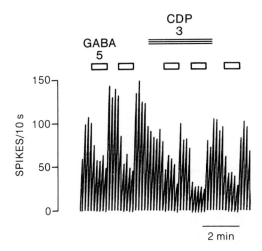

Fig. 8   Integrated firing rate histogram of a CA$_1$ pyramidal neuron activated with a low current of ACh (2 nA) showing that its response to GABA is not substantially modified by concurrent microiontophoretic application of chlordiazepoxide (CDP).

If an enhanced GABA activity were responsible for the selective effect of BZD on KA activation of CA$_1$ pyramidal neurons, one could expect GABA to reduce the KA-induced excitation much more readily than that produced by GLU and ACh. Contrarily to this prediction, microiontophoretic applications of GABA had very similar effects on the activation of CA$_1$ pyramidal neurons produced by KA, ACh and GLU (Table 3 and Fig. 9).

TABLE 3: Effect of GABA on kainate (KA)-, acetylcholine (ACh)- and glutamate (GLU)-induced activations of CA$_1$ pyramidal neurons[+]

Iontophoretic currents (nA) (mean ± s.e.m.)	Number of neurons tested	Rate of firing (Hz) (mean ± s.e.m.)		
		before GABA	during GABA	after GABA
KA 13.3 ± 0.9	19	14.1 ± 2.1	6.3 ± 1.4 (55%)	11.8 ± 2.1
ACh 8.9 ± 0.9	13	15.8 ± 1.5	6.0 ± 1.3 (62%)	15.6 ± 3.1
GLU 2.7 ± 0.7	11	10.5 ± 2.5	5.2 ± 1.6 (51%)	8.1 ± 2.0

[+] GABA was applied with a current of 5.6 ± 0.4 nA (mean ± s.e.m.). The degrees of reduction by GABA (indicated in brackets) of the activations produced by KA, ACh and GLU were not statistically different.

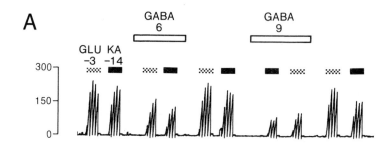

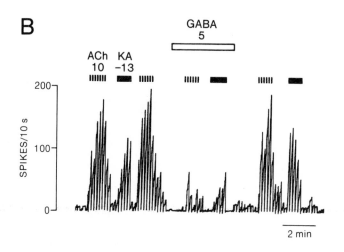

Fig. 9   Integrated firing rate histograms of two CA$_1$ pyramidal neurons showing that microiontophoretic applications of GABA have a similar effect on KA-, GLU- and ACh-induced activations.

DISCUSSION

Several observations made during the present studies are in agreement with the excitotoxic hypothesis: 1) the greater excitatory potency of KA as compared to GLU (in both CA_1 and CA_3) is consistent with its greater neurotoxicity (Kizer et al. 1978; 2) the exquisite sensitivity of CA_3 pyramidal neurons to the excitatory action of KA is congruent with the extreme susceptibility of these neurons to its neurotoxic action (Nadler et al., 1978); 3) the selective blockade of KA excitatory action in the CA_1 region by BZD is consistent with the protection afforded by DZP against KA neurotoxicity in this region (Fuller and Olney, 1979). Several other observations, such as the insensitivity of trigeminal mesencephalic neurons to both the neurotoxic and neuroexcitatory actions of KA (de Montigny and Lund, 1980), also suggest that excessive excitation of target neurons by neurotoxic amino acids might play an important role in inducing neuronal death. It remains to be established to which extent neuroexcitation contributes to the neuronal loss seen in certain types of epilepsy or in Huntington's chorea.

Radioligand binding studies (Simon et al., 1976; Baudry and Lynch, 1979; Henke and Cuenod, 1979; London and Coyle, 1979) have already suggested that GLU and KA bind to different receptor sites. Several observations in the present studies concur with this conclusion: 1) the clear dissociation between the relative excitatory potencies of these amino acids in CA_1 and CA_3; 2) the appearance of a depolarization block at lower frequencies with GLU applications than with KA; 3) the differential effect of BZD on these amino acids.

The extreme regional variation of the excitatory action of KA is strongly suggestive of a receptor-mediated effect, although it cannot be ascertained if "KA-sensitive" receptors are located on presynaptic terminals or on postsynaptic membranes (or on both). The specific and selective blockade of KA-induced excitation by BZD constitutes a further suggestion that KA activation is receptor-mediated. The implication of this pharmacological effect of BZD in their clinical anxiolytic efficacy is first suggested by the fact that it was obtained with low and clinically relevant doses. Moreover, the 4:1 ratio of LOR:DZP potencies in blocking KA-induced activation corresponds to that of their clinical anxiolytic potencies. The failure of phenobarbital and chlorpromazine to exert a similar effect suggests that the anticonvulsant and sedative properties of BZD might not be related to their ability to block KA-induced activation.

One striking feature of these observations is the clear regional selectivity of the action of BZD on KA activation. The molecular basis for this regional selectivity is unknown. It is however noteworthy that the hippocampus has been reported to possess two pharmacological distinct BZD binding sites, one of which differs from the site present in cerebral cortex and cerebellum (Volicer and Biagioni, 1982; Williams et al., 1980). Since the outstanding characteristic of BZD is a selective removal of emotional inhibition, leading to a reinforcement of instrumental behavior (Haefely, 1978), a selective blockade of a yet unidentified endogenous ligand of "KA-sensitive" receptors in the limbic system would be conceptually appealing to account for their anxiolytic action in humans.

Numerous studies have disclosed the intimate interaction between BZD and GABA (see Tallman et al., 1980). The present results indicate that the blockade of KA activation of CA_1 neurons by BZD cannot be attributed to enhancement of the GABAergic neurotransmission: 1) GABA did not exert any selective suppression of KA activation; 2) low intravenous doses of LOR and low current microiontophoretic applications of CDP (which both markedly reduce KA activation) failed to potentiate the depressant effect of GABA. Klepner et al. (1979), using triazolopyridazines, have reported the presence of two distinct BZD binding sites in the rat CNS, one of which would not be coupled to GABA receptors and proposed that this latter site might mediate the anxiolytic action of BZD. It is thus possible that the selective action of BZD on KA-activation might be mediated by these receptors.

More than 10 years ago, Olds and Olds (1969) have made the observation that low doses of BZD reduced the unitary activity in the hippocampus but not in other brain regions of the unanesthetized unrestained rat. The powerful supressant action of BZD on spontaneous and evoked activity in the hippocampus has been confirmed by other groups of investigators (Chou and Wang, 1977; Jalfre et al., 1971). As speculative as it may be, it is tempting to imagine that an endoge- nous ligand for the "KA-sensitive" receptor contributes to the physiological activation of CA_1 pyramidal neurons and that its action is blocked by BZD. Whatis certain however is that the disclosure of an endogenous ligand for these "KA-sensitive" receptors would certainly activate many investigators interested in the pathophysiology of behavioral phenomena as diverse as epilepsy, Huntington's chorea and anxiety.

ACKNOWLEDGMENTS

We thank M. Lerebours and L. Ruel for their help in preparing the manuscript and D. Cyr and G. Filosi for the illustrations. Supported by a Canadian Medical Research Council grant and a scholarship from the Fonds de la Recherche en Santé du Québec to C. de M.

REFERENCES

Baimbridge, K.G. and J.J. Miller (1981). Neurosci. Abst. 7, 188.2
Baudry, M., and G. Lynch (1979). Eur. J. Pharmacol. 57, 283-285.
Ben-Ari, Y., E. Tremblay, O.P. Ottersen and B.S. Meldrum (1980). Brain Res. 191, 79-97.
Braestrup, C. and R.F. Squires (1978). Eur. J. Pharmacol. 48, 263-270.
Chou, D.T. and S.C. Wang (1977). Brain Res. 12, 427-440.
Coyle, J.T. and R. Schwarcz (1976). Nature 263, 244-246.
Darragh, A., M. Scully, R. Lambe and I. Brick (1981). Lancet ii, 8-10
De Bonnel, G. and C. de Montigny (1982). Submitted.
De Montigny, C. and J.P. Lund (1980). Neuroscience 5, 1621-1678.
De Montigny, C. and D. Tardif (1981). Life Science 29, 2103-2111.
Foster, A.C., E.E. Mena, D.T. Monaghan and C.W. Cotman (1981). Nature 289, 73-75.
Fuller, T.A. and J.W. Olney (1979). Neurosci. Abst. 5, 1880.
Haefely, W.E. (1978). In M.A. Lipton, A. Di Mascio and K.F. Killam (Eds.). Psychophamacology: A generation of Progress, Raven Press, New York, pp. 1359-1374.
Henke, H. and M. Cuenod (1979). Neurosci. Lett. 11, 341-345.
Hunkeler, W., H. Möhler, H., L. Pieri, P. Pole, E.P. Bonetti, R. Cumin, R. Schaffner and W. Haefely (1981). Nature 290, 514-516.
Jalfre, M., M.A. Monachon and W. Haefely (1971). Naunyn Schmiedeberg's Arch. Pharmacol. 270, 180-191.
Johnston, G.A.R. (1973). Biochem. Pharmacol. 22, 137-140.
Kandel, E.R. and A. Spencer (1961). J. Neurophysiol. 24, 243-259.
Kizer, J.S., C.B. Nemeroff and W.W. Youngblood (1978). Pharmacol. Rev. 29, 301-318.
Klepner, C.A., A.S. Lippa, D.I. Benson, M.C. Sano and B. Beer (1979). Pharmacol. Biochem. Behav. 11, 457-462.
London, E.D. and J.T. Coyle (1979). Molec. Pharmacol. 15, 492-505.
Mason, S.T., P.R. Sanberg and H.C. Fiberger (1978). Science 201, 352-355.
Möhler, H. and J.G. Richards (1981). Brit. J. Pharmacol. 74, 813P-814P.

Nadler, J.V. (1981). Life Sci. 29, 2031-2042.
Nadler, J.V. and G.J. Cuthbertson (1980). Brain Res. 195, 47-56.
Nadler, J.V., B.W. Perry, and C.W. Patman (1978). Nature 271, 276-277.
Olds, M.E. and J. Olds (1969). Int. J. Neuropharmacol. 8, 87-103.
Olney, J.W., O. Lan Ho and V. Rhee (1971). Exp. Brain Res. 14, 61-76.
Polc, P., J.-P. Laurent, R. Scherschlicht, and W. Haefely (1981). Naunyn-Schmiedeberg's Arch. Pharmacol. 316, 317-325.
Simon, J.R., J.F. Contrera and M.J. Kuhar (1976). J. Neurochem. 76, 141-147.
Tallman, J.F., S.M. Paul, P. Skolnick and D. Gallager (1980). Science 207, 274-281.
Volicer, L. and T.M. Biagioni (1982). J. Neurochem. 38, 591-593.
Williams, E.F., K.C. Rice, S.M. Paul and P. Skolnick (1980). J. Neurochem. 55, 591-5976.
Zaczek, R., M.F. Nelson and J.T. Coyle (1978). Eur. J. Pharmacol. 52, 323-327.

AN ANALYSIS OF BIOELECTRICAL PHENOMENA EVOKED BY MICROIONTOPHORETICALLY APPLIED EXCITOTOXIC AMINO-ACIDS IN THE FELINE SPINAL CORD

I. ENGBERG, J. A. FLATMAN, J. D. C. LAMBERT and AMY LINDSAY

Institute of Physiology, University of Aarhus, DK–8000 Aarhus C, Denmark

KEYWORDS

Excitotoxic amino-acids; motoneurones; membrane conductance; focal potential; extracellular potassium; extracellular space; barbiturates; calcium channels.

INTRODUCTION

Diacidic amino acids with the appropriate molecular configuration (Watkins, 1978) depolarize and excite most types of neurone. Most, if not all, of these agents applied topically in sufficient quantities will act as neurotoxins - irreversible damage ultimately occurs followed by neuronal death and necrosis. Thus, the term "excitotoxic" amino-acids has been coined by Olney (1978).

Neuronal death only occurs at sites where "receptors" for the amino-acids exist. Thus, most soma-dendritic areas are susceptible, while fibres and glia are often spared (Olney, 1978; Herndon and Coyle, 1978). These properties have resulted in the use of amino-acid induced lesions in neuroanatomical and behavioural studies for which the reader is referred to other chapters of this book. Kainic acid is the most widely used excitotoxin, but lesions have also been induced with a variety of other analogues - e.g. N-methyl-D-aspartate, Ibotenate and AMPA (Olney, 1978; Arnt, 1981).

During the past seven years we have investigated the physiological phenomena underlying responses to microiontophoretic application of a range of excitatory amino-acids in the feline lumbo-sacral grey matter. Our results disclose some of the mechanisms in the neurotoxic action of these analogues. The following items will be discussed:

1. Characteristics of the amino-acid evoked depolarization, changes in membrane conductance and firing of action potentials.

2. Interaction of barbiturates and calcium blockers with amino-acid responses.

3. Changes in the intra- and extracellular potentials during amino-acid action. The difference between these potentials gives the effective transmembrane potential of the neurone.

4. Spread of drug action following micro-iontophoretic application of various analogues.

5. Changes in extracellular K^+-activity and estimates of changes in the size of the extracellular volume during amino-acid action.

170

RESULTS AND DISCUSSION

It was originally thought that all excitatory amino-acid analogues interacted with a single common receptor (Curtis, Duggan, Johnston, Tebécis and Watkins, 1972). Excitation was assumed to be mediated by a ubiquitous mechanism involving an increase in the membrane permeability for Na^+ and K^+ and having a reversal potential of around -30 mV (see McLennan, 1975).

Subsequently, pharmacological support for at least three excitatory amino-acid receptors has accumulated (Watkins and Evans, 1981). We have shown that, in terms of response shape, repetitive firing and G_M changes, there are qualitative differences in motoneuronal responses to the excitatory analogues (Lambert, Flatman and Engberg, 1981).

The following results are based on intracellular recordings made from lumbo-sacral motoneurones in barbiturate anaesthetized cats (unless otherwise stated). Electrodes were usually of the concentric recording-iontophoretic type (Engberg, Flatman and Lambert, 1979a). G_M was measured by injecting constant current pulses through the central, screened intra-cellular electrode (Engberg et al, 1975). We are aware that this technique of measuring G_M may inherently cause the activation/inactivation of various ionic currents. Thus, the term apparent G_M is to be preferred. Further, to obtain a true value for the net G_M change, the G_M measured during agonist application should be compared with that pertaining at the same level of potential for a current depolarized membrane. Possible contributions of membrane "rectification" are thereby accounted for. Thus the action of an agent which is accompanied by a net decrease in G_M cannot be fully accounted for by postulating activation of electrotonically distant (dendritic) receptors and a passive depolarization of the soma.

Abbreviations

AMPA: α-amino-3-hydroxy-5-methyl-4-isoxazolepropionate, NMDA: N-methyl-D-aspartate, DLH: DL-homocysteate, G_M: Membrane conductance, aK^+: K^+-activity (extracellular), aCh^+: Choline$^+$-activity (extracellular), E_M: Intracellular potential, E_{TM}: Transmembrane potential, AP: Action potential, FP: Focal potential, ECV: Extracellular volume.

Characteristics of neuronal responses

Motoneurones in barbiturate anaesthetized cats are usually silent. Adequate applications of excitatory amino-acid analogues depolarize the neurone to a point where repetitive firing starts. The net G_M change during the initial depolarizing phase depends on the analogue used and varies from a marked decrease to a marked increase. The decrease in G_M seen with short applications of NMDA and ibotenate is shown in fig. 1. Analogues may be roughly grouped according to the apparent G_M change (Lambert et al, 1981), as shown in Table 1, below.

Net G_M change	Analogue
Decrease	NMDA, Ibotenate*, D-homocysteate
Little change	L-glutamate, L-aspartate, L-homocysteate
Increase	Kainate, AMPA.

*The first application of ibotenate is accompanied by a marked decrease in G_M. Thereafter follows a slowly developing, long-lasting inhibitory phase (see below).

The firing pattern evoked is also dependent on the analogue applied. In general, the greater the G_M decrease accompanying the initial depolarization, the more stable the repetitive firing and the lower the firing threshold (Lambert et al, 1981). Thus, NMDA and D-homocysteate could evoke repetitive firing lasting many minutes (Lambert et al, 1978; Engberg et al, 1978). Kainate and AMPA depolarizations were frequently silent. However, a short period of firing may be evoked with these agents during the rising phase of the depolarization.

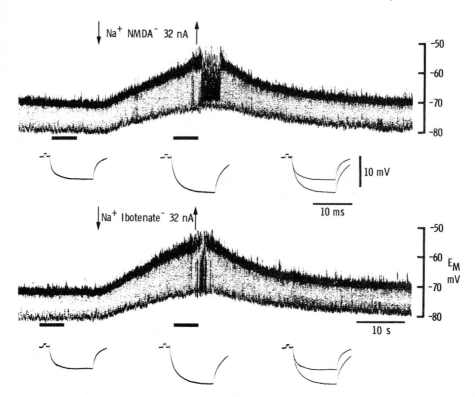

Fig. 1. NMDA and ibotenate depolarizations accompanied by a decrease in G_M. Both responses are from the same neurone in a barbiturate anaesthetized cat. (NB. This was the first application of ibotenate to this neurone.) The high fidelity membrane potential recording is modulated by transients evoked by -3 nA G_M measuring pulses. Fifty voltage transients were averaged and are shown beneath the heavy bars marking when they were taken and superimposed to the right. The two agonists (current balanced applications between the arrows) were approximately equipotent and both responses were accompanied by a decrease in G_M. G_M was measured just before the evoked firing (AHPs visible on trace).

The G_M decrease typical for NMDA and D-homocysteate is largest just before the repetitive firing starts - it is then obscured by the action potentials. When AP generation is blocked by local anaesthetics (Flatman, Lambert and Engberg, 1983) there is an enormous decrease in apparent G_M during the period previously obscured by firing. In sufficiently large and longlasting doses even these amino-acids cause a G_M increase after the initial phase of low G_M and firing. When the firing stops, G_M is very high, and the neurone becomes heavily depolarized, often with a sudden jump.

Similar changes of E_M and G_M, in response to aspartate or NMDA, have been seen in cultured murine spinal cord neurones (MacDonald, Porietis and Wojtowicz, 1982) and in neurones of feline somatosensory cortex (Flatman, Schwindt, Crill and Stafstrom, 1982). It appears that the bistable E_M behaviour and G_M changes can be partly explained by the opening of voltage-dependent conductance channels for Na^+ (and possibly other ions) by aspartate and NMDA. The operation of such channels produces a negative slope region on the I/V relation of the cell membrane.

Although we usually apply agonists for relatively short durations (a few minutes at most), it is relevant to report that we do not see evidence of desensitization. The depolarization is

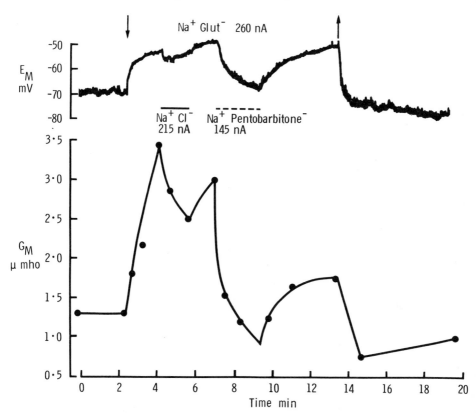

Fig. 2. The effect of iontophoretically applied pentobarbitone on the E_M and G_M response to glutamate in an anaemically decorticated cat after the anaesthesia had worn off. The initial phase of the glutamate depolarization was accompanied by a ca 2.5 times increase in G_M. A "worst case control" (Lambert and Flatman, 1981) application of NaCl was then made, during which the glutamate depolarization was decreased by about 3 mV with a concurrent fall in G_M. During the subsequent application of Na pentobarbitone the E_M and G_M fell much more - to near control levels. After pentobarbitone - but still during glutamate - the G_M remained markedly depressed despite the nearly complete recovery of E_M. (From Lambert and Flatman, 1981).

maintained throughout the application. The time course of the responses, however, varies with the analogues. A substance like glutamate, which is very quickly taken up and removed from the ECV, causes a fast on - fast off response. Even after large longlasting doses, the control situation is quickly reestablished. Kainate is the very opposite; with small doses its actions are slow in onset and last for some minutes or longer after the application. With large doses, kainate actions are irreversible. AMPA is about as potent as kainate, but the neurones recover more quickly - probably because AMPA can cross the blood-brain barrier (Krogsgaard-Larsen, Schulz, Mikkelsen and Hansen, 1981).

Barbiturate anaesthetics and calcium blockers

Using anaemically decorticated cats, we have investigated the interaction of barbiturate anaesthetics with excitatory amino-acid responses (Lambert et al, 1980a; Lambert and Flatman, 1981). Pentobarbitone or thiopentone were applied intravenously, or, directly onto the neurone under study by iontophoresis. Our two main findings were: a) The depolarizations to analogues which caused a marked decrease in G_M (e.g. DLH and NMDA) were reduced by the barbiturates. b) The slowly developing increase in G_M, which accompanies large, longlasting applications of L-glutamate, was markedly reduced - G_M often returning to levels close to the pre-glutamate value (fig. 2).

Both these observations infer that barbiturate anaesthetics will afford some protection against the excitotoxic action of the excitatory amino-acids (cf. Di Chiara, Morelli, Imperato, Faa, Fossarello and Porceddu, 1981). Furthermore, when barbiturates are present a potent, inhibitory phase develops after ibotenate applications (Lambert et al, 1980b). The inhibition is probably mediated by the GABA-analogue muscimol, which is derived from decarboxylation of ibotenate (Curtis, Lodge and McLennan, 1979). This inhibitory wave - during which responses to other excitatory analogues are reduced - would also be expected to protect against the neurotoxic action of ibotenate. The inhibition was not seen during and following application of methyl-ibotenate which is not degraded to muscimol in the CNS (Lambert et al., in preparation).

Padgen and Smith (1981) have shown that a Ca^{++} influx accompanies all excitatory amino-acid responses in the frog spinal cord (the size of the Ca^{++} current probably depending upon which receptor is activated). This correlates with studies in the sensorimotor cortex, where a dramatic fall in extracelullar Ca^{++} is seen during amino-acid action (Heinemann and Pumain, 1981). We have long been aware that an inwardly directed Ca^{++} current may be involved in the genesis of amino-acid responses which are accompanied by an apparent decrease in G_M. Experiments where the interaction of Ca^{++} antagonists with DLH responses was tested gave inconclusive results (Engberg et al, 1979b). D600 only slightly depressed DLH responses. Co^{++} was more reliable in depressing the DLH depolarization (fig. 3), but increases were also seen, especially when Co^{++} itself caused a hyperpolarization. More disconcertingly, Ca^{++} itself often caused small decreases (fig. 3). The lack of consistency in our results may be correlated with the fact that only about 40% of motoneurones show a net inward current on depolarization (Schwindt and Crill, 1980). This current is very susceptible to neurone damage and is probably carried by Ca^{++} ions.

We have recently noted that when the "classical" voltage-dependent Na^+ and K^+ conductances are inhibited by iontophoretically applied lignocaine, NMDA evokes rhythmic oscillations of E_M (Flatman et al, 1982). This was most clearly seen in motoneurones of the posterior tibial nerve. The oscillations consisted of a prepotential followed by a spike of low amplitude (< 30 mV) and long duration (ca 50 ms) which resembled Ca^{++}-dependent spikes in other neurones. Similar Ca^{++}-dependent spikes have been demonstrated in neurones of the cat somatosensory cortex during application of NMDA (Flatman et al, 1982 and in preparation).

Further evidence supporting the possible participation of an increased P_{Ca} in the action of excitatory amino acids on spinal cord neurones has been forwarded by Sonnhof and Bührle (1980) and by Padgen and Smith (1981), both groups studying the action of glutamate on the isolated, spinal cord of frog. However, Shapovalov, Shiriaev and Velumian (1978) have shown that the action of glutamate on the same preparation is unaltered when the preparation is bathed in Ca-free medium.

Intra- and extracellular potentials

It has long been appreciated that the potential of the extracellular environment may alter under certain circumstances - e.g. spreading depression (Leão, 1947), hypoxia (van Harreveld and Bierstecker, 1964), following ortho- and antidromic activation (Hubbard, Llinás and Quastel, 1969) and during iontophoretic drug application (McCance and Phillis, 1968; Krnjević, 1971). The necessity of subtracting the extra- from the intracellularly recorded events in order to obtain the effective neuronal transmembrane potential has long been realized for e.g. synaptic events. This procedure has yet to win wide acceptance for events evoked by drug addition (but see Krnjević and Schwartz, 1967). It is, however, crucial when, for example, reversal potentials are being measured. Ignoring the fact that the extracelullar environment may be moving negatively by tens of mV can obviously lead to erroneous conclusions.

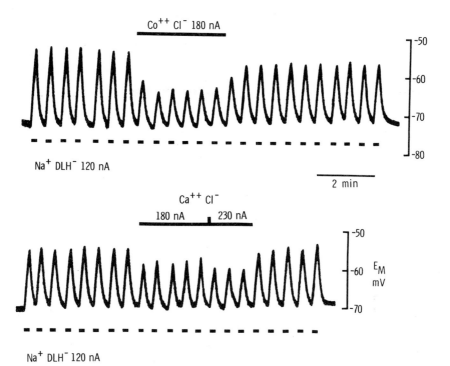

Fig. 3. The interaction of Co++ and Ca++ ions with DLH depolarizations. The slow, low fidelity E_M recording is modulated by responses to regular current balanced applications of DLH. Upper trace: during a current balanced application of Co++Cl-, DLH responses are reduced to ca 45% of control. Recovery after Co++ was not complete (to ca 75% of control). This result was fairly typical for neurones with high (> -70 mV) membrane potentials. Lower trace: later during the same impalement DLH responses were also reduced during a current balanced application of Ca++ Cl- (to ca. 60% of control during 230 nA).

The results so far described were obtained with the "classical" technique of referring the potential recorded from an intracellular electrode to a distant reference electrode (a large Ag/AgCl electrode buried in the musculature). In 1978 we became aware that the extracellular potential in the grey matter became negative during iontophoretic application of amino-acids (Focal Potential (FP), Flatman and Lambert, 1979). The FPs could have considerable size (up to -50 mV) and range. That these FPs are manifestations of neuronal responses to the excitatory analogues, and not technical artifacts has been established (Flatman and Lambert, 1979).

Thus during iontophoretic application of excitatory amino-acids two simultaneous potential changes are occurring - the intracellular electrode becomes less negative with respect to the distant indifferent electrode, while the extracellular environment becomes more negative. Transmembrane potential (E_{TM}) is obtained by electronically subtracting the potential recorded just extracellularly from one of the barrels of the iontophoretic electrode from that recorded intracellularly. (These experiments are technically difficult since recording in the vicinity of current passing iontophoretic barrels is often complicated by "coupling" artifacts, despite attempts to obtain accurately current-balanced iontophoretic ejections). An experiment of this type is shown in fig. 4.

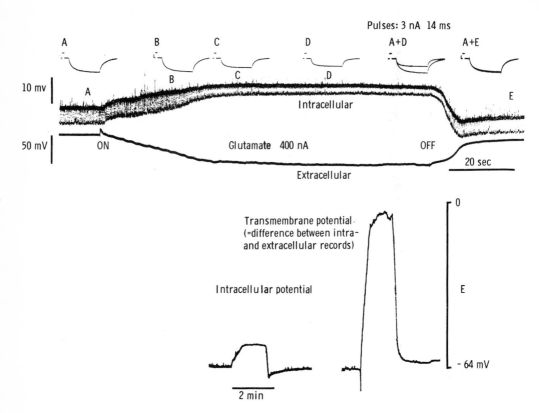

Fig. 4. Upper part: Simultaneous intra- and just extracellular recording of potential changes evoked by glutamate. The intracellular trace is modulated by G_M measuring pulses, examples of which are shown above (A-E; the letters also indicate when these were recorded). Lower part: The same intracellular potential change as shown above, but on a slow time scale, compared to E_{TM} obtained via a differential amplifier.

Our experiments with measurements of E_{TM} have revealed that all excitatory analogues - irrespective of their grouping in Table 1 - can cause complete depolarization with E_{TM} values close to 0mV. This transition from resting membrane potential to complete depolarization was relatively smooth for kainate and AMPA. The responses to these agents are similar in that the depolarizing phase is slow and accompanied by a net increase in G_M with little, if any, firing (see above and Lambert, Hansen, Engberg and Flatman, 1982). When a maximum response has been attained, the E_M is usually between -30 and -50 mV, while E_{TM} shows a complete depolarization (fig. 5). The membrane is then essentially short circuited.

For the analogues which evoke stable RF (e.g. NMDA and DLH) E_M remains relatively stable during firing, while the FP continues to increase. If the agonist dose is sufficient, the neurone suddenly stops firing, and this is accompanied by a sudden depolarizing jump in the E_M record. The G_M is then very high, also with these analogues.

Spread of drug action

The extent to which an E_{TM} measurement applies for a whole motoneurone (whose dendritic tree may have a radius > 1 mm) is debateable. Clearly the E_{TM} for an agent whose effects (in terms of FP) can be detected at a great distance (e.g. kainate, NMDA) will be more or

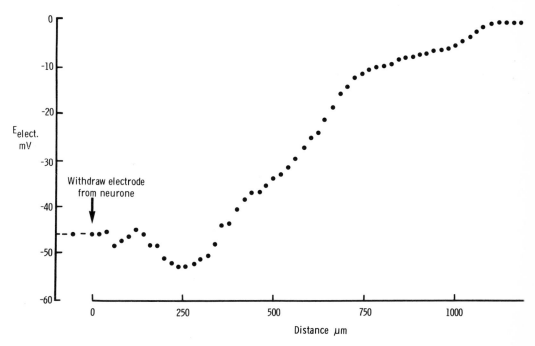

Fig. 5. The spread of focal potential in the grey matter following a heavy iontophoretic application of kainate (11 min at 60 nA). The Na+ kainate application was terminated shortly before the start of this figure. The intracellular electrode was then withdrawn in 20 §m steps. The potential recorded by the electrode (E_{elect}) is plotted as a function of distance. On withdrawing the electrode from the neurone there was no positive jump indicating that E_{TM} = 0 mV and E_M = FP = -46 mV. A region of even greater negativity (max. -53 mV) was seen 0.25 mm away from the impalement site. Thereafter, potential declined with distance. Negativity could be detected a little more than 1 mm away from the impaled motoneurone.

less representative for the whole neurone. For other agents where the FP falls steeply with distance (e.g. L-glutamate) the E_{TM} value is likely to be correct for the part of the membrane onto which the agonist is applied, but will certainly not pertain for the distal dendrites.

The range of a kainate evoked FP is shown in fig. 5. On withdrawing the intracellular electrode, the intra- and extracellular potentials (with respect to a distant indifferent electrode) were identical (i.e. E_M = FP = about 45 mV; E_{TM} = about 0 mV). The negativity could still be detected > 1 mm from the site of impalement.

Where excitotoxic amino-acids are used to produce lesions, simply monitoring the extracellular potential will give an indication of the spread from the lesion site.

Tissue resistance, aK+ and ECV

We have observed three phenomena accompanying the FP: a) Increase in tissue resistivity, b) Increase in extracellular K+-activity and c) Decrease in extracellular volume.

a) Tissue resistance, as measured by voltage transients evoked by the injection of current pulses through the extracellular FP recording electrode, is increased during the amino-acid action as illustrated in fig. 6. When measured with a microelectrode having a tip resistance

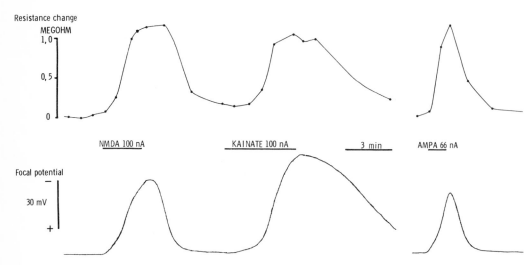

Fig. 6. Examples of tissue resistance changes and FPs caused by iontophoresis of NMDA, kainate and AMPA. The upper curves are plotted from measurements of averaged short trains of resistance measuring pulses recorded simultaneously with the FPs shown below. The microelectrode had a tip resistance of 5 megohms at the start of the recording. There is a short interval in the recording after the kainate response.

of 5 megohms before drug application, an increase of about 1 megohm is typical with FPs of about -50 mV. The resistance rise follows the time course of the FP, while the recovery appears to be somewhat slower. Since no resistance change is detected in the white matter or in the CSF, we conclude that the resistance increase is a consequence of changes in tissue resistivity rather than an alteration of electrode properties. We have no detailed information on the topographical relationship between the resistivity change and the FP. However, measurements with larger tipped NaCl filled microelectrodes (1 megohm instead of 5 megohms) show a much smaller increase in resistance, which indicates that some of the resistance change is located just outside the electrode tip.

b) The extracellular aK^+, close to the site of drug application, was measured with a K^+-sensitive microelectrode (Corning resin n:o 477317) inserted in the central canal of the multibarrelled iontophoresis unit. The tip separation was kept at 5-10 §m. One of the "drug" barrels containing NaCl was used to record the FP and thus also served as potential reference for the ionsensitive electrode. As illustrated in fig. 7, there is a substantial increase in aK^+ when kainate is applied. Although the responses to repetitive K^+-ejections from one of the drug barrels are superimposed on the curves, it is clear that the time course of the baseline aK^+-rise mirrors that of the FP very closely. The small dose of kainate was chosen to allow demonstration of the simultaneous decay of FP and aK^+. Glutamate and NMDA also increase aK^+ with a time course parallel to that of the FP (cf. fig. 8 for NMDA).

The similarity of the two curves is, indeed, striking. In fact, when the potential of a good K^+ electrode was recorded with reference to a distant ground (instead of the local reference electrode), the curve was nearly flat; i.e. the FP and K^+-signal were of equal size. This, of course invites the idea that the FP merely represents a K^+-diffusion potential in the ECV. Although this may be true for areas with acute heavy cell damage, it cannot be the entire explanation in the present situation where living neurone processes and glial structures extend from the region of drug action into its surroundings.

c) The responses to the K^+-pulses also change in relation to the FP. The pulses were originally used in order to check the electrode performance during the experiment, but the

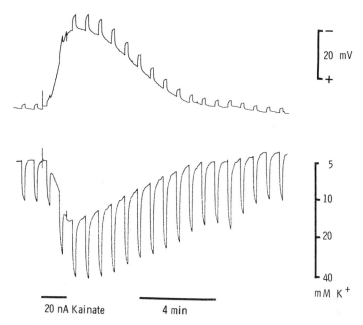

Fig. 7. Extracellular aK+ and FP responses to a kainate ejection. The upper (FP) and the lower (aK+) traces are both modulated by responses to short ejections of K+ from another barrel of the iontophoresis electrode.

increase in their responses during kainate action gave them another role. Together with the increase in tissue resistivity they indicate a decrease in ECV. This indication we followed with the use of choline ions (Ch+) to monitor changes in ECV. Neuronal membranes have a very low permeability to Ch+-ions. The use of Ch+ in ECV measurements was suggested by Hansen and Olsen 1980, because aCh+ can easily be measured with ionsensitive electrodes. The K+-electrodes used in their and our work are very sensitive to tetralkylammonium ions (Neher and Lux, 1973). Typical calibration curves for K+ and Ch+ from the present experiments show that the electrodes are about 100 times more sensitive to Ch+ than to K+.

The responses to repetitive ejection of short Ch+-pulses from one of the drug barrels increased markedly upon kainate application (fig. 8). The sizes of the Ch+-responses before and during kainate action cannot be directly compared in the figure, since the latter are superimposed on the K+-response. A calculation based on the calibration curves for the electrode and taking the K+-response into account, gives a peak aCh+ during the maximal kainate response about nine times as high as the control peak. This means that the volume in which Ch+ is distributed - mainly the ECV - is enormously reduced. Similar to the change in tissue resistance, the reduction of ECV seems to be slightly more longlasting than the FP. This is not surprising since the resistance change is probably a reflexion of the volume change (cf. Freygang and Landau, 1955).

The extracellular rise in aK+ may be an important factor in the amino-acid action (cf. Sonnhof and Bührle, 1980). As shown in the cortex by Dietzel, Heinemann, Hofmeier and Lux (1982a) such a rise - whether due to local epileptiform discharges, iontophoresis of K+ or destruction of cells - is followed by a decrease of the ECV concomitant with a negative field potential. These authors present a model, in which a local extracellular aK+ elevation depolarizes adjacent glial membranes (causing an inward K+-flow). Due to the extension of the glial structures (by continuity or coupling) the intracellular depolarization spreads to peripheral areas with normal aK+, where K+ leaves the glia. This creates a current loop; extracellularly the current is carried back to the central area by Na+ and Cl-. The different

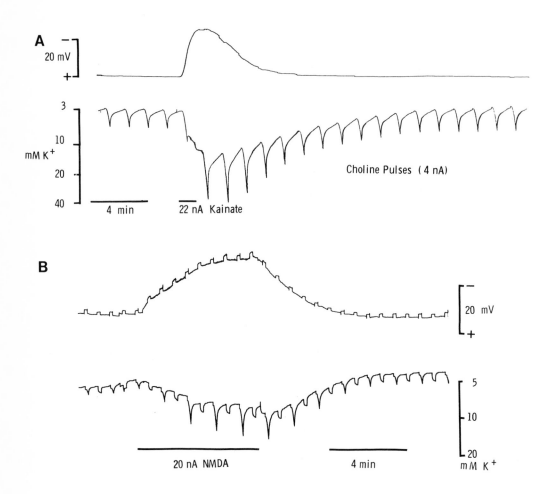

Fig. 8. Similar records to those of fig. 7 obtained during kainate (A) and NMDA (B) actions. The lower trace in A is modulated by responses to short Ch+ ejections, that in B by both Ch+ and K+ ejections (the ionsensitive electrode used was about 100 times more sensitive to Ch+ than to K+, the calibration shown is only for the latter ion). Note the increase in the Ch+ responses indicating a vast reduction in ECV, which is slightly more longlasting than the FP.

transport numbers of the current carrying ions in the different compartments, will cause osmotic changes leading to the reduction in ECV. A judgement of the applicability of this model to the situation in the spinal cord has to await further studies of the ionic changes, which occur with iontophoresis of the different analogues. However, glutamate with its shortlasting local action may give an excitation of neurones that creates a situation similar to that of the stimulus-induced epileptiform discharges. Low doses of NMDA, which give intense repetitive firing without shortcircuiting the neurones, may do this even more readily. On the other hand, with the enormous and longlasting changes that can be evoked by kainate, there is far more K+ liberated and much larger ECV reduction than during the epileptic seizures. These findings are more compatible with what is seen during spreading depression and ischemia, when metabolic changes and gross movement of NaCl into cells are also involved (cf. Nicholson and Kraig, 1981, Hansen and Olsen, 1980, and the discussion by Dietzel et al, 1982b).

GENERAL DISCUSSION

The in vivo nervous system, consisting of tightly packed neuronal elements in a three dimensional matrix, is not the ideal preparation in which to investigate the discrete mechanisms by which excitatory amino-acids evoke depolarizations. There are technical and interpretative problems. Technical difficulties include: a) The impaled neurone cannot be visualized. The exact site of impalement in a geometrically complex structure with uneven receptor distribution is unknown (though electrophysiological characteristics of the AP sometimes may permit an educated guess). b) Most agents have to be applied by iontophoresis with its inherent problems. c) It is difficult to alter the ionic environment in a quantified manner when attempting to investigate the ionic dependency of the response.

The interpretative problems are, perhaps, more important and not so well appreciated. In an earlier study (Engberg et al, 1979a) we investigated the potential and ionic dependency of the DLH evoked depolarization. The depolarization decreased in size on increasing aK_o and appeared to have a null potential in the vicinity of where E_K would be expected to lie. We tentatively concluded that a decrease in conductance of potential dependent K^+ channels was (at least in part) responsible for the depolarization. At that time, we were unaware of the significance of FPs, which are also generated by neighbouring neurones within range of the agonist application. Thus, a more accurate assessment of the reversal potential is probably made by examining the E_{TM} record. At the reversal level, i.e. when the E_{TM} does not change during agonist application, the E_M record would be negative going and exactly duplicate the FP record. In fact, we never managed convincingly to reverse the polarity of the DLH response with hyperpolarizing current injections (fig. 15, Engberg et al, 1979a). An explanation of these results may be that DLH opens or closes voltage-dependent conductance channels which are inoperable at very high membrane potentials.

Because the causal and secondary effects of excitatory amino-acid application are so inextricably linked it is dubious as to whether any significance can be attributed to the demonstration of a "reversal potential" for an amino-acid evoked depolarization - especially when long, large doses are used. All the excitotoxic amino-acids will, in sufficient doses, cause a complete depolarization (E_{TM}) of the membrane (see RESULTS) with a very high G_M. This zero potential can then be assumed to be the "reversal potential", but the cells are swollen, and the ionic gradients across the membrane bear no resemblance to those at rest. At this point one is investigating the final excitotoxic effect of the amino-acid rather than the mechanism producing the depolarization. These cautionary notes should be borne in mind when attempts are made to compare $E_{putative\ transmitter}$ with $E_{synaptic\ event}$.

The problems of investigating "reversal potentials" in vivo are not even resolved by using very small doses of agonists. In fig. 8 it can be seen that aK^+ increases significantly even during the early part of the response to a very modest dose of NMDA, at a time when G_M is known to be very much reduced.

Although the intact nervous system is inappropriate for studying the primary events underlying amino-acid induced excitation, it is obvious that the neurotoxic action is best studied in the intact nervous system. Changes in the ionic gradients, extracellular composition and osmolarity are clearly involved in the toxic action. Thus topical applications of excitotoxic amino-acids in sufficient doses will lead to a complete depolarization accompanied by a complete break-down of the membrane resistance. The normal ionic regulatory mechanisms will be unable to cope. If this situation is allowed to continue for any length of time, neuronal death will result. This aciton will be independent of which receptor (Watkins and Evans, 1981) is initially activated.

Cultured mammalian neurones represent a preparation where the membrane is in intimate contact with the bathing medium (Ransom, Neale, Henkart, Bullock and Nelson, 1977) and thus are suitable for fundamental mechanistic studies. Responses of cultured spinal cord neurones to excitatory amino-acid analogues often bear little qualitative resemblance to those seen in the in vivo spinal cord (Nielsen and Lambert, 1981). For example, L-glutamate is a very potent excitor of cultured neurones - possibly because the application site is not surrounded by neuronal elements which are very efficient in removing the amino-acid. Kainate is relatively impotent on cultured neurones, and responses to this agent recover rapidly and completely, which is in stark contrast to its effects in the ventral horn grey matter, where it accumulates. When using an electrode placed just outside a cultured neurone, we have not been able to detect significant shifts of the extracellular potential (Lambert, unpublished observations). In this preparation K^+ will not accumulate in the extracellular space and will therefore not contribute to the depolarization.

Nevertheless, MacDonald et al. (1982) have shown that cultured spinal cord neurones can respond to excitatory amino acids in a manner analogous to that seen in cat spinal motoneurones or neocortical neurones and have been able to identify the conductance changes underlying, for example, the action of aspartate.

CONCLUDING REMARKS

We are still not able to identify the ionic mechanisms underlying the action of even an excitatory amino acid like NMDA which presumably acts mostly at one class of receptor (Watkins and Evans, 1981). The response to NMDA of some cultured spinal cord neurones and neocortical neurones in vitro is similar to motoneuronal responses (see earlier). From our results and these in vitro experiments it would appear that the action of excitatory amino acids is highly complex, involving voltage-sensitive channels for Na^+ and an increase in Ca^{++} influx. Around resting E_M a decrease in G_K is probably also important. Obviously, as depolarization develops, many voltage-dependent conductances can be affected, thus, for example, increasing K^+ efflux.

It is unfortunate that the experimental manipulations needed to identify the amino-acid-operated ionophores require Draconian modification of the extracellular ionic composition and the addition of powerful pharmacological agents. It is always difficult to exclude the possibility that these manipulations radically alter the normal pattern of membrane response to excitatory amino acids.

ACKNOWLEDGEMENTS

The authors wish to thank Marianne Stürup-Johansen, Susanne Andersen, Finn Marquard and Robert Langley for technical assistance. Karen Damgaard Ottesen is greatfully acknowledged for preparing a Camera-Ready typescript. This work was supported by the Danish Medical Research Council.

REFERENCES

Arnt, J. (1981). Neurosci. Lett. 23, 337-342.
Curtis, D.R., A.W. Duggan, D. Felix, G.A.R. Johnston, A.K. Tebecis and J.C. Watkins (1972). Brain Res. 41, 283-301.
Curtis, D.R., D. Lodge and H. McLennan (1979). J. Physiol. 291, 19-28.
Di Chiara, G., M. Morelli, A. Imperato, G. Faa, M. Fossarello and M.L. Porceddu (1981). In: Glutamate as a Neurotransmitter, G. Di Chiara and G. L. Gessa (eds), Raven Press, New York, 355-373.
Dietzel, I., U. Heinemann, G. Hofmeier and H.D. Lux (1982a). In: Physiology and Pharmacology of Epileptopgenic Phenomena, M.R. Klee et al. (eds), Raven Press, New York.
Dietzel, I., U. Heinemann, G. Hofmeier and H.D. Lux (1982b). Exp. Brain Res. 46, 73-84.
Engberg, I., J.A. Flatman and J.D.C. Lambert (1975). Br. J. Pharm. 55, 312-313P.
Engberg, I., J.A. Flatman and J.D.C. Lambert (1978). Br. J. Pharm. 64, 384-385P.
Engberg, I., J.A. Flatman and J.D.C. Lambert (1979a). J. Physiol. 288, 227-261.
Engberg, I., J.A. Flatman and J.D.C. Lambert (1979b). J. Physiol. 296, 96-97P.
Flatman, J.A., I. Engberg and J.D.C. Lambert (1982). Neuroscience 7, S71.
Flatman, J.A. and J.D.C. Lambert (1979). J. Neurosci. Meth. 1, 205-218.
Flatman, J.A., J.D.C. Lambert and I. Engberg (1983). In preparation.

Flatman, J.A., P.C. Schwindt, W.E. Crill and C.E. Stafstrom (1982). Soc. Neurosci.Abstr.8, in press.
Freygang, W.H. Jr. and W.M. Landau (1955). J. Cell. Physiol. 45, 377-392.
Hansen, A.J. and C.E. Olsen (1980). Acta Physiol. Scand. 108, 355-365.
Harreveld, A. van and P.A. Bierstecker (1964). Amer. J. Physiol. 206, 8-13.
Heinemann, U. and R. Pumain (1981). Neurosci. Lett. 21, 87-91.
Herndon, R.M. and J.T. Coyle (1978). In: Kainic Acid as a Tool in Neurobiology, E.G. McGeer, J.W. Olney and P.L. McGeer (eds), 189-200.
Hubbard, J.I., R. Llinas and D.M.J. Quastel (1969). Electrophysiological Analysis of Synaptic Transmission. Monographs of the Physiological Society, Number 19. Edward Arnold, London.
Krnjevic, K. (1971). In: Methods of Neurochemistry, Vol. 1, R. Fried (ed.), Marcel Dekker Inc. New York, 129-172.
Krnjevic, K. and S. Schwartz (1967). Exp. Brain Res. 3, 306-319.
Krogsgaard-Larsen, P., B. Schultz, H. Mikkelsen and J.J. Hansen (1981). Abstract of presentation of 181st ABS National Meeting Atlanta, Georgia.
Lambert, J.D.C. and J.A. Flatman (1981). Neuropharmacology 20, 227-240.
Lambert, J.D.C., J.A. Flatman and I. Engberg (1978). In: Iontophoresis and Transmitter Mechanisms in the Mammalian Central Nervous System, R.W. Ryall and J.S. Kelly (eds), Elsevier/North-Holland Biomedical Press, 375-377.
Lambert, J.D.C., J.A. Flatman and I. Engberg (1980a). Acta Physiol. Scand. 108, 14A.
Lambert, J.D.C., J.A. Flatman and I. Engberg (1980b). Neurosci. Lett., Suppl. 5, S81.
Lambert, J.D.C., J.A. Flatman and I. Engberg (1981). In: Glutamate as a Neurotransmitter, G. Di Chiara and G. L. Gessa (eds), Raven Press, New York, 205-216.
Lambert, J.D.C., J.J. Hansen, I. Engberg and J.A. Flatman (1982). Neuroscience 7, S126.
Leao, A.A.P. (1947), J. Neurophysiol. 10, 409.
MacDonald, J.F., A.V. Porietis and J.M. Wojtowicz (1982). Brain Res. 237, 248-253.
MacDonald, J.F. and J.M. Wojtowicz (1982). Can. J. Physiol. Pharmacol. 60, 282-296.
McCance, I. and J.W. Phillis (1968). Int. J. Neuropharmacol. 7, 447-462.
McLennan, H. (1975). In: Handbook of Psychopharmacology, Vol. 4, L.L. Iversen, S.D. Iversen and S.H. Snyder (eds), Plenum Press, New York, 211-228.
Neher, E. and H.D. Lux (1973). J. Gen. Physiol. 61, 385-399.
Nicholson, C. and Kraig, R.P. (1981). In: The Application of Ion Sensitive Microelectrodes, T. Zeuthen (ed.), Elsevier/North Holland Biomedical Press.
Nielsen, F.B. and J.D.C. Lambert (1981). Neurosci. Lett. Suppl. 7, S352.
Olney, J.W. (1978). In: Kainic Acid as a Tool in Neurobiology, E.G. McGeer, J.W. Olney and P.L. McGeer (eds), Raven Press, New York, 95-121.
Padjen, A.L. and P.A. Smith (1981). In: Amino Acid Neurotransmitters, F.V. DeFeudis and P. Mandel (eds), Raven Press, New York, 271-279.
Ransom, B.R., E. Neale, M. Henkart, P.N. Bullock and P.G. Nelson (1977). J. Neurophysiol. 40, 1132-1150.
Schwindt, P. and W. Crill (1980). J. Neurophysiol. 43, 1700-1724.
Shapovalov, A.I., B.I. Shiriaev and A.A. Velumian (1978). J. Physiol. 279, 437-455.
Sonnhof, U. and Ch. Ph. Bührle (1980). Pflügers Arch. 388, 101-109.
Watkins, J.C. (1978). In: Kainic Acid as a Tool in Neurobiology, E.G. McGeer, J.W. Olney and P.L. McGeer (eds), Raven Press, New York, 37-69.
Watkins, J.C. and R.H. Evans (1981). Ann. Rev. Pharmacol. Toxicol. 21, 165-204.

THE ROLE OF SEIZURES IN KAINIC ACID INDUCED BRAIN DAMAGE

Y. BEN-ARI

Lab. Physiol. Nerv., C.N.R.S. 91190–Gif-sur-Yvette, France

ABSTRACT

Focal injection of kainic acid in a number of brain structures produces in addition to the damage at the site of injection, pathological alterations in "distant" structures in particular in the hippocampal formation and other limbic structures. There is now good evidence that the in adequate experimental conditions the distant damage is largely due to the spread of paroxysmal discharge and not to a direct action of the toxin (by diffusion). The usefulness of KA to study the relationship between epilepsy and brain pathology is reviewed and the possible causes of the particular vulnerability of the ammon's horn to epilepsy is discussed.

KEYWORDS

Kainic acid induced limbic seizures ; ammon's horn sclerosis ; local and distant brain damage ; lability of GABAergic inhibition - intracellular Ca^{++}.

INTRODUCTION

One of the most consistent effects of systemic, intracerebroventricular or local injections of kainic acid (KA) in a number of brain structures is to elicit recurrent motor seizures having a typical limbic aetiology and subsequent pathological alterations in the brain which involve the hippocampal formation, amygdala and other limbic or closely related structures (Ben-Ari et al., 1981 ; Nadler, 1981 ; Coyle et al., 1981). The gradient of vulnerability is of particular interest since it is reminiscent of that seen in chronic epileptics (ibid).
A few years ago, we provided direct evidence that following intra-amygdaloid injections of KA in freely moving rats, epileptiform activity was first generated at the site of injection and rapidly propagated to the ipsilateral ammon's horn (Ben-Ari et al., 1979a). Since administration of an anticonvulsant blocked the epileptiform activity in the hippocampus as well as the subsequent damage and not that seen at the site of injection we suggested (Ben-Ari et al., 1979b) that the damage inflicted upon the brain by focal KA has a two-fold aetiology : direct toxic action of KA at the site of injection and "distant" brain damage produced by the spread of seizure activity (and not by a direct action of KA by diffusion). This hypothesis has received further support more recently and evidence has been obtained which further stress the important role played by seizure activity in mediating the limbic brain damage in other experimental situations (see below).

In the present report, the relationship between epilepsy and brain damage
produced by KA is reviewed.

Systemic administration of KA

Clinical effects : The time course of the clinical patterns following
systemic administration of KA is of particular interest. In adult, freely moving
animals, following i.p. (Ben-Ari et al., 1981) or i.v. (Lothmans and Collins,
1981) administration, even when high (subsequently lethal) doses are given, the
drug has relatively little motor effects during the first 15-20 minutes, wet-
shakes start at this time, reach a peak after 40 minutes before subsiding when
the limbic motor seizures start. The motor signs which characterize the limbic
motor seizures (LMS) are similar to those seen after repeated electrical stimulation of the amygdala or other limbic structures (i.e. Goddard et al., 1969 ;
Racine, 1972). They include sniffing, masticatory movements, head nodding,
rearing and forepaw tremor, rearing and loss of postural control. Since some of
these symptoms and their organization are remarkably similar to those described
earlier during amygdaloid "kindling" (in Racine, 1972) ; we have used the same
five stages terminology. Like direct intracerebral injections, systemic KA never
produces tonico-clinic generalized convulsions (such as these induced by pentetrazole or bicuculline (see below). Recurrent LMS and status epilepticus are
manifested for several hours, these can be readily blocked by diazepam (Fuller
and Olney, 1979 ; Ben-Ari et al., 1980b).

Electrographic effects : Cortical and deep recordings have consistently revealed that the epileptiform events start (10-20 minutes after i.p. or i.v.
injections i.e. Ben-Ari et al., 1981 ; Lothmans and Collins, 1981) in the
temporal hippocampal formation and in particular in the entorhinal and subicular
cortices. Paroxysmal activity rapidly propagates to the rest of the hippocampal
formation in a caudato-rostral direction before invading the lateral septum and
other limbic structures. Initially there is little or no paroxysmal events in
the cortical mantle. Therefore the onset and spread of epileptiform events
implies a central role to the limbic system, as also suggested by the nature of
the clinical events.

Metabolic alterations : Using the 2-deoxyglucose technique (i.e.
Sokoloff, 1978), a remarkable parallelism between the electrographic and
clinical data and the subsequent metabolic changes has been demonstrated
(Ben-Ari et al., 1981 ; Lothmans and Collins, 1981). The increase in glucose
consumption starts exclusively in the caudal hippocampal formation (fig. 1) ;
by administriving lower doses of KA or by reducing the severity of the seizure
with diazepam (Ibid) it can be shown that the caudal regio-inferior-entorhinal
and subicular cortices are probably the most susceptible structures. At longer
delays the rise in metabolism involves the lateral septum and at still longer
delays 1 h or more,when the LMS are manifested,the rise in radioactive material
is seen to involve a large number of structures which are part of or strongly
interconnected with the limbic system, such as the medial thalamic structures
and associated rostral limbic frontal cortex, the amygdaloid complex and closely
related areas of the pyriform lobe and ventral putamen (i.e. fig. 2). Following
2-3 days, again in keeping with the electrographic events, high levels of metabolism remain restricted to the amygdala (Ben-Ari et al., 1981).

*Figure 1 : Alterations in local glucose consumption following
systemic KA administration. Case D 53, 55 minutes after KA, the animal had not
displayed any limbic motor seizure. Note in the frontal sections the increase
labeling in the hippocampal formation and lateral septum. Also note that the
labeling in the amygdala is not increased at this stage.*

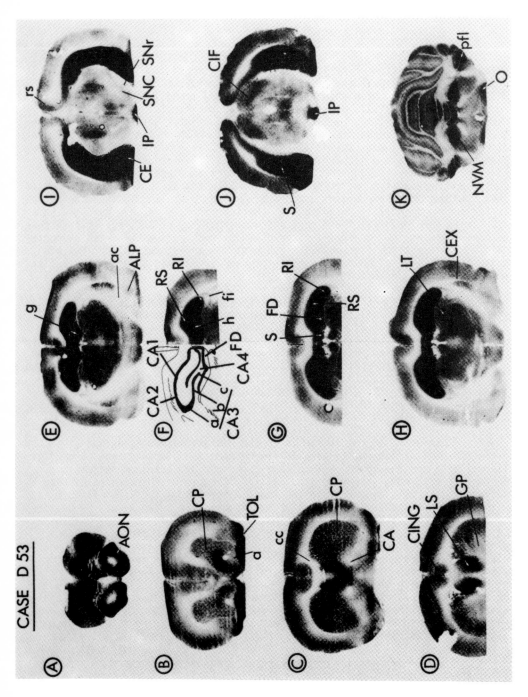

fig. 1

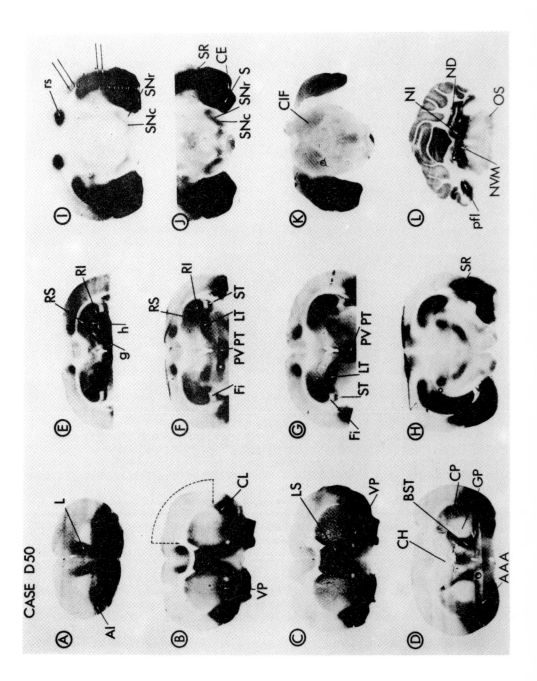

fig.2

Interestingly, there is a concomittant decrease in regional metabolism in the neocortex and several deep (non-limbic) structures (i.e. fig. 2) ; the metabolic maps are therefore almost opposite to those seen after bicuculline or pentetrazole (rise in neocortex, cerebellum, etc ... and fall in hippocampus and other limbic structures, Ben-Ari et al., 1981).

    Pathological sequelae : With a few exception, there is also a remarkable parallelism between the maps of pathological sequelae and the regions of increased metabolism (Ben-Ari et al., 1981, also see Schwob et al., 1980). With the Fink-Heimer stain, argyrophylic neurons are consistently encountered in the hippocampal formation in particular in the CA3-CA4 region, entorhinal cortex, claustrum amygdala, lateral septum, etc ... This striking correlation strongly suggest that the development of cell damage in limbic structures is intimately related to the excessive increase in neuronal activity and metabolism (see below).

General comments about the systemic KA model of temporal lobe epilepsy

It is clear that limbic structures are preferentially involved in the sequelae induced by systemic injections of KA. Since a) spontaneous recurrent LMS are readily observed at long term (1-3 months, Tremblay and Ben-Ari, unpublished observations) , b) the pathological alterations are reminiscent of ammon's horn sclerosis in man ;systemic KA provides a useful tool to induce temporal lobe epilepsy in particular since the temporal pattern of events enables to study in good conditions the spread of epileptiform of activity in the brain and its pathological sequelae. In this model, the entorhinal-subicular cortices are activated first by KA, the epileptiform activity then rapidly spreads along well described anatomical routes to involve the fascia-dentata, ammon's horn and other limbic structures and plays an important role in the damage seen subsequently (see below). It is important to emphasize that in keeping with anatomical observations lesion experiments or studies made with focal injections of KA (see below), the motor seizures are manifested only when the limbic circuitry and most particularly the amygdaloid complex is fully activated. There is as a matter of fact some evidence that during the 1 h delay between KA administration and the occurence of the first limbic motor seizures there is more sort of "kindling" of this circuitry (in preparation). However, we still have little information concerning the sites of direct action of systemic KA and the permeability of the blood brain barrier to KA ; furthermore, it is not clear whether the barrier is disrupted in relation to epileptic episodes, in keeping for instance with bicuculline induced generalized convulsions (i.e. Johansson and Nilsson, 1977). This type of information is clearly necessary in order to better differentiate between the "toxic" (direct) action of KA and those due to the seizures produced by KA.

    Figure 2 : Alterations in local glucose consumption following systemic KA administration. Case D50, 4 h after KA, the animal had displayed more than 20 limbic motor seizures and almost 20 minutes status epilepticus. Note the increase in radioactivity in the ammon's horn (Regio inferior (RI) and superior (RS), entorhinal cortex (CE), infra and prelimbic cortices (L), claustrum (CL), septum (LS) and ventral pallidum (VP), amygdala and bed nucleus of the stria terminalis (BST), paraventricular and paraventricular nuclei (PV-PT) and retrosplenial cortex (NS) as well lateral nucleus of the thalamus (LT). In contrast the labelling is decreased in most neocortical areas (see Ben-Ari et al., 1981).

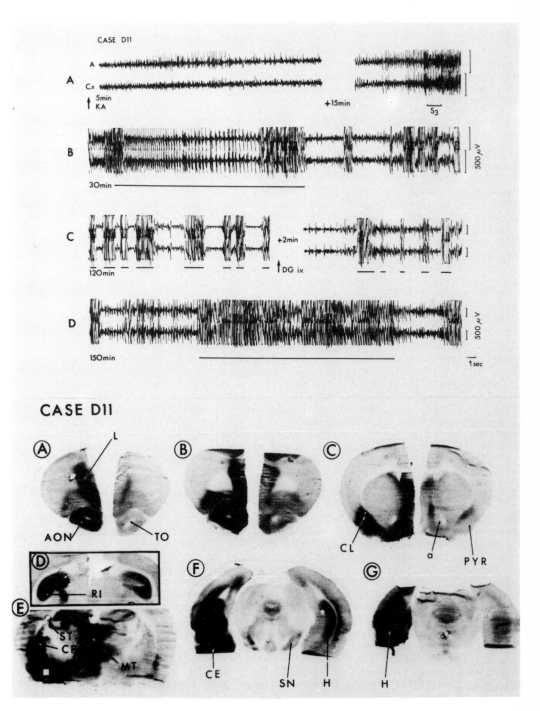

fig.3

Figure 3 : Regional glucose utilization in case D11 which received and intra-amygdaloid injection of KA in chronic unanaesthetized conditions. The animal displayed several individual limbic motor seizures (but not status epilepticus) before sacrifice;the electrographic records obtained at the site of injection (A-amygdala) and cortical EEG are depicted. In photomicrograph, the white quadrangle represents the site of injection. The pattern of labelling is largely similar to that seen after systemic KA although it is primarily unilateral.

Local injections of KA

Local injection of KA in a large number of brain structures have been shown to induce various abnormal motor behaviors and pathological alterations in "distant" brain structures often with a regional distribution similar to that described above (i.e. Wurthele et al., 1978 ; Ben-Ari et al., 1979b,1980a,b ; Zaczek et al., 1980 ; and reviews in Nadler, 1981 ; Coyle et al., 1981). However, the electrographic and metabolic patterns following such manipulations and the role of epileptic activity in the "distant" damage has been largely studied in relation with intra-amygdaloid injections of the toxin (i.e. Ben-Ari et al., 1980b). The effects of such injections can be briefly summarized as follows : In chronic unanaesthetized rats, epileptiform activity is first apparent at the site of injection (fig. 3), following various delays (often 5-10 minutes). These propagate to the ipsilateral ammon's horn and the contralateral amygdala. Typical motor seizures are observed after short delays (often 5-20 minutes) for several hours (i.e. Ben-Ari et al., 1981a,b). With the 2-deoxy-glucose treatment (Tremblay et al., 1982), the autoradiographs reveal an increased glucose uptake somewhat similar (although it is largely unilateral) to that seen following systemic KA. Labelled areas include (i.e. case D11, fig. 3) the deep layers of the infra and prelimbic cortices in the ipsilateral frontal cortex (fig. 3A,B) and the hippocampal rudiment (fig. 3B,C) ; the posterior cingulate cortex, the agranular insular and prepyriform cortices and the cortex adjacent to the rhinal sulcus (fig. 3). In addition, an increased metabolism is noticed in septal area, the claustrum and ventral pallidum, the insula calleja magna, the mediodorsal and reuniens nuclei of the thalamus as well as the parataenial and paraventricular nuclei. In the caudal allocortical areas, there is an increased metabolism over the ammon's horn, subicular and entorhinal cortices,parasubiculum and area 29b of the retrosplenial cortex (i.e. fig. 3).

By superimposing the autoradiographs on the stained sections (see Tremblay et al., 1982), the pattern of metabolic alterations can be analyzed with greater detail. Whereas in control conditions the highest level of labelling is present in the molecular layer of the fascia dentata (i.e. fig. 4A,C) following systemic (fig. 4B,D,E or F) or intra-amygdaloid KA (not illustrated) the highest grain density in the hippocampal formation is noticed in the lacunosum moleculare area of the regio inferior and in the stratum lucidum. In keeping with lesion experiments (i.e. Nadler and Cuthberson, 1981 ; Nadler this volume) this stresses the importance of the mossy fibers in mediating the epileptiform discharge and its pathological outcome. Furthermore the earliest pathological alterations are noticed in the CA3a,b region. The damage involves in addition to the pyramidal layer,the stratum lucidum (which appears vacuolated fig. 5A) and the stratum lacunosum moleculare (which is intensely argyrophylic with the Fink-Heimer stain (fig. 5 A,B). In the hippocampal formation the pathological alterations are also observed in the hilus (i.e. CA4 in figure 5B) whereas the granular layer is particularly resistant to the experimental procedure (ibid). The pattern of damage in other brain structures is also almost identical to the regional distribution of increased glucose consumption (i.e. Tremblay et al., 1982).

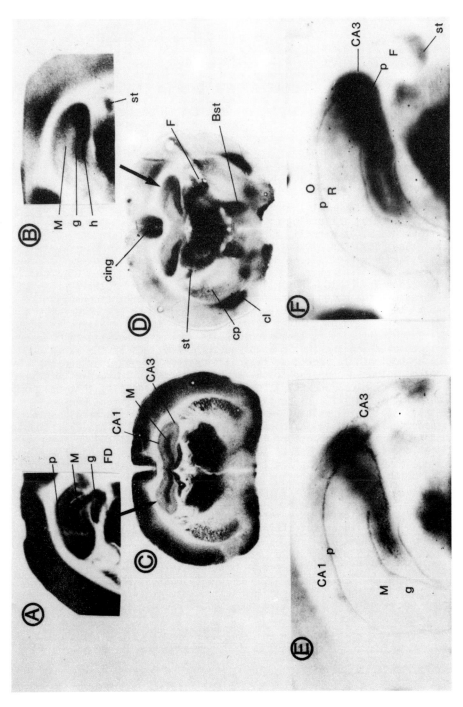

fig.4

Figure 4 : *Pattern of regional glucose consumption in a control*
(A-C) and KA treated case (B,D,E and F). The latter received systemically KA
and displayed recurrent(LMS)and status epilepticus before sacrifice. B,C and D :
photomicrographs of a frontal sections of the control and KA treated animals
respectively. The alterations in labelling are similar to those described in
fig. 2. A higher magnification of the hippocampal formation area of the KA
case is shown in B. A,E,F : To increase the anatomical resolution, the auto-
radiographs were put on top of the mounted cresyl violet-stained section from
which the autoradiograph was originally obtained. Care was taken to ensure a
precise alignment between the autoradiograph and the section. A picture was
taken by focussing on the stained section A-E or on the 2 D-G film (F). It
is evident that in the KA labelled animal, the strong labelling involves the
hilus and regio inferior along a pattern which corresponds to the mossy fiber
system and stratum lacunosum moleculare of CA3 (i.e. Tremblay et al., 1982).

Several observations suggest that the distant lesions noted in the ammon's horn
are in fact caused by the prolonged and intense limbic seizure activity that KA
initiates and not by KA directly (i.e. via diffusion or uptake and release).
There have been discussed elsewhere (Ben-Ari et al., 1980b ; Ben-Ari, 1981 ;
Nadler, 1981 and Coyle et al., 1981) will be only briefly summarized below :
a) there is an excellent correlation between the severity of epileptiform
discharge recorded in situ -in particular in terms of post-ictal depression-
and the damage in the ammon's horn ; b) administration of anticonvulsants
reduces both the epileptiform discharge and the damage in the ammon's horn
and not in the injected amygdala ; c) damage in the medial thalamus is often
more severe contralateral to the injected site than the ipsilateral one ;
d) injections of KA in the septum or preoptic bed nucleus of the stria terminalis area do not readily reproduce typical limbic motor seizures and the hippocampal pathology when compared to the amygdala (this is in keeping with extensive anatomical, clinical and physiological evidence suggesting that the amygdala
is anodal point for eliciting the typical limbic seizures, i.e. Ben-Ari,
1981 ; Wada, 1980) ; in contrast small injections in the entorhinal cortex
readily produces the typical hippocampal damage (Schwob et al., 1981) ; e) in
the ammon's horn the damage occurs earlier and often is limited to the rostral
(septal) pole and not the adjacent temporal pole ; f) transection of the perforant path abolishes distant but not local damage, in contrast similar procedure
does not abolish the damage obtained after ventricular injection (Nadler and
Cuthberson, 1981 ; Nadler, this volume).

There are several indications that the local (toxic) and distant (epilepsy
related) damage have important different characteristics. Thus a) there are
clear cut morphological differences -in particular in terms of the rapid microglial invasion at the site of injection- (Ben-Ari et al., 1980 a,b) ; b) the
distant and not the local damage cab be obtained in various experimental
conditions including local microiontophoretic injections of KA in the hippocampus (Ruth, 1982) and intra-amygdaloid injections of folates (Olney et al.,
1981) ; c) Zaczek et al. (1981) have reported pharmacological differences
between distant and local damage.

Intra-cerebroventricular (i.c.v.) injections of KA

The pathological sequelae of i.c.v. injections of KA have been extensively investigated by Nadler and co-workers (Nadler et al., 1980 ; Nadler, this volume). The
clinical effects of i.c.v. administration include (in anaesthetized preparation)
exophtalmos, vibrissae and body tremor, foaming, mydryasis and rigidity of trunk
musculature i.e. Nadler et al., 1978 ; Ben-Ari et al., 1980b) ; at longer delays
recurrent convulsive episodes are also observed. The electrographic effects or

A

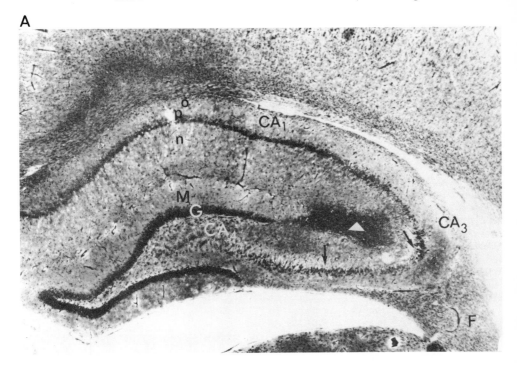

B

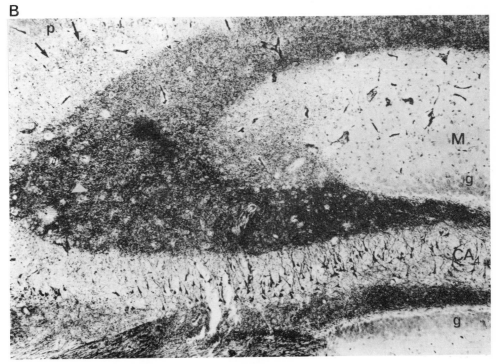

fig.5

Figure 5 : Pathological alterations produced by intra-amygdaloid injections of KA. Fink-Heimer stains. Note the strong argyrophilia of the lacunosum area (triangles in A and B). Also note in B the damage produced in CA4 ; in contrast the granule cells (g) and pyramidal neurons of CA1-CA2 (p) are not affected.

metabolic sequelae of i.c.v. injections of KA have not been studied. The pathological alterations include lesions with a distribution and gradient somewhat similar to that described above (i.e. CA3 > CA1 > granules in the hippocampal formation, damage in the amygdala and other limbic structures. However in addition the entire pyriform, prepyriform and entorhinal cortices (bilaterally) display severe neuronal loss without gliosis extending through all cell layers. There are several indications that the brain damage is at least partly related to the paroxysmal activity induced by KA and cannot be solely explained by a direct action of the toxin. Thus, administration of an anticonvulsant reduce the motor disturbances produced by i.c.v. KA (in contrast to the exophtalmos and mydriasis which are not reduced) as well as the "distant" damage, in particular in the pyriform and entorhinal cortices (i.e. Ben-Ari et al., 1980 b). Furthermore, lesion experiments suggest that the critical pathways for destruction of neurons by local (intra-hippocampal) and i.c.v. injections of KA are completely different (i.e. Nadler and Cuthberson, 1981 ; Nadler, 1981 ; Nadler, this volume).

GENERAL DISCUSSION

Why are limbic structures so vulnerable to recurrent seizure episodes ?

Since limbic structures are vulnerable to a variety of deleterious conditions the possibility that systemic physiological disturbances associated with the seizures episodes could contribute to the damage must be considered. Such a contribution however appears most unlikely since : a) following systemic KA in rats, neuronal damage develops in animals with mild motor seizures and can be obtained with doses which do not produce clear cut systemic metabolic derangements (Lothmans and Collins, 1981) ; b) the typical brain damage can be obtained in experimental conditions in which motor convulsions are not induced (i.e. Ruth, 198 2 ; Sloviter and Damiano, 1981a,b) ; c) in experiments currently performed, we have obtained direct evidence by means of direct measurement of the (local) hippocampal PO_2, PCO_2 and blood flow that the damage is not explicable in terms of a local hypoxia or hypercapnia (in preparation). These observations as well as the predominant role of fiber pathways in mediating the distant brain damage and the observation that in anaesthetized rats repetitive electrical stimulation of the perforant path can reproduce a similar pattern of damage (Sloviter and Damiano, 1981a) points on the paroxysmal discharge per se as a critical cause of the distant damage. The reasons for the selective vulnerability of hippocampal (and other limbic) neurons to an excessive rise in neuronal discharge and metabolism are poorly understood. Several recent experiments suggest that an excessive rise in intracellular Ca^{++} could be an important factor in the neurotic changes produced in a variety of conditions ; if the internal protein sequestring capacity would be exceeded proteolytic enzymes may be directly activated (i.e. Schanne et al., 1979 ; Drayton et al., 1973). Direct measurement of Ca^{++} concentrations in the ammon's horn reveal indeed a particularly prominent reduction of the extracellular Ca^{++} in the pyramidal layer during electrically induced seizures (Krnjevic et al., 1980). Using red alizarine preliminary histochemical evidence in keeping with this hypothesis has been obtained in this laboratory (in preparation).

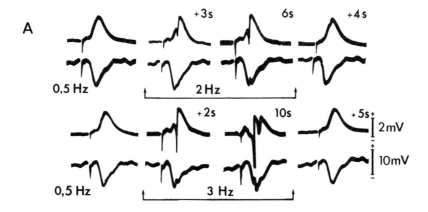

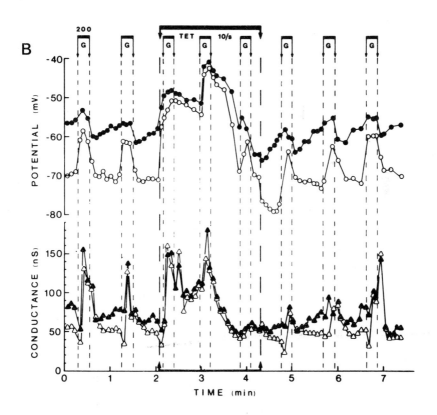

fig.6

Figure 6 : A. *Concomittant recording in situ of the field potentials generated by a stimulation of the hippocampal commissure in the pyramidal (top) and dendritic (bottom) layers of the ammon's horn (CA1) in situ. Note that when the frequency of stimulation is increased to 2 or 5 Hz (top or bottom pair of records) population spikes are generated in the pyramidal layer without significant changes in the typical negative waves (field EPSP) recorded concomittantly with a twin-set of microelectrodes from the dendrites (see Cherubini et al., 1982). B. Effects of application of GABA on the IPSP and associated conductance changes. Intracellular record from the pyramidal layer in situ and extracellular application of GABA (i.e. Ben-Ari et al., 1981b). Commissural stimulation at 1 Hz elicited prominent IPSP (top of the figure, depolarization is due to Cl⁻ leakage from the electrode) and a conductance increase (bottom of the figure). Extracellular applications of GABA (200 nA, arrows) depresses the IPSP and its underlying conductance increase. This effect is not observed during or shortly after a brief tetanus (i.e. Ben-Ari et al., 1979c).*

Why are epileptiform discharges so readily elicited in limbic structures ?

In addition to their particular vulnerability to the pathological sequelae of seizures episodes, in both man and experimental animals, limbic structures are also particularly susceptible to epilepgogenic procedures. Seizure activity is more readily elicited in the hippocampus and amygdala than in any other brain structure ; furthermore within the hippocampal formation seizure activity is more readily elicited in CA3 than in CA1 (Schwartzkroin and Prince, 1978) thus in parallel to the greater histological vulnerability of CA3 to seizure episodes.

Whereas earlier studies had emphasized the importance of the enhancement of excitatory drive as a seizure inducing mechanism, recent observations suggest that the lability of the recurrent GABAergic inhibition in the hippocampus may be a particularly important factor in epileptogenesis (Ben-Ari et al., 1981b). Thus, intracellular observations have shown that the normally powerful GABAergic inhibition is surprisingly labile particularly at frequencies of stimulation above 2-3 Hz ; the inhibition is rapidly diminished during such stimulation both in terms of the IPSP and their associated conductance changes (Ben-Ari et al., 1979c, 1981b). A major reason for this loss of sensitivity is diminished sensitivity to GABA (fig. 6B). These observations suggest that post-synaptic desensitization of GABA receptors is an important factor in this lability of inhibition. As shown in fig. 6A, concomittant recording of the dendritic field EPSP and the somatic population spikes reveal that during such stimulation bursts of spikes can be generated in the pyramidal layer without observing significant changes in the excitatory drive (also see Cherubini et al., 1982).

It is therefore of particular interest to note that following systemic administration of KA in anaesthetized preparations, the recurrent GABAergic inhibition as measured by the paired pulse technique is completely blocked (Sloviter and Damiano, 1981b). Furthermore, hilar interneurones which, in addition to the pyramidal shaped cell bodies lying in the granular layer, mediate the recurrent GABAergic inhibition (i.e. Andersen et al., 1966) appear to be particularly vulnerable to systemic KA (Sloviter and Damiano, 1981b, also see fig.5 and Ben-Ari et al. 1981). Therefore an impairement of recurrent inhibition perhaps resulting first from a desensitization of GABA receptors and upon maintained exacerbated enhancement of neuronal discharge from a permanent damage of the interneurones, may well play a central role in the induction of the epileptiform discharge and its pathological outcome. Further studies are however required to test this hypothesis and in particular to confirm by immunocytochemical means the GABAergic nature of the vulnerable neurones.

To conclude, there is little doubt that KA has powerful seizure eliciting properties in addition to its "neurotoxic" characteristics. Furthermore the epileptiform activity generated by KA plays an important role in the brain damage produced by the neurotoxin since in appropriate conditions, lesions in a number of brain sites -in particular within the limbic system- can be produced with little "direct" contributions of KA. However, since the extent of both the direct and "remote" (epilepsy related) damage depend on the experimental paradigms (dose, volume, anaesthetics, site of injection, etc ...) the respective contribution of the two actions of KA must be assessed in each experimental condition using a multidisciplinary approach including appropriate electrophysiological observations.

REFERENCES

Andersen, P., Holmqvist, B., and Voorhoeve, P.E. (1966). Acta Physiol. Scand., 66, 448-460.
Ben-Ari, Y. (Ed.) The Amygdaloid Complex, Elsevier-North/Holland, Amsterdam, (1981) 514pp.
Ben-Ari, Y., Lagowska, Y., Tremblay, E., and Le Gal La Salle, G. (1979a). Brain Res., 163, 186-180.
Ben-Ari, Y., Tremblay, E., Ottersen, O.P., and Naquet, R. (1979b), Brain Res., 165, 362-365.
Ben-Ari, Y., Krnjević, K., and Reinhardt, W. (1979c). Can. J. Physiol. and Pharmacol., 57, 1462-1466.
Ben-Ari, Y., Tremblay, E., and Ottersen, O.P. (1980a). Neuroscience, 5, 515-527.
Ben-Ari, Y., Tremblay, E., Ottersen, O.P. and Meldrum, B.S. (1980b). Brain Res., 191, 79-97.
Ben-Ari, Y., Tremblay, E., Riche, D., Ghilini, G., and Naquet, R. (1981a). Neuroscience, 6, 1361-1391.
Ben-Ari, Y., Krnjević, K., Reiffeinstein, R., and Reinhardt, W. (1981b). Neuroscience, 6, 2445-2463.
Cherubini, E., Rovira, C., Padjen, A. and Ben-Ari, Y. (1982). Neuroscience Letters, in press.
Coyle, J.T., Bird, S.J., Evans, R.H., Gulley, R.L., Nadler, J.V., Nicklas, W.J., and Olney, J.W. (1981). Excitatory amino-acid neurotoxins : selectivity, specificity and mechanisms of action - NRP research program. 19, 427pp.
Drayton, W.R., Reville, W.J., Goll, D.E., and Stroner, M.H. (1973). Biochem., 15, 2156-2167.
Fuller, T., and Olney, J.W. (1979). Soc. Neurosc., Abstr., 5, 556.
Goddard, G.V., Mc Intyre, D.C., and Leech, C.K. (1969). Exptl. Neurol., 25, 295-330.
Johansson, B., and Nilsson, B. (1977). Acta Neuropathol. (Berlin), 38, 153-158.
Krnjević, K., Morris, M., and Reiffenstein, R. (1980). Can. J. Physiol. Pharmacol., 58, 579-583.
Lothman, E.W., and Collins, R.C. (1981). Brain Res., 218, 299-318.
Nadler, J.V., Perry, B.W., and Cotman, C.W. (1978). Nature, 271, 676-677.
Nadler, J.V., and Cuthberson, G.J. (1980), Brain Res., 197, 47-56.
Nadler, J.V., Perry, B.W., Gentry, C., and Cotman, C.W. (1980). J. Comp. Neurol., 192, 333-359.
Nadler, J.V. (1981). Life Sciences, 29, 2031-2042.
Olney, J.W., Fuller, T.A., and De Gubareff, T. (1981). Nature, 292, 165-166.
Racine, R. (1972). Electroenceph. clin. Neurophysiol., 32, 281-294.
Ruth, R.E. (1982). Exptl. Neurol., 76, 508-527.
Schanne, F.A.Y., Kane A.B., Young, E.E., and Farber, J.L. (1979). Science, 206, 700-702.
Schwob, J.E., Fuller, T., Price, J.L., and Olney, J.W. (1980). Neuroscience, 5, 991-1014.

Schwartzkroin, P.A., and Prince, D.A. (1978). Brain Res., 147, 117-130.
Sloviter, R.S., and Damiano, B.P. (1981a). Neuroscience Letters, 24, 279-284.
Sloviter, R.S., and Damiano, B.P. (1981b). Neuropharmacol., 20, 1003-1011.
Sokoloff, L. (1980). Brain, 102, 653-668.
Tremblay, E., Ottersen, O.P., Rovira, C., and Ben-Ari, Y. (1982). Neuroscience, in press.
Wada, J.A. (1981). Kindling II. Raven Press, New York.
Wuerthele, W.M., Lovell, K.L., Jones, M.Z., and Moore, K.E. (1978). Brain Res., 149, 489-492.
Zaczek, R., Simonton, S., and Coyle, J.T. (1980). J. Neuropath. Exp. Neurol., 39, 245-264.
Zaczek, R., Nelson, M.F., and Coyle, J.T. (1981). Neuropharmacol., 20, 183-199.

EXCITATORY AMINO ACID TRANSMITTERS IN CEREBELLUM AND OPTIC TECTUM

M. CUÉNOD, A. DILBER, H. HENKE, G. TOGGENBURGER, L. WIKLUND
and M. WOLFENSBERGER

Brain Research Institute, University of Zurich, August Forel-Strasse 1, 8029 Zurich/Switzerland

ABSTRACT

This review presents evidence which favors a special role of aspartate in the climbing fibers of the rat cerebellum and of glutamate and aspartate in some fibers of the pigeon optic nerve. The localisation and properties of kainic acid binding sites in the cerebellum are also discussed.

KEYWORDS

Aspartate; glutamate; kainic acid; ethanolamine; olivo-climbing fiber neurons; retino-tectal neurons.

INTRODUCTION

While much is known about the inhibitory transmitters, there are still many uncertainties about the excitatory transmitters, in spite of their importance, in the vertebrate brain. In this paper, recent work performed in our laboratory on in vitro and in vivo release of glutamate and aspartate, on kainic acid binding-sites and on selective retrograde labeling with D-[^{3}H]-aspartate will be reviewed.

CEREBELLUM

The afferent input to the cerebellar cortex consists of (a) the climbing fibers, which originate in the inferior olive and forms excitatory synaptic contacts with the Purkinje cells, and (b) the mossy fibers, which arise from various sources in the spinal cord and the brainstem and, via the granule cells and their parallel fibers, activate the Purkinje cells. In the first one, evidence supporting a special role of aspartate will be presented.

In vitro release of endogenous amino acids and effect of olive
destruction by 3-acetylpyridine treatment. Toggenburger, et al. (1983)
observed a Ca^{2+}-dependent, K^+-induced release of endogenous aspartate,
glutamate, GABA and glycine from slices of rat cerebellar hemispheres,
while threonine, serine, asparagine, glutamine, alanine, isoleucine,
leucine, thyrosine, phenylalanine, lysine, histidine and arginine
were not affected by the depolarisation. GABA is likely to be the inhibitory transmitter in part at least of the Purkinje cells and in
interneurons of the cerebellar cortex (Fonnum, et al., 1970; Curtis
and Felix, 1971; Hökfelt and Ljungdahl, 1972; Fonnum and Walberg,
1973), while glycine has been associated with some Golgi neurons
(Wilkin, et al., 1981). Glutamate has been related to the granule
cells on the basis of pool, release and uptake studies (Young, et al.,
1974; Hudson, et al., 1976; McBride, et al., 1976a, 1976b; Sandoval
and Cotman, 1978). In what concerns aspartate, Nadi, et al. (1977)
noted a drop in cerebellar tissue level following degeneration of
the inferior olive cells and climbing fibers induced by 3-acetylpyri-
dine, without change in glutamate. We have also treated rats with
3-acetylpyridine (3-AP) in order to destroy the olivo-cerebellar
climbing fiber system (Desclin and Escubi, 1974; Llinas, et al.,
1975). Quantitative estimation two weeks after 3-AP injection revealed
that only 0.7 % of the olivary neurons had survived in those areas
projecting to the cerebellar hemispheres, thus allowing to optimally
select the tissue for the in vitro experiments (Wiklund, et al., 1982;
Toggenburger et al., 1983). In slices of cerebellar hemispheres, the
Ca^{2+}-dependent K^+-induced release of aspartate was significantly
reduced by 26% in the 3-AP treated animals as compared to control,
suggesting that the climbing fibers projecting to the hemisphere contribute to the aspartate efflux. The decreases in glutamate (14%),
GABA (9%) and glycine did not reach significance. A contribution of
the climbing fibers to glutamate release remains possible, however,
on the basis of this observation, since its massive release, presumably from parallel fibers, may obscure an effect induced by the 3-AP
treatment. Thus, the present evidence supports the idea that aspartate, possibly associated with glutamate, is released from the climbing fiber terminals in the hemispheric cerebellar cortex. This conclusion is supported by similar experiments, in which the cerebellar
slices, before depolarisation, were preincubated with D-$[^3H]$-aspar-
tate, L-$[^3H]$-aspartate or L-$[^3H]$-glutamate. For both D-$[^3H]$-aspartate
and L-$[^3H]$-glutamate a massive Ca^{2+}-dependent K^+-induced release was
observed, reduced by 27% and 38% respectively in slices from climbing
fiber deprived animals. In contrast, incubation with L-$[^3H]$-aspar-
tate led to very low release, not significantly decreased in 3-AP
treated animals. Thus, as shown in table 1 L-$[^3H]$-aspartate and
L-$[^3H]$-glutamate behaved differently in rat cerebellar slices in many
respects: (a) the uptake was 4 times larger for L-$[^3H]$-glutamate than
L-$[^3H]$-aspartate after incubation at the same substrate concentration
of 0.5 µM. (b) The fractional rate constant of release was about 5
times higher for L-$[^3H]$-glutamate. (c) The fraction of release which
was Ca^{2+}-dependent was higher for L-$[^3H]$-glutamate (84%) than for
L-$[^3H]$-aspartate (50%) and (d) the relative specific activity of the
released amino acid relative to that of tissue stores is 1.1 for L-
$[^3H]$-aspartate and 3.5 for L-$[^3H]$-glutamate. These observations favor
the hypothesis of a different compartmentation in cerebellar slices

TABLE 1

Parameters of L-[^{3}H]-aspartate and L-[^{3}H]-glutamate in rat
cerebellar slices

	L-[^{3}H]-aspartate	L-[^{3}H]-glutamate
uptake (pmol / mg protein . min)	0.45 ± 0.05 (n=11)	1.88 ± 0.22 (n=10)
fractional rate constant of release (% . min^{-1})		
50 mM K$^+$, 2 mM Ca^{2+}	2.8 ± 0.8 (n=6)	14.4 ± 2.0 (n=6)
5 mM K$^+$, 2 mM Ca^{2+}	0.4 ± 0.06 (n=3)	
degree of Ca^{2+}-dependence = $\dfrac{[\text{release with 50 mM K}^+, 2\text{ mM Ca}^{2+}]}{[\text{release with 50 mM K}^+, 0.1\text{ mM Ca}^{2+}, 12\text{ mM Mg}^{2+}]}$	2.0 ± 0.6 (n=4)	6.3 ± 0.7 (n=4)
$\dfrac{\text{specific activity in eluate during 50 mM K}^+ \text{ stimulation}}{\text{specific activity in tissue}}$	1.1 ± 0.3 (n=10)	3.5 ± 0.2 (n=10)

Slices were incubated during 4 minutes (37°C) with either L-[^{3}H]-aspartate or L-[^{3}H]-glutamate at a concentration of 0.5 μM in Earle's physiological salt solution. Then they were washed and for uptake measurements immediately frozen on dry ice. For release they were transferred to superfusion chambers and depolarized by increasing the K$^+$ concentration to 50 mM after a 40 minute superfusion period (for details see Toggenburger et al., 1982). Ca^{2+} dependence was determined by comparing release in the presence of 2 mM Ca^{2+} with that at low Ca^{2+}, high Mg^{2+} concentration.

To determine tissue content of amino acids, slices were homogenised in 10% (w/v) trichloroacetic acid, centrifuged and the supernatant used for amino acid analysis. The endogenous and radiolabeled amino acids from tissue or collected during release were separated by ion-exchange chromatography (Durum DC-4A resin column, analyzer from Biotronik, Munich) and quantified by the fluorescence of the corresponding O-phthalaldehyde derivative.

(from Toggenburger et al., 1983)

for the two amino acids, the glutamate releasable compartment(s) being larger than the aspartate one(s) and less connected with the non-releasable pools. Indeed, the aspartate uptake amounts to 24% of the glutamate uptake, while its release is only about 3% of the glutamate one, suggesting that a larger part of the aspartate does not reach or leave the releasable pool, a conclusion also supported by the high relative specific activity of the released [^{3}H]-glutamate.

D-[^{3}H]-aspartate retrograde labeling of the olivary-climbing fiber system. We have suggested that certain transmitters (or related molecules), after having been selectively taken up in the nerve terminals which use them, are transported retrogradely to the cell body. Thus, when a molecule such as tritiated glycine, GABA, D-aspartate, choline, dopamine or serotonin is injected in a given zone of terminals, autoradiograms performed after an appropriate survival time reveal the labeling of the fibers and cell bodies of origin of the respective projections, presumably glycinergic, GABAergic, glutamate or aspartatergic, cholinergic, dopaminergic or serotonergic (Streit, et al., 1979; review in Cuénod, et al., 1982).

D-[^{3}H]-aspartate which is transported by the same high affinity uptake system as L-aspartate and L-glutamate, but is not metabolised, has been successfully applied to selectively labeled neurons presumably using glutamate or aspartate as transmitter, first in cortico-striate neurons (Streit, 1980), then in cortico-thalamic (Baughman and Gilbert, 1981) and cortico-dorsal-column-nuclei neurons (Rustioni and Cuénod, 1982) as well as on retino-tectal ganglion cells (Beaudet, et al., 1981).

Wiklund, et al. (1982, 1983) applied, either by injection or by superfusion, D-[^{3}H]-aspartate in various regions of the cerebellar cortex and deep nuclei, and observed a selective retrograde labeling of the corresponding part of the inferior olive. All the neurons and their axons were intensely labeled, while the mossy fiber sources in the brainstem or spinal cord remained free of label. Granule cells also were unlabeled by D-[^{3}H]-aspartate, an observation which is surprising in view of the strong evidence that they use glutamate as transmitter, but might be related to the fact that parallel fiber terminals do not seem to possess high affinity uptake for their presumed transmitter. At any rate, the very intense selective retrograde labeling of the olivary-climbing system with D-[^{3}H]-aspartate correlates well with the reduction of L-aspartate release in climbing fibers depleted cerebellar as reported above.

Kainic acid binding-sites. Kainic acid is a structural analogue of glutamic acid. Its binding and histotoxicity have been related to the excitatory amino acid transmitters and extensively studied in the mammalian neostriatum. In cerebellar membranes, specific [^{3}H]-kainic acid binding at 50 μM concentration has been measured in many species: in most mammals, the amount of kainic acid bound is 200 to 300 fmol/mg protein, while in birds (pigeon, hen) it is 15'000 fmol/mg and in the trout it reaches 42'000 fmol/mg. The kinetic studies of [^{3}H]-kainic acid binding in the rat cerebellum reveals a K_d of 18 nM and B_{max} of 300 fmol/mg protein, while in the pigeon, the data are best interpreted by assuming two binding-sites, characterized respectively by a K_d of 30 and 330 nM and a B_{max} of 2'600 and 106'000 fmol/mg protein. The low affinity binding-site has a Hill-coefficient of 2.2 and shows a positive cooperativity (Henke and Cuénod, 1980). The high binding capacity of the pigeon cerebellum made it possible to perform successfully autoradiographs of histological sections exposed to 1.5 nM $[^3H]$-kainic acid. They revealed a predominant location of the silver grains over the molecular layer of the cerebellar cortex (Henke, et al., 1981).

In the striatum, the evidence favors a postsynaptic location of the binding site (Henke and Cuénod, 1979), relative to the cortico-striatal input, in which the putative transmitters are glutamate and aspartate. In the cerebellum, however, the situation might be different. Griesser, et al. (1982) determined the $[^3H]$-kainic acid binding in cerebellar membranes of various mice cerebellar mutant strains. The expectation was that the binding site would be associated predominantly with Purkinje cell membranes, which is postsynaptic to the parallel and climbing fiber input, both assumed to use excitatory amino acid transmitters. It turned out that the binding was little or not affected in the cerebellum of Purkinje cell degeneration (Pcd, 80% of control, expressed per mg protein) and nervous (nr, 66%) mice, which are primarily missing Purkinje cells, but was markedly reduced weaver (wv, 34%) and realer (rl, 6%), which are characterized by a paucity of granule cells and parallel fibers. The strongest deficit in binding, however, was observed in the staggerer cerebellum (sg, 5% of control), which is almost devoid of parallel fiber - Purkinje cell synaptic contacts. Therefore, it seems unlikely that the bulk of the kainate binding sites are localized on Purkinje cell membranes, but they could be related to the granule cell - parallel fiber system and particularly their synapses with the Purkinje cells. Such an interpretation would also be compatible with the location, in the molecular layer, of the radioactivity, in autoradiographs of rat cerebellar sections incubated with $[^3H]$-kainic acid (Henke, et al., 1981).

Encouraged by the large amount of kainic acid binding-sites in the pigeon cerebellum and by its selective localisation in the molecular layer of the cerebellar cortex (Henke and Cuénod, 1980; Henke, et al., 1981), we decided to attempt the isolation of that binding-site. Dilber, et al. (1982) succeeded in solubilising it, using Triton X-100. At a concentration of 0.25%, the low affinity binding site is predominantly extracted, while a 1% Triton X-100 extracts both the high and low affinity ones. The binding and pharmacological properties remain present in the solubilized form.

OPTIC TECTUM

The retino-tectal pathway has been used as a model to study the in vivo release of transmitters, or of related compounds. Earlier investigations had shown that retinal ablation induces in two to four weeks a decrease of glutamate and aspartate in the tectal layers containing the degenerated optic nerve fibers (Fonnum and Henke, 1982) and of glutamate uptake in tectal synaptosomes (Henke,

et al., 1976). Kainic acid, injected in the tectum, induces a dendritic and somatic lesion which can be prevented by previous degeneration of the optic nerve (Streit, et al., 1980). Furthermore,
application of [^{3}H]-D-aspartate to the optic tectum led to retrograde labeling of a small proportion of retinal ganglion cells
(Beaudet, et al., 1981). Using a push-pull cannula implanted in the
optic tectum, the perfusion fluid can be collected and has been analysed by gas chromatography and mass fragmentography (Wolfensberger,
in press; Wolfensberger and Amsler, 1982; Wolfensberger, et al.,
1982a). Modification in perfusion composition presumably reflects
changes in composition of the extracellular space, which take place
during synaptic activity. Thus, electrical stimulation of the optic
nerve at 40 Hz for 5 minutes induced a 2.5 fold increase in aspartate
and a 1.5 fold increase in glutamate as compared to resting periods
(Canzek, et al., 1981). This tectal elevation of endogenous aspartate
and glutamate during optic nerve activity suggests that these amino
acids are released during synaptic transmission, and, in view of the
data mentioned above, that they originate from a population of optic
nerve terminals. It remains, however, possible that aspartate and
glutamate are metabolites of compounds which would be released at
the synapse, or that they are coming from other compartments. It
should be mentioned, however, that after degeneration of one optic
nerve, the in vitro Ca^{2+}-dependent K$^+$-induced release of endogenous
glutamate and aspartate as well as of exogenous D-[^{3}H]-aspartate is
increased in the degenerated tectum and possibly decreased in the
opposite tectum, as compared to normal animals (Toggenburger, et al.,
in preparation). This surprising result implies a transcellular
effect of the optic nerve degeneration.

Furthermore, we have also observed a 2 to 3 fold increase of 2-amino-
ethanol (ethanolamine) collected from the optic tectum during optic
nerve stimulation (Wolfensberger, et al., 1982b), possibly reflecting
a base-exchange reaction of membranes phospholipids (Porcellati, et
al., 1971; Kanfer, 1972) induced by synaptic and/or axonal activity.
Microiontophoretic application of ethanolamine alone did not affect
the discharge pattern of tectal neurons, but in conjunction with
glutamate or GABA, it did potentiate their respective excitatory or
inhibitory effects (Wolfensberger et al., 1982b). This modulatory
effect of ethanolamine could be due to reduction of amino acid uptake or to an action on the receptors, enhancing their efficacy.

Tectal slices, exposed to high K$^+$ concentration or to veratridine,
release beside GABA, β-alanine, which has a strychnine sensitive inhibitory action on tectal neurons (Toggenburger, et al., 1981).
Finally, a release of proline has been observed in tectal slices,
induced by K$^+$ depolarisation, in a Ca^{2+}-dependent manner (Wolfensberger, et al., 1982c), a finding supporting the idea that proline,
or a related compound, might play a transmitter role in the optic
tectum, as well as in other structures (see Felix and Künzle, 1976).

CONCLUSION

Evidence has been reviewed which favors a transmitter role of aspartate in the rat cerebellar climbing fibers and of glutamate and

aspartate in the pigeon optic nerve. The kainic acid binding site in the cerebellum appears to involve the parallel fiber-Purkinje cell synapse. However, although the amino acids glutamate and aspartate are serious candidates as excitatory central transmitters, they are probably not the only ones, and one might even doubt that they are always the substances effectively released: indeed they might turn out to be, in some cases, metabolites of the real transmitters. The problem of the receptors is also complex and far from being solved, as three or four different receptor-types have been identified on the basis of agonist and antagonist properties. Watkins and colla-borators have proposed the existence of N-methyl-D-aspartate, quis-qualate and a kainate receptors, and possibly other types of recep-tors. In view of these many uncertainties, a precise attribution of excitatory transmitters to specific nervous pathways meets with diffi-culties. However, information resting on presynaptic markers such as pool, uptake and release of glutamate and aspartate in normal tissue and after degeneration of specific afferents led to the description of "glutamatergic" or "aspartatergic" pathways (see Fonnum, this symposium). This has been extended in a few cases to the collection, in vivo, of endogenous transmitter released upon stimulation of spe-cific pathways. Furthermore, retrograde labeling with D-[^{3}H]-aspar-tate, when present, supports the hypothesis that a pathway uses excitatory amino acid transmitters. The importance of such characte-risation of pathways according to their transmitter is evident, and will also allow to define models on which basic research on central excitatory transmission can be followed up.

ACKNOWLEDGEMENT

This work was supported by grants 3.408.78, 3.505.79 and 3.506.79 of the Swiss National Science Foundation and the Dr. Eric Slack-Gyr-Foundation.

REFERENCES

Baughman, R.W. and C.D. Gilbert (1981). J. Neuroscience, 1, 427-439.
Beaudet, A., A. Burkhalter, J.C. Reubi and M. Cuénod (1981). Neuro-science, 6, 2021-2034.
Canzek, V., M. Wolfensberger, U. Amsler and M. Cuénod (1981). Nature, 293, 572-574.
Cuénod, M., P. Bagnoli, A. Beaudet, A. Rustioni, L. Wiklund and P. Streit (1982). Cytochemical Methods in Neuroanatomy, Alan R. Liss, New York, pp. 17-44.
Curtis, D.R. and D. Felix (1971). Brain Res., 34, 301-321.
Desclin, J.C. and J. Escubi (1974). Brain Res., 77, 349-364.
Dilber, A., M. Cuénod, K. Winterhalter, H. Henke and R.W. Olsen (1982). Neurosc. Lett. Suppl. 10, S. 147
Felix, D. and H. Künzle (1976). Advances in Biochemical Psychopharma-cology, Raven Press, New York, pp. 165-173.
Fonnum, F. and H. Henke (1982). J. Neurochem., 38, 1130-1134.
Fonnum, F., J. Storm-Mathisen and F. Walberg (1970). Brain Res., 20, 259-275.
Fonnum, F. and F. Walberg (1973). Brain Res., 54, 115-127.

Griesser, C.A.V., M. Cuénod and H. Henke (1982). Brain Res. 246, 265-271.

Henke, H., A. Beaudet and M. Cuénod (1981). Brain Res., 219, 95-105.

Henke, H. and M. Cuénod (1979). Neurosci. Lett., 11, 341-345.

Henke, H. and M. Cuénod (1980). Neurotransmitters and their Receptors, John Wiley & Sons, New York, pp. 373-390.

Henke, H., T.M. Schenker and M. Cuénod (1976). J. Neurochem., 26, 131-134.

Hökfelt, T. and A. Ljungdahl (1972). Adv. Biochem. Psychopharmacol., 6, 1-36.

Hudson, D.B., T. Valcana, G. Bean and P.S. Timiras (1976). Neurochem. Res., 1, 73-81.

Kanfer, J.N. (1972). J. Lipid Res., 13, 468-476.

Llinas, R., K. Walton, D.E. Hillman and C. Sotelo (1975). Science, 190, 1230-1231.

McBride, W.J., M.H. Aprison and K. Kusano (1976a). J. Neurochem., 26, 867-870.

McBride, W.J., N.S. Nadi, J. Altman and M.H. Aprison (1976b). Neurochem. Res., 1, 141-152.

Nadi, N.S., D. Kauter, W.J. McBride and M.H. Aprison (1977). J. Neurochem., 28, 661-662.

Porcellati, G., G. Arienti, M.G. Pirotta and D. Giorgini (1971). J. Neurochem., 18, 1395-1417.

Rustioni, A. and M. Cuénod (1982). Brain Res., 236, 143-155.

Sandoval, M.E. and C.W. Cotman (1978). Neuroscience, 3, 199-206.

Streit, P. (1980). J. Comp. Neurol., 191, 429-463.

Streit, P., E. Knecht and M. Cuénod (1979). Science, 205, 306-308.

Streit, P., M. Stella and M. Cuénod (1980). Brain Res., 187, 47-57.

Toggenburger, G., D. Felix, M. Cuénod and H. Henke (1982). J. Neurochem., 39, 176-183.

Toggenburger, G., L. Wiklund, H. Henke and M. Cuénod (1983). subm.

Wiklund, L., G. Toggenburger and M. Cuénod (1982). Science, 216, 78-80.

Wiklund, L., G. Toggenburger and M. Cuénod (1983). submitted.

Wilkin, G.P., A. Csillag, R. Balazs, A.E. Kingsbury, J.E. Wilson and A.L. Johnson (1981). Brain Res., 216, 11-33.

Wolfensberger, M. (in press). In Measurement of Neurotransmitter Release in Vivo, John Wiley & Sons, New York.

Wolfensberger, M. and U. Amsler (1982). J. Neurochem., 38, 451-457.

Wolfensberger, M., U. Amsler, V. Canzek and M. Cuénod (1982a). J. Neurosc. Meth., 5, 253-260.

Wolfensberger, M., D. Felix and M. Cuénod (1982b). Neurosci. Lett., in press.

Wolfensberger, M., G. Toggenburger and M. Cuénod (1982c). Neurosc. Lett. Suppl. 10, S. 524/5.

Young, A.B., M.L. Oster-Granite, R.M. Herndon and S.H. Snyder (1974). Brain Res., 73, 1-13.

MECHANISMS OF EXCITOTOXINS EXAMINED IN ORGANOTYPIC CULTURES OF RAT CENTRAL NERVOUS SYSTEM

*WILLIAM O. WHETSELL, Jr., and **ROBERT SCHWARCZ

*Division of Neuropathology, University of Tennessee Center for the Health Sciences,
Memphis, TN 38163
**Maryland Psychiatric Research Center, University of Maryland School of Medicine,
Baltimore, MD 21228

INTRODUCTION

Six years ago, Coyle and Schwarcz (1976) and McGeer and McGeer (1976) reported that intrastriatal injections of the potent neuroexcitotoxin (see Olney, 1980), kainic acid (KA), produce axon-sparing neurodegenerative lesions in the striatum of the rat. Ablation of corticostriatal fibers before such injections abolished the neurotoxic effects of KA (McGeer et al, 1978; Biziere and Coyle, 1978). The consequences of KA administration have now been widely studied and the striatal lesion has been construed to represent an animal model for the neurodegenerative disorder, Huntington's disease (HD; Coyle et al, 1977; Fibiger, 1978). Our studies (Whetsell et al, 1979; Whetsell, 1979; Whetsell and Nicklas, 1980) in organotypic cultures of rat striatum (CA), striatum-plus-frontal cortex (CA-CX) and frontal cortex alone (CX), have demonstrated that the neurotoxic effects of KA can be observed only in CA-CX and CX cultures.

Because of certain structural similarities to KA, we have recently begun to evaluate, in vivo (Schwarcz et al, 1982; Schwarcz et al, this volume) and in vitro (present study and Whetsell and Schwarcz, 1982), the neurotoxic effects of the endogenous dicarboxylic amino acid, quinolinic acid (QUIN). This agent is an hepatic tryptophan metabolite with excitotoxic and convulsant properties (Lapin, 1978; Stone and Perkins, 1981; Schwarcz et al, 1982). The studies described here were designed to (a) investigate, in a comparative fashion, the neurotoxic qualities of KA and QUIN in organotypic cultures derived from different parts of the rat brain and (b) to examine whether the anti-neurotoxic properties of (-)2-amino-7-phosphonoheptanoic acid (-APH) which we have observed in the whole animal (Schwarcz et al, this volume) vis-a-vis QUIN, can be noted in vitro. In more general terms, the experiments reported in this paper were intended to explore the mechanisms involved in the specific neurotoxicity of KA and QUIN in our tissue culture systems and to critically evaluate the applicability of this in vitro model of nervous system for detailed scrutiny of excitotoxic actions.

METHODS

Preparation and handling of tissue cultures: Organotypic cultures of CA, CX,
CA-CX or hippocampus (HIP) were prepared from brains of newborn (12-24 hours old)
Sprague-Dawley rats. Animals were sacrificed by etherization, soaked in 80% ethanol for 10 minutes, and rinsed in two changes of balanced salt solution (Earle's
BSS). Brains were removed under sterile conditions and rinsed in Eagle's minimal
essential medium (MEM). A single complete coronal cut was made through the cerebrum with a No. 11 scalpel blade beginning on the dorsal aspect of the cerebrum
at the junction of the anterior and middle thirds. The anterior third of the
cerebrum was removed and discarded. On the cut surface of the remaining two-
thirds, the lateral ventricle, CA, centrum semiovale (immature), and overlying
CX of either cerebral hemisphere were clearly visible. The CA and an elongated
piece of the overlying CX were dissected out separately from either side and
placed in separate dissecting dishes in pools of MEM. These portions were then
further dissected under the dissecting microscope into smaller cube-shaped pieces,
each approximately 0.5 - 1.0 mm^3. Confirmation of proper dissection of CA could
be established by visualizing the distinctly striated microscopic appearance of
the individual cubes of tissue. CX could be separated from the underlying structures, including immature subcortical white matter, so that it was clear that the
CX cubes to be explanted were composed entirely of soft, homogeneous opalescent
densely cellular tissue in which no fibrous component was microscopically visible.

Dissection of HIP was carried out by lifting away the remaining CX from the hemisphere to expose the thalamus, bilaterally, and the caudal end of the HIP on the
lateral aspect of each thalamus. The HIP on either side was followed downward
and laterally with a blunt dissecting probe and scalpel. When the entire HIP had
been identified, the caudal (medial) end was severed, and the entire structure
was gently rolled away from the thalamus and cut free from its attachments along
the lateral ventricular wall. The cortex overlying the hippocampal formation
itself was next dissected away so that the hippocampal formation was then isolated.
It, like the CA and CX, was placed into a separate dissecting dish containing MEM.
Then cross-sections of HIP, each approximately 0.5 mm thick, were made across its
long axis. The characteristic sea-horse shape of each piece indicated the accuracy of the dissection. Only pieces showing that shape were used for culture.

After pieces of CA, CX and HIP were dissected, individual cultures were prepared
by placing dissected pieces in the desired combinations on individual round-glass
coverslips coated on one side with reconstituted rat-tail collagen. Each coverslip carried 0.05 ml of feeding medium composed of 10% 9-day chick embryo extract,
60% Eagle's MEM with glutamine added, 30% heat-inactivated human placental serum
and 0.6 % glucose (final concentration). The different kinds of cultures established were: CX cultures consisting of two pieces of CX only approximately 2 mm
apart; CA cultures made of two pieces of CA alone approximately 2 mm apart; CA-CX
cultures composed of one piece of CX centered on the coverslip and two pieces of
CA approximately 1 mm to either side of the central CX explant; and HIP cultures,
two pieces of HIP approximately 2 mm apart. Each coverslip carrying the explants
in feeding medium was then placed into a Maximow double-coverslip assembly, exposed to 5% CO_2 -95% room air mixture for five minutes, sealed and incubated at
34.5^{o}C. After five days incubation, the cultures were refed with nutritive medium and subsequently fed twice weekly. All cultures were studied sequentially
during development by direct light microscopic visualization (bright field optics).
They were washed only when there was visible evidence of significant sloughing of
cells as is occasionally observed with excessively large explants; generally this
procedure was not necessary.

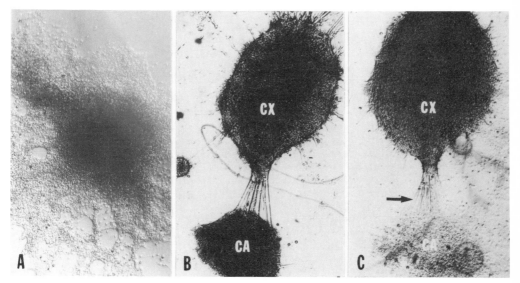

FIGURE 1: A. Light microscopic view of living CA culture. B. Light
microscopic appearance of CA–CX culture at five days in vitro.
(Mag. 260 X). Note fiber bridges between CX and CA. A single prominent fiber cable is seen between CX and a small fragment of CA,inadver-
tently broken away from larger CA during explantation. Mag. 260 X.
C. Same CA–CX culture at 21 days in vitro. CA has shown more spreading
and thinning than CX. Arrow denotes appearance of fiber bridges at
this age. (Mag. 260 X).

FIGURE 2: A. Light microscopic appearance of living HIP culture at 21
days in vitro. Light C–shaped zone (arrow) is interpreted as pyramidal
cell layer. Mag. 640 X. B. Higher magnification of HIP culture in
A. showing detail of pyramidal cell layer in living state. C. Appearance of HIP culture (whole-mount) stained with cresyl violet. Larger
arrow indicates pyramidal cell layer; smaller arrow indicates granule
cell layer. Mag. 200 X.

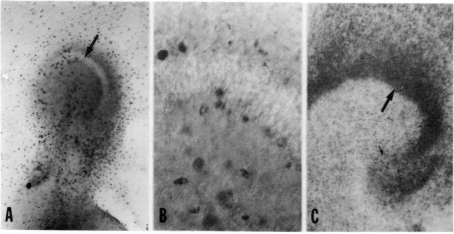

During development or after experimental treatment, cultures to be studied by
light microscopic histologic techniques were fixed by direct immersion of the
round glass coverslip (with culture attached) into a 10% buffered formalin solution at room temperature. These cultures were stained as whole-mount preparations
by taking the coverslip and its culture through appropriate procedures for Nissl
stain (cresyl violet), Palmgren's silver impregnation (Ecob-Johnson et al, 1978),
or Golgi stain (Toran-Allerand, 1976). Cultures to be studied by electron microscopy were fixed by immersion of culture-bearing coverslips into 2% glutaraldehyde
in phosphate buffer at 4°C (two hours), and post-fixed in 1% OsO_4 in phosphate
buffer at 4°C(one hour). They were dehydrated and embedded in Spurr embedding
medium (Polysciences, Warrington, PA.) still attached to the glass coverslips.
After polymerization of the epoxy resin, glass coverslips were removed. The embedded cultures were viewed by dissecting microscope and oriented for ultrami-
crotomy. In all cases individual explants were separated for sectioning so that
the individual regional components of the cultures, i.e., CA, CX or HIP could be
studied. Thick sections (0.5 microns) were cut and stained on glass slides with
0.1% aqueous toluidine blue stain for light microscopy, or thin sections (500 Å)
were cut, collected on copper grids, and stained with uranyl acetate-lead citrate
for electron microscopy. The sections for electron microscopy were always made
in the flat plane of the cultures so that larger areas could be studied and so
that the orientation of the sections was the same as that for the living cultures
or the whole-mount preparations.

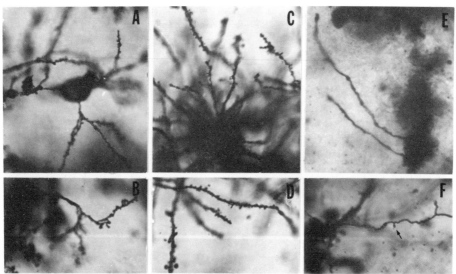

FIGURE 3: A. Light microscopic appearance of Golgi-stained neuron and
processes from CA of CA-CX culture at 21 days in vitro. Spiny projections on processes are interpreted as dendritic spines. B. Appearance
of Golgi-stained processes in CX portion of CA-CX culture at 21-days in
vitro. Dendritic spines are prominent on most Golgi-positive fibers.
C.& D. Golgi-stained fibers in two regions of a HIP culture at 20 days
in vitro.
E. & F. Appearance of Golgi-stained fibers from two different CA cultures
at 21 days in vitro. Poorly branched fibers show irregular surfaces but
only rare projections compatible with dendritic spines (arrow). Mag. of
all photographs = 600 X.

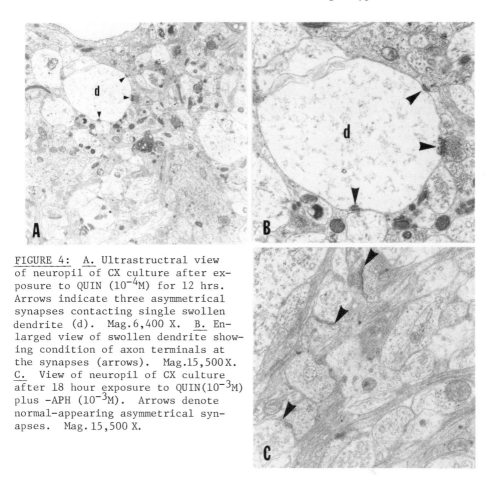

FIGURE 4: A. Ultrastructral view
of neuropil of CX culture after exposure to QUIN (10^{-4}M) for 12 hrs.
Arrows indicate three asymmetrical
synapses contacting single swollen
dendrite (d). Mag.6,400 X. B. Enlarged view of swollen dendrite showing condition of axon terminals at
the synapses (arrows). Mag.15,500X.
C. View of neuropil of CX culture
after 18 hour exposure to QUIN(10^{-3}M)
plus -APH (10^{-3}M). Arrows denote
normal-appearing asymmetrical synapses. Mag.15,500 X.

Experimental procedures: At 21 to 25 days in vitro, cultures were selected for
experimental exposure to either QUIN (10^{-3}, 10^{-4}or 10^{-5}M), nicotinic acid *(NIC,
10^{-3}, 10^{-4}or 10^{-5}M) or KA (10^{-4}). The amino acids were incorporated into the
usual nutritive medium, and selected cultures received the experimental solutions
by usual feeding procedures. Sibling control cultures received only nutritive
medium at the same time and under the same conditions as the experimental cultures.
When the cultures had received the experimental solution, they were replaced into
Maximow chambers and reincubated at 34.5°C for 1, 8, 12, 18 or 24 hours. At the
end of each of these time periods, some cultures were fixed and prepared for either
light or electron microscopic study. Two groups of cultures of CA-CX were incubated in QUIN ($10^{-3}$and 10^{-4}M) and KA (10^{-4}M) at seven days in vitro in order to
perform preliminary comparisons of the responses of less mature cultures to the
effects of these two amino acids. These cultures were studied only by electron
microscopy.

Other groups of 21 day-old cultures of CX, CA-CX and HIP were incubated in feeding
medium containing QUIN (10^{-3}or 10^{-4}M) plus equimolar or ten-fold less amounts of

----

*NIC, the major metabolite of QUIN, differs structurally from QUIN only in the loss
of one carboxyl group. It was used as a control for specificity of QUIN neurotoxicity.

-APH (kindly supplied by Dr. James Collins, London). These cultures were fixed and prepared for either light or electron microscopy at the same time intervals and by the same procedures as cultures incubated in either QUIN, NIC or KA alone.

RESULTS

Growth and development of cultures: Each of the different components of the cultures, i.e., CX, CA or HIP, showed different characteristic architectural growth patterns. As we have previously described (Whetsell et al, 1979), CA cultures showed a tendency to flatten into an irregular aggregate of closely-packed small round or ovoid cells with occasional stubby bundles of fibers projecting for short distances in a mat-like arrangement around the central explant (Fig. 1A). The CX cultures did not show as great a tendency to flatten and spread and instead retained a somewhat thicker, more dense central explant in which cellular detail was less distinct. At the edges, numerous neurites projected around the CX explant in a fine-fibrillar sun-burst array growing out as much as 1 mm by four to five days in vitro. In the combination CA-CX cultures, in as few as four days in vitro, fibers originating in the CX cultures approached and penetrated the edges of the CA cultures, bridging the approximately 1 mm distance between the explants. CX fibers appeared to grow directly to the CA explants (Fig. 1B), often to the apparent exclusion of the more generalized outgrowth in all directions which was seen in cultures of CX alone. It is not clear whether CA outgrowth fibers make contact with CX explants in CA-CX cultures since fiber crossings from CA to CX were never seen to develop before CX fibers had crossed to CA. After the initial bridging occurred in these cultures, the space between the explants was quickly (two days) filled with an indistinct fiber network (see also Fig. 1C).

In HIP cultures, throughout the development, explants retained the characteristic sea-horse configuration while fiber outgrowth occurred all around the explant in a radiation of long, thin neurites; bundles of fibers were not observed to develop around the explants. From the time of explanatation, a distinct C-shaped lighter zone could be observed in the living cultures which, by 21 days in vitro, could be distinguished as a zone of closely-packed well-developed large, pyramidal-shaped cells, considered to represent the pyramidal cell layer of the hippocampus (Fig. 2 A & B). A distinct zone representing granule cells of the HIP could not be identified in the living cultures.

Histologic studies: Fixed whole-mount preparations of CA cultures stained for Nissl substance (cresyl violet stain) demonstrated abundant closely-packed Nissl-positive cells compatible with the appearance of nerve cells of different sizes. Palmgren's silver stain confirmed the presence of abundant nerve cells and neurites (Whetsell et al, 1979). Likewise, CX cultures stained with cresyl violet displayed thick aggregates of Nissl-positive cells, but individual cellular detail

FIGURE 5: A. Electron microscopic appearance of neuropil of CA portion of 21-day CA-CX culture after 18 hours exposure to QUIN (10^{-4}M)·Mag.6,400X. Arrows show asymmetrical synapses associated with swollen dendrites (d). B. Detail of synapse of one swollen dendrite (d) from A. Mag. 15,000X. C. Detail for swollen dentrite (d) and associated asymmetrical synapse (arrow) in CA portion of CA-CX culture exposed to KA (10^{-4}M) for one hour. Mag. 15,000X. D. Appearance of CA portion of CA-CX culture at 21 days in vitro following 18 hours exposure to NIC (10^{-4}M). Mag. 15,000X. E. Appearance of neuropil of CA portion of 21-day CA-CX culture following exposure to QUIN (10^{-4}M) plus -APH (10^{-4}M) for 18 hours. Appearance is identical to that of normal control not shown. Arrows indicate most of the asymmetrical synapses found in this field. F. Enlarged view of neuropil from E. showing detail of asymmetrical synapses (arrows). Mag. 15,000X.

FIGURE 5

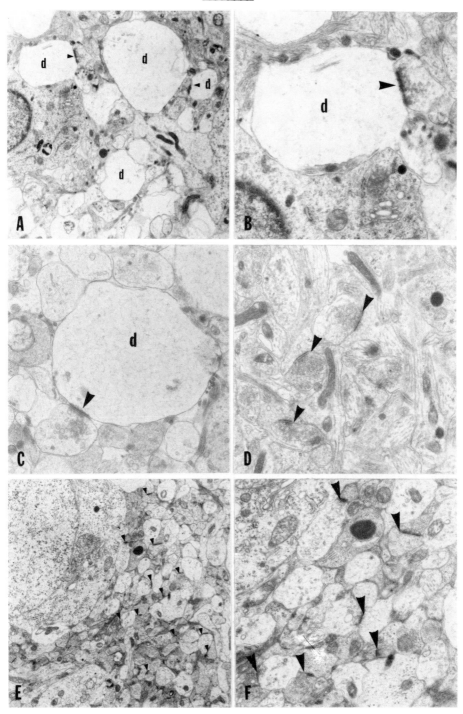

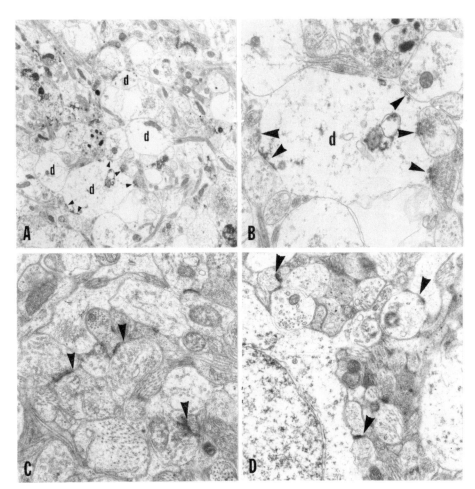

FIGURE 6: A. Ultrastructural appearance of neuropil of HIP culture
following exposure to QUIN (10^{-4}M) for 12 hours. Arrows point out
synapses on a swollen dendrite (d). Mag. 6,400 X. B. Detail of swollen
dendrite in A. Arrows denote five asymmetrical synapses with undisturbed
axon terminals. Mag. 15,500X. C. Appearance of HIP culture neuropil
after 24 hrs. incubation in NIC (10^{-4}M). Arrows show asymmetrical synapses of normal appearance. Top arrow demonstrates a probable axospinous
synapse. Mag. 15,000X. D. HIP culture after 18 hours exposure to QUIN
(10^{-3}M) and -APH (10^{-3}M). Mag. 15,500X. Arrows indicate asymmetrical synapses.

was not as distinct in the thicker CX cultures. Nissl stain of HIP cultures demonstrated at least two distinct zones of Nissl-positive cells each forming a more
or less C-shaped line, the C-shaped lines roughly interlocking in most cultures
(Fig. 2C). Of these two lines of cells, one was always more prominent because
of the larger size and the abundance of the cells composing it. This line of
larger more distinct cells was interpreted in these preparations as the pyramidal
cell layer corresponding to the pyramidal cell layer observed in the living cultures.

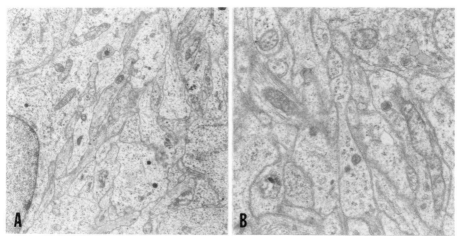

FIGURE 7:   A. General ultrastructural view of untreated CA culture.
Mag. 6,400 X.   B.   Appearance of CA culture neuropil after incubation
in QUIN (10^{-3}M) for 18 hours. Mag.15,500X. Note lack of synaptic
complexes in either view.

In the Golgi preparations of CX, CA-CX and HIP cultures, impregnation of nerve
cells and processes clearly showed presence of well-developed dendritic branching
and dendritic spines (Fig. 3A, B, C, D).   In contrast, cultures of CA alone demonstrated a paucity of Golgi-stained fibers, the most prominent of which appeared
as smooth, poorly-branched processes.   The processes that were present showed
some irregularity, but clear patterns indicating dendritic spines were rarely observed (Fig. 3E, F).

Ultrastructural studies: Electron microscopic study, limited in this description
to observations in neuropil, showed abundant synapse formation in CX, CA-CX(both
components) and HIP cultures (Fig. 4,5,6).   However, in CA cultures alone, there
was a severe reduction, by comparison, in the number of synaptic complexes(Fig.7A).
Closer study of synapses in all types of cultures disclosed abundant asymmetrical
synapses,in some cases clearly axospinous, in CX, CA-CX and HIP cultures while the
occasional synapses seen in the cultures of CA alone appeared as axodendritic or
axosomatic synapses.

Effects of exposure to amino acids: Our previous studies of effects of KA upon
CA, CX or CA-CX cultures (Whetsell et al, 1979; Whetsell & Nicklas, 1980) have
indicated that while exposure to KA for up to 48 hours produced severe disruption
in CX and CA-CX cultures, no such changes were observed in cultures of CA alone
either by light or electron microscopy. As shown here, shorter (as little as one
hour) exposure to KA (10^{-4}M), resulted in swelling and clearing of the postsynaptic elements at asymmetrical synapses in the CX or CA-CX cultures as the first
sign of disruption (Fig 5C).   At later times (12, 18 or 24 hours), tissue disruption was so severe that identification of synapses or other normal components
of neuropil was not possible (not shown here).   HIP cultures exposed to KA (10^{-4}M)
for one to five hours showed changes in neuropil like those seen in CX and CA-CX
cultures after one hour, specifically postsynaptic swelling involving asymmetrical
synapses (Fig. 6A, B).   After 12, 18, or 24 hours, HIP cultures appeared to be so
generally disrupted that only rare synaptic profiles could be identified.   When
they were seen, the postsynaptic element showed marked swelling or sometimes rup-
ture while the presynaptic component was still relatively intact (not shown here).

Similar severe disruption and swelling of neuropil structures in CX, CA-CX and
HIP cultures was seen at 24 hours exposure to QUIN (10^{-3}, 10^{-4} or 10^{-5}M). However,
at 12 hours incubation in QUIN (10^{-4} or 10^{-5}M), it was clear that the most pronounced change from the normal ultrastructural appearance of the neuropil in CX,
CA-CX or HIP cultures was a prominent dendritic swelling and clearing at asymmetrical synapses while the presynaptic elements in these cultures were usually
undisturbed(Fig. 4A&B, 5A&B, 6A&B). The appearance was identical to that seen in
such cultures exposed to KA for one to five hours in that the axon terminal, the
synaptic cleft and the postsynaptic density were still morphologically intact
while the dendrite itself was severely altered by swelling. Occasionally, dilated
cisternal structures similar to those observed in whole animal (Schwarcz et al,
this volume) could be observed in the swollen dendrites, but no clearly identi-
fiable characteristics of dendritic spines could be seen. Cultures of CA alone,
exposed to QUIN for the same periods showed no detectable alterations compared to
control sibling cultures of CA alone (Fig. 7B). Cultures of CX, CA-CX and CA
alone and HIP exposed to NIC (10^{-3}M or lower) for up to 24 hours showed no evidence of disruption. Synaptic structures as well as the rest of the neuropil
showed no morphologic changes compared to control sibling cultures (Fig. 5D,6C).

Though a thorough comparison of the relative potencies of the neurotoxicity of
KA and QUIN in cultures at three weeks of age is incomplete, it can be said that
the earlist evidence for neurotoxicity of KA (10^{-4}M), described above, was visible ultrastructurally after one hour's incubation. The same morphological changes
also described above, in response to QUIN (10^{-3} or 10^{-4}M) were not distinct until
12 hours of incubation; for QUIN (10^{-5}M), earliest changes occurred between 12 and
18 hours.

Cultures which were simultaneously exposed to QUIN (10^{-3}M) and -APH (10^{-3} or 10^{-4}M)
showed no detectable ultrastructural changes (see Fig. 6,7). Careful scrutiny
of numerous synaptic complexes in CX, CA-CX and HIP cultures produced no evidence
of morphological alterations from the normal appearance.

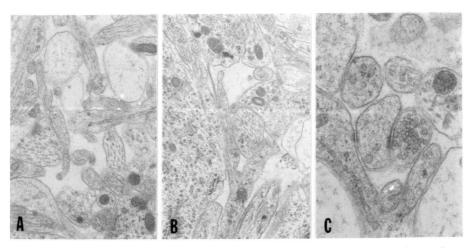

FIGURE 8: A. Ultrastructural appearance of CA portion of seven-day culture
of CA-CX after 16 hours of incubation in QUIN (10^{-4}M). Mag.14,600 X.
B. Appearance of CX in same CA-CX culture shown in A. Note that no appar-
ent disturbance of normal but immature morphology can be observed.
Mag.14,600X. C. Detail of one of the rare immature synapses observed in
CX but not CA of the culture shown in A. and B. Mag.34,000X.

Preliminary studies on immature cultures of CA-CX have been begun. In seven-day old cultures of CA-CX in which connecting fiber bridges originating from the CX explant had been distinctly observed, exposure to KA (10^{-4}M) or to QUIN (10^{-3}or 10^{-4}M) for sixteen hours resulted in no detectable disruption of neuropil of either CA (Fig. 8A) or CX (Fig. 8B). In the CA portion of these cultures no clear evidence of synaptogenesis was observed morphologically. In the CX portions of these cultures, occasional immature synapses could be found (Fig. 8C) in which vesicles were beginning to aggregate and a thin but definite postsynaptic thickening could be seen.

DISCUSSION

In organotypic cultures of different parts of the mammalian (rat) central nervous system (CNS), we have studied the effects of two structurally closely related dicarboxylic amino acids, KA and QUIN. Organotypic nerve tissue culture techniques seem particularly well-suited for these studies since they permit interaction and experimental manipulation of living and developing, yet isolated and controllable, regions of CNS. Because of the relative inaccessibility of the intact animal nervous system, organotypic cultures of central or peripheral nervous tissues have been considered to constitute an important experimental model for the investigation of certain neurobiological and neuropathological questions (Bornstein, 1973; Raine, 1973; Whetsell, 1979).

In the course of the present study, a new concept regarding the mechanism of neurotoxicity of excitatory amino acids has begun to emerge through the use of this tissue culture model: evidence is presented here for the dependency of KA- and QUIN-neurotoxicity upon the presence of normal synaptic patterns. An additional observation which has evolved in these studies is that the development of normal synaptogenesis may depend upon appropriate interaction of tissue components, presumably neurons.

Analysis of our tissue culture systems at the light microscopic level has indicated that when isolated from input from other parts of the CNS, CA of the rat shows a deficiency in the development of dendritic spines. Analysis of the same systems by electron microscopy demonstrates the while CX, CA-CX and HIP develop extensive normal-appearing synaptic complexes, CA grown in isolation shows a paucity of synaptic development. Furthermore, in all cultures except CA alone, many synaptic complexes show an appearance compatible with that of axospinous synapses.

In whole animal studies of rat, cat and monkey, it has been shown that a large number of the presynaptic elements within the striatum originate extrastriatally, namely in cerebral cortex, thalamus and substantia nigra (Kemp and Powell, 1971; Hattori and McGeer, 1973; Carpenter, 1975; Pasik et al, 1976). Kemp and Powell (1971) have indicated that synapses showing symmetrical contacts ultrastructurally are formed by intrinsic presynaptic elements while extrinsic presynaptic elements may form either symmetrical or asymmetrical contacts. In quantative morphological studies in the striatum of the monkey, 82% of synapses were axospinous (Pasik et al, 1976); further, 92% of axospinous synapses were found to be asymmetrical. Hattori and McGeer (1973) showed that in the developing striatum of the rat, only rare asymmetrical synapses are present until about two weeks after birth. Therefore, the observation that there is abnormal synaptogenesis in CA isolated during development from extrinsic input (Whetsell et al, 1979; Panula et al, 1979) is not surprising. The observation suggests that extrastriatal regions of the brain, for example the cerebral cortex, may influence the normal development of the complex synaptic structure in the striatum. It is intriguing to speculate about the role of the putative neurotransmitter glutamate (GLU) in this phenomenon: GLU-containing nerve cells, apparently not intrinsic in but projecting to the striatum from the cerebral cortex (Divac et al, 1977; Kim et al, 1977), may exert some influence upon the process of synaptogenesis. In our cultures, CX cultures, probably containing glutamatergic neurons, as well as HIP cultures, also probably containing glutamatergic neurons even if isolated from CX (Cotman and Nadler, 1981), are capable of developing normal synapses in vitro. In contrast, the typical synaptic appearance of striatum was accorded to CA in vitro only when it was permitted to develop in combination with CX. Our preliminary studies of CA and CX in CA-CX cultures at seven days in vitro show no demonstrable synapse formation in CA but early synapse formation in CX, observations compatible with the in vitro findings of Hattori and McGeer (1973).

It is the postsynaptic element in these various culture systems which seems to show the earliest degenerative change following exposure to either KA or QUIN. According to the excitotoxic hypothesis (see Olney, 1980), postsynaptic receptors are involved in initiation of the neurotoxic effects of KA and related amino acids. Our observations suggest that a similar mechanism may be involved following exposure to QUIN. Since neither KA- nor QUIN-induced neurodegenerative changes were observed in CA cultures or in seven-day old CA-CX cultures in which there is little or no mature synapse formation, it appears that the presence of the synaptic complexes and perhaps in particular those of the axospinous type, may be necessary in order for the neurotoxic effects of either of the two compounds to occur. It therefore seems reasonable to postulate that certain synaptic complexes develop a selective postsynaptic vulnerability to KA and QUIN as a function of their normal development.

Tissue culture systems have been previously employed to study the possible relationship between KA-neurotoxicity and GLU or GLU receptors (Seil et al, 1981). While it had originally been suggested that KA and GLU interact with the same receptors (Simon et al, 1976), multiple evidence against this concept has accumulated since (see Watkins, 1981, for review). Our recent data (Schwarcz et al, this volume) indicates that QUIN, too, lacks affinity to GLU receptors and that it appears to be equally inactive at specific binding sites for ^{3}H-kainate. The present results, using the selective amino acid anagonist -APH (Perkins et al, 1981; Evans et al, 1982), suggest that QUIN acts at a specific postsynaptic site which is pharmacologically closely related to the well-established N-methyl-D-asparate receptor (Watkins, 1981). However, because of its possible roles in synaptogenesis (see above) and in the mediation of KA-neurotoxicity (McGeer et al, 1978; Biziere and Coyle, 1978), a synergistic action of GLU and QUIN at QUIN receptors must also be taken into consideration. Such interactions have been shown to exist between KA and GLU in the cerebellum (London and Coyle, 1979; Foster and Roberts, 1981) and would certainly conform conceptually to the data presented here.

In summary,our in vitro studies indicate that the neurotoxicity of both KA and QUIN is intimately related to appropriate synaptogenesis in regions in which these agents induce a neurodegenerative effect. Taken together with our in vivo studies (Schwarcz et al, this volume), the evidence suggests that the endogenous tryptophan metabolite, QUIN, should be considered for further investigation as an endogenous agent capable of inducing selective neurodegeneration morphologically similar to that observed with the exogenous experimental agent, KA, and to that seen in the human neurodgenerative disorder, HD. Additionally, the potent antagonism of QUIN by -APH, both in vitro and in vivo, indicates that the mechanisms related to the prevention of excitotoxic nerve cell degeneration may be successfully investigated in our test systems.

ACKNOWLEDGEMENTS

This work is supported by USPHS grant number NS-16941. The authors gratefully acknowledge the expert assistance of Ms. Jana Brady, Ms. Mary Margaret James, Mr. Frank Moretta and Ms. Alice Rome.

REFERENCES

Biziere, K., and J.T. Coyle (1978): Neurosci. Lett., 8:303-310.
Bornstein, M.D. (1973): In: Progress in Neuropathology (H. Zimmerman, ed.). Vol. II, pp. 69-90, Grune & Stratton, New York.
Carpenter, M.B. (1976): In: Human Neuroanatomy. Seventh edition, pp. 496-520, Waverly, Baltimore.
Cotman, C.W., and J.V. Nadler (1981): In: Glutamate: Transmitter in the Central Nervous System (P.J. Roberts, J. Storm-Mathisen and G.A.R. Johnston, eds.), pp. 117-154, Wiley, New York.
Coyle, J.T., and R. Schwarcz (1976): Nature, 263:244-246.
Coyle, J.T., R. Schwarcz, J.P. Bennett and P. Campochiaro (1977): Progr. Neuro-Psychopharmac., 1:13-30.
Divac, O., F. Fonnum and J. Storm-Mathisen (1977): Nature, 266:377-388.
Ecob-Johnston, M.S., J. Schwarcz, T.S. Elizan and W.O. Whetsell, Jr. (1978): J. Neuropath. Exp. Neurol., 37(5):518-530.
Evans, R.H., A.A. Francis, A.W. Jones, D.A.S. Smith and J.C. Watkins (1982): Br. J. Pharmac., 75:65-75.
Fibiger, H.C. (1978): In: Kainic Acid as a Tool in Neurobiology (D.G. McGeer, J.W. Olney and P.L. McGeer, eds.), pp. 161-176, Raven, New York.
Foster, G.A., and P.J. Roberts (1981): Neurosci. Lett., 23:67-70.
Hattori, T., and E.G. McGeer (1977): Brain Res., 129:174-180.
Kemp, J.M., and T.P.S. Powell (1971): Philos. Trans. R. Soc. Land. (Biol.), 262:413-427.
Kim, J.S., R. Hassler, P. Haug and K.S. Paik (1977): Brain Res., 132:370-374.
Lapin, I.P. (1978): J. Neural Transm. 42:37-43, 1978.
London, E.D., and J.T. Coyle (1979): Eur. J. Pharmac., 56:287-290.
McGeer, E.G., and P.L. McGeer (1976): Nature, 263:517-519.
McGeer, E.G., P.L. McGeer P.L. and K. Singh (1978): Brain Res., 139:381-383.
Olney, J.W. (1980): In: Experimental and Clinical Neurotoxicology (P.S. Spencer and J.H. Schaumburg, eds.), pp. 272-294. Williams & Wilkins, Baltimore.
Panula P., L. Rechardt and H. Hervonen (1979): Neuroscience, 4:1441-1452.
Pasik, P., T. Pasik and M. Difiglia (1976): In: ARNMD Research Publications, Vol. 55: The Basal Ganglia (Yahr, M.D., ed), pp. 57-89, Raven,New York.
Perkins, M.N., T.W. Stone, J.F. Collins and K. Curry (1981): Neurosci. Lett., 23:333-336.
Raine, C. (1973): In: Advances in Neuropathology (H. Zimmerman, ed.), Vol.II, pp. 27-68, Grune and Stratton, New York.
Schwarcz, R., W.O. Whetsell, Jr. and R.M. Mangano (1982): Science, in press.
Seil, F.J., N.K. Blank, W.R. Woodward and A.L. Leiman (1981): Adv. Biochem. Psychopharmac., 27:347-354.
Simon, J.R., J.F. Contera and M.J. Kuhar (1976): J. Neurochem., 26:141-147.
Stone, T.W., and M.N. Perkins (1981): Eur. J. Pharmac., 72:411-412.
Toran-Allerand, C.D. (1976): Brain Res., 118:293-298.
Watkins, J.C. (1981): In: Glutamate: Transmitter in the Central Nervous System, (P.J. Roberts, J. Storm-Mathisen and G.A.R. Johnston, eds.), pp. 1-24, Wiley, New York.
Whetsell, W.O., Jr., M.S.Ecob-Johnston and W.J. Nicklas (1979): Advances in Neurol., 23:645-654.
Whetsell, W.O., Jr. (1979): In: Proceedings of Fifth Science Symposium, Food and Drug Admin., pp. 117-125.
Whetsell, W.O., Jr. and R. Schwarcz (1982): Soc. Neurosci. abstr., 8(1):404.
Whetsell, W.O., Jr. and W.J. Nicklas (1980): J. Neuropath. Exp. Neurol., 39:395.

Session III

EXCITOTOXINS AS TOOLS IN NEUROSCIENCE

Chairman: J. T. Coyle

IBOTENATE AS A TOOL IN NEUROBIOLOGY. STUDIES ON DOPAMINERGIC AND CHOLECYSTOKININ IMMUNOREACTIVE NEURONS AFTER IBOTENATE INDUCED LESIONS

K. FUXE[*], L. F. AGNATI[**], P. FREY[***], C. KÖHLER[*****], M. F. CELANI[*], K. ANDERSSON[*], N. BATTISTINI[**], C. FARABEGOLI[**] and R. SCHWARCZ[****]

[*]Department of Histology, Karolinska Institute, Stockholm, Sweden
[**]Departments of Human Physiology and Endocrinology, University of Modena, Modena, Italy
[***]Wander Research Institute, (a Sandoz Research Unit) Bern, Switzerland
[****]Maryland Psych., Res. Center, Neurosci. Program, Baltimore, Maryland, U.S.A.
[*****]Astra Res. Lab. Södertälje, Sweden

ABSTRACT

Ibotenate striatal pyriform and hippocampal lesions have again been shown to produce highly localized lesions with absence of distant lesions. The results amplify the view that the use of ibotenate lesions in combination with biochemistry, quantitative microfluorimetry and receptor autoradiography open up new ways to morphofunctional characterize central neurons under normal and experimental conditions as illustrated in the present analysis on DA and CCK immunoreactive neurons.

KEYWORDS

Ibotenic acid; kainic acid; dopamine; CCK-8; CCK-4; receptor autoradiography; dopamine receptors; glutamate receptors; aminefluorescence histochemistry

INTRODUCTION

Previous studies in this laboratory (Schwarcz et al., 1979a,b,d) have shown that ibotenic acid may represent a new tool in the morphological and functional characterization of central neuron systems. Thus, as a neurotoxin ibotenic acid unlike kainic acid, does not produce distant lesions and it possesses less general toxicity than kainic acid. Therefore, it has been possible to obtain very restricted lesions by intracerebral injections of ibotenic acid, which like kainic acid does not damage axons of passage and nerve terminals of extrincic origin. A large number of studies indicate that the neurotoxic mechanism of ibotenic acid is different from that of kainic acid (Köhler et al., 1971a,b, Coyle et al., 1981, Roberts et al., 1981). Studies on ^{3}H-kainic acid binding sites (Schwarcz and Fuxe 1979, Coyle et al., 1981) have e.g., shown that while ibotenic acid has little affinity for these binding sites, it shows unlike kainic acid a substantial affinity for the ^{3}H-glutamate binding sites (see Roberts et al., 1981). Furthermore, studies on the hippocampus have provided histological evidence that ibotenic acid, produces degeneration of CA-3 and CA-4 pyramidal cells and of granule cells to an equal extent (Köhler et al., 1979), which is in contrast to the selective vulnerability of CA-3/CA-4 cells to kainic acid

223

toxicity. Furthermore, unlike kainic acid, ibotenic acid is not dependent upon an intact glutamatergic transmission in order to produce its toxic effects. In view of these findings it has been suggested that ibotenic acid may produce its neurotoxic activity through interfering directly with the glutamate receptor (see Coyle et al., 1981).

Previous studies have shown that striatal kainic lesions may provide an animal model for Huntington's disease (Coyle and Schwarcz 1976, McGeer and McGeer, 1976). We have been especially interested in the changes in pre- and postsynaptic mechanisms in striatal dopamine (DA) nerve terminal systems following such lesions in view of previous suggestions that dopaminergic hyperactivity may be the main factor in producing the involuntary movements of Huntington's disease. Previous studies have shown that two days following the lesion striatal DA turnover and levels are increased (Andersson et al., 1980, Schwarcz et al., 1979c). Ten days following the lesion striatal DA turnover is instead reduced on both the intact and on the lesioned side following unilateral kainic acid induced striatal lesions. Thus, a compensatory biological change has taken place. Such mechanisms can in part be responsible for the maintenance of symmetrical motor behaviour in unilaterally lesioned animals (see Andersson et al., 1980). However, following striatal lesions with KA there is a marked reduction in the number of DA receptors and a very marked reduction in the DA sensitive adenylate cyclase activity (see Schwarcz et al., 1978, Govini et al., 1978), Therefore, changes in DA release cannot be the only mechanism involved in the return of symmetry following striatal lesions with KA. In view of the demonstrated loss of DA receptors following striatal kainate lesions dopaminergic hyperactivity can probably only induce choreatic movements in the early phase of Huntington's disease, when DA receptors are still present and DA turnover is enhanced.

In the present paper we have analyzed if striatal ibotenate lesions produce a similar time-course of changes in DA activity in the striatum as seen after kainic acid (see above). Ibotenate induced lesions have also been used to further characterize the cholecystokinin (CCK) immunoreactive neurons of the brain. This problem has been evaluated by studying if ibotenate induced lesions in the pyriform cortex and in the s triatum can differentially effect CCK-8, nonsulfated CCK-8 and CCK-4 levels in striatum and pyriform cortex (Dockray et al., 1978, Rehfeld et al., 1978, Frey 1982). Finally, it has also been tested by means of receptor autoradiography if ibotenate induced lesions of the piriform cortex and of the dorsal hippocampus change the postsynaptic properties of striatal DA neurons and glutamate pathways respectively, by the use of the radioligands, ^{3}H-spiperone and ^{3}H-N-propylnorapomorphine (^{3}H-NPA) for DA receptors and ^{3}H-glutamate receptors.

MATERIAL AND METHODS

Male specific pathogen free Sprague-Dawley rats were used. They were given food pellets and water ad libitum and were kept under regular day and night conditions (lights on at 6.00 a.m. and off at 8.00 p.m.). The following types of experiments have been performed:

1. The Effects of unilateral ibotenate striatal lesions on DA levels and turnover

Ten days before the experiment a group of 12 rats was injected with ibotenic acid dissolved in phosphate buffered saline (PBS) (10 µg/µl). 0.5 µl was injected at four different positions within the striatum using the following coordinates: A 9.0; L: 3.0; V: +2.0 and 0.0 and A: 8.0; L: 3,0; V: +1.5 and -0.5 (see Fuxe et al., 1979). In another group of 12 rats the solvent was injected in the same way. Ten days after the lesion the rats were decapitated and the telencephalon disected out and taken to aminefluorescence histochemistry (see Fuxe et al., 1980). The DA fluorescence observed in sections of the telencephalon was measured by means of quantitative microfluorimetry (Löfström et al., 1976, Agnati et al., 1979) making it possible to determine DA levels in discrete areas of the striatum and express them into pmol/g wet weight. The measurements were made at the level A 8500 according to König and Klippel (1963). The striatal DA stores were measured in the marginal zone, in the medial part and in the central part of the caudate. The measurements were made both on the lesioned and on the contralateral side. The same type of measurements were also made in animals injected with solvent on one side. A possible change in DA turnover was studied by means of the tyrosine hydroxylase inhibition model. α-methyl tyrosine methylester (H44/68, 250 mg/kg, i.p.) was administered 2 h before killing in half of the lesioned animals and in half of the animals injected with PBS.

For comparison the effects of unilateral kainate striatal lesions have been studied on DA levels and turnover on the lesioned and contralateral side (see Andersson et al., 1980). Briefly, kainic acid (1µg in 0.5 µl phosphate buffered saline, pH 7.4) was infused unilaterally into the neostriatum (coordinates: 7.9 A; 2.6 L; 4.8 V) (see Andersson et al., 1980). The rats were killed 2 and 10 days after the lesion. The telecephalon was processed for the cellular demonstration of catecholamines as described above. After the measurements of DA fluorescence had taken place, the sections were stained with cresyl violet to evaluate the extent of the lesion in the light microscope.

2. Effects of ibotenate striatal lesions and ibotenate pyriform lesions on the CCK contents in the striatum

The striatal ibotenate lesions were performed unilaterally as described above and the rats were killed 10 days following the operation. 16 rats were injected with ibotenic acid and 16 rats were injected with PBS. The CCK peptides were extracted by homogenization in 5 - 10 parts (W/V) of icecold 90 % methanol using a teflon potter homogenizer. The homogenate was centrifuged and evaporated under nitrogen. The method of Frey (1982) was used to separate different CCK peptides (CCK-8, CCK-8 nonsulfated and CCK-4) on HPLC and to measure their concentration by radioimmunoassay (RIA).

The unilateral pyriform ibotenate lesions were performed stereotaxically by infusing into the piriform cortex ibotenate (5 µg in 0.5 µl phosphate buffered saline, pH 7.4) at each of the following locations: 7.4 A; 4.7 L; -2.7 V (coordinates according to König and Klippel), 6.6 A; 5.0 L; -3.0 V and 4.6 A; 5.0 L; -3.2 V. 10 days after the operation the rats were decapitated. The striatum and the pyriform cortex were rapidly dissected out, and the CCK peptides were separated by HPLC and their concentrations measured by RIA as described above (Frey, 1982). As controls served rats which were injected with PBS alone as described above. The extent of the pyriform lesion was determined by processing some brains for morphological analysis by light microscopy using a cresyl violet staining procedure to study the nerve cell bodies.

CCK immunoreactivity in the pyriform cortex was also studied by means of immunohistochemistry, using antibodies raised against CCK-8 and the PAP technique (see Köhler et al., 1982). The rats were perfused through the ascending aorta with a 5% (W/V) surcrose-buffer solution immediately followed by a fixative (500 ml) consisting of 4% paraformaldehyde in 0.1 M phosphate buffer (pH 7.4). The fixed brains were cut on a Vibratom (Oxford instruments) and individual 70-120 µm thick sections were collected in test-tubes containing phosphate buffered saline (PBS). After extensive washing the sections were incubated free floating with an antiserum to CCK-8. (Immunonuclear corporation), diluted 1:1800 in PBS containing 1% goat serum (in PBS) for 2-3 days. Control sections were incubated either with non-immune serum or CCK-8 antiserum preabsorbed with CCK-8 (Peninsula laboratories). (100 μg/CCK-8/ml diluted antiserum). The antibody-antigen complex was visualized using the peroxidase-antiperoxidase (PAP) method of Sternberger (1979). After reaction with diaminobenzidine and H_2O_2 the sections were defatted and coverslipped.

3. Effects of unilateral pyriform ibotenate lesions on ^{3}H-NPA binding and ^{3}H-spiperone binding in the striatum as evaluated by receptor autoradiography

The ibotenate lesions of the pyriform cortex were made as described above. 10 days following the lesion the rats were perfused with 0.1 M phosphate buffer containing 0.1 % formaldehyde. Coronal sections of the telencephalon were cut in a cryostat (Dittes, Heidelberg) immediately following the perfusion. 14 μm thick coronal sections were made and incubated with ^{3}H-spiperone (30.0 Ci/mmol, NEN, Boston, Massachussetts, U.S.A) to label the DA receptors of the D_2 type (see Seeman, 1980). The concentration used was 0.75 nM. The sections were incubated for 10 min at +37° C. For details on the assay buffer used, see Creese et al., (1977). Unspecific binding was determined by assessing autoradiograms of adjacent sections after incubation with ^{3}H-spiperone in the presence of 10^{-6} M (+)butaclamol. The sections were rapidly washed in cold buffer (2 washes) followed by a last wash in distilled water. The sections were taken from various rostrocaudal levels of the teldiencephalon (see Results). Other coronal sections taken at various rostrocaudal levels were incubated with ^{3}H-NPA (60.0 Ci/mmol, NEN, Boston, Masachussetts, U.S.A) in a concentration of 1.3 nM in order to label the agonist prefering sites of the DA receptors (see Seeman, 1980). Incubation with ^{3}H-NPA took place during 30 min at room temperature. Washing was performed as described above.

The slides in the dried labelled sections were fixed onto the inner surface of a 10 x 12 inch large Siemens-Elema film cassette by means of a double sided Scotch brand tape. ^{3}H-Ultrofilm (LKB, Stockholm, Sweden) was opposed to the object glasses under dark conditions, after which the film cassette was stored at +4° C for a period of 3 weeks. Development was made at +20° C for 5 min using a D-19 Kodak developer (undiluted). After rinsing, fixation was made by immersion of the film in a Kodak rapid fixer at room temperature for 5 min. The films were then again rinsed for about 20 min at room temperature and dried.

4. Effects of unilateral ibotenate hippocampal lesions on ^{3}H-glutamate binding in the hippocampus as evaluated by receptor autoradiography

Ibotenic acid was injected stereotaxically into the hippocampus in a concentration of 5 μg/0.5 μl. Two injections were made at the following coordinates (250 g rats): -1.8 behind bregma; 1.5 mm from the midline; 3.2 beneath the dura mater, and 2.5 mm behind bregma; 3.4 below dura mater. The rats were perfused with icecold 0.1 M phosphate buffer containing 0.1 % formaldehyde. Immediately after the perfusion the diencephalon was cut in a cryostat (Dittes, Heidelberg) as described above. The sections were incubated with a solution contaning ^{3}H-glutamate (44 Ci/mmol; Amersham, England) in a concentration of 100 nM. Tris-HCl buffer (50 mM; pH 7.4) containing 1 mM of calcium chloride was used, and the sections were incubated for 15 min at room temperature (see Roberts, 1981). Unspecific binding was defined as the binding in the presence of l-glutamate in a concentration of 10^{-4} M. A very rapid washing of the sections was performed with cold buffer. For the preparations of the autoradiograms, see above.

The extent of the ibotenate lesions was evaluated by staining the sections with cresyl violet after the receptor autoradiographical studies had been completed.

RESULTS

1. Effects of striatal ibotenate lesions on DA levels and turnover

As seen in fig. 1 the DA levels are increased on the ibotenate lesioned side compared with the PBS injected side only in the marginal zone of the caudate nucleus, while the DA levels in the medial and central caudate are not significantly affected. Furthermore, no significant changes in DA levels are found on the side contralateral to the lesion when compared with the side contralateral to the PBS injected side. In the H 44/68 experiment a trend for an increase of DA turnover was observed in the medial caudate. Such a trend was not observed on the contralateral side (fig. 1).

As seen in table 1 kainate striatal lesions 10 days after the operation did not produce any significant changes in the striatal DA levels and in contrast, led to a reduction of DA turnover both on the ipsi- and contralateral side (see Andersson et al., 1980). Furthermore, it must be pointed out that the morphology in the central caudate following a 10 day kainate lesion was so deteriorated that it was not possible to make any measurements of DA fluorescence in this area. These results underline the view that kainate lesions produce a larger degree of unspecific damage than ibotenic acid (table 1). Instead, kainate induced lesions produced a clearcut increase of DA levels in the marginal zone and in the medial and central caudate as evaluated 2 days following the lesion when DA levels can still be measured in the central caudate. At this time interval also a significant increase of DA turnover could be observed both in the medial and central caudate, but not within the marginal zone of the caudate. In view of these findings it seems possible that kainate induces a much more rapid destruction of striatal tissue, which leads to an early activation of DA turnover, which 10 days later has been replaced by a bilateral compensatory reduction of DA turnover. It seems possible that ibotenate striatal lesions are less toxic to the animals and produce a slower nerve cell degenration than kainic acid, which may lead to the prolonged activation of the intact striatal DA nerve terminal systems after ibotenate lesions. A compensatory reduction of DA turnover on the intact side may therefore not be necessary at this time interval to maintain striatal synaptic assymetry.

2. Effects of striatal and pyriform ibotenate lesions on the CCK immunoreactive neurons

As seen in fig. 2 ibotenate pyriform lesions produce a marked reduction of the CCK-8 levels in the pyriform cortex as well as of the nonsulfated CCK-8 levels and of the CCK-4 levels. Injections of PBS into the pyriform cortex have no effect on the levels of these CCK peptides. As also seen in fig. 2 the levels of CCK-8, nonsulfated CCK-8 and CCK-4 in the ipsilateral striatum are not changed by this type of pyriform lesion on the lesioned side. The light microscopical analysis of the lesions show that beside the pyriform cortex also large parts of the amygdaloid cortex and of the supragenual cortex are damaged by the ibotenate injections into the pyriform cortex.

These results indicate that there exists no major CCK immunoreactive pathway from the pyriform cortex and the amygdaloid area into the striatum, although highly localized projections may well exist. The dramatic reductions of the levels of the CCK peptides in the pyriform cortex itself give evidence that the various CCK peptides are stored within interneurons of this cortical region. The

TABLE 1

The effects of unilateral kainate striatal lesions on the DA levels and turnover in various parts of the caudate nucleus of the ipsi- and contralateral side in relation to DA levels and turnover in intact controls

DA levels are shown in per cent of normal control value. In the turnover experiment with H 44/68 the values are expressed as means±s.e.m. in per cent of the respective DA levels at the time of H 44/68 injection. Number of rats within parenthesis. *= p< 0.05; **= p< 0.01. Mann-Whitney U-test.

| | | 2 day treatment | | | 10 day treatment | | |
| | | Kainic acid injected | | | Kainic acid injected | | |
		Ipsi %	Contra %	Normals %	Ipsi %	Contra %	Normals %
Cma		165±7** (4)	130±9 (4)	100±4 (4)	108±12	104±10	100±4
Cme		130±8* (4)	110±6 (4)	100±7 (4)	118±9	116±9	100±3
Cce		162±9* (4)	101±8 (4)	100±7 (4)	–	–	–
Cma	0 h	100±4 (4)	100±7 (4)	100±4 (4)	100±12	100±10	100±4
H 44/68	1 h	85±7 (4)	86±8 (3)	75±4 (5)	69±10 (5)	82±12(5)	75±4 (5)
	2 h	47±6 (5)	62±5 (5)	57±2 (5)	69±12	78±12	57±2
Cme	0 h	100±6 (4)	100±6 (4)	100±7 (4)	100±8	100±8	100±3
H 44/68	1 h	54±4** (5)	77±7 (5)	76±3 (5)	92±9* (5)	80±10(5)	76±3 (5)
	2 h	42±6**	63±4 (4)	58±3 (5)	77±11	78±12	58±3
Cce	0 h	100±6 (4)	100±8 (4)	100±7 (4)	–	–	–
	1 h	54±7* (5)	76±7 (5)	75±3 (5)	–	–	–
	2 h	45±3** (5)	62±6 (5)	54±2 (5)	–	–	–

results further imply that CCK-4 and nonsulfated CCK-8 may be stored together with CCK-8 in this part of the brain.

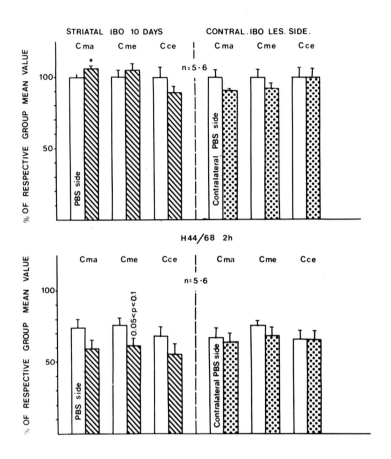

Fig. 1. Effects of striatal ibotenate lesions on the DA levels and turnover in the striatum of rats 10 days after the lesion. For details on treatment, see text. Means $\pm$ s.e.m. are shown out of 4-6 rats. Values are given in per cent of respective group mean value. In H 44/68 results are expressed in per cent of the values at the time of injection of the tyrosine hydroxylase inhibitor. Mann-Whitney U-test was used. *= p< 0.05. Cma= marginal zone; Cme= medial caudate zone; Cce= central caudate.

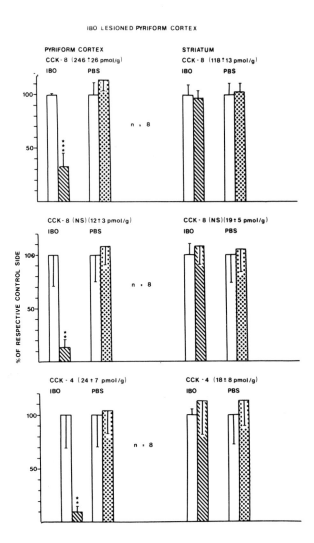

Fig. 2. Effects of unilateral ibotenate pyriform lesions on the CCK-8, CCK-8 nonsulfated and CCK-4 levels in the pyriform cortex and in the striatum of the lesioned and unlesioned side. Means ± s.e.m. are shown. n= 8. The values are expressed in per cent of respective control side mean value. The left pairs of the columns represent the results obtained on the ibotenate lesioned side. The right pair of the columns represent the results obtained following injection of phosphate buffered saline (PBS). Mann–Whitney U-test was used. **= p< 0.01; ***= p< 0.001.

Fig. 3. CCK-8 immunoreactive mediumsized, bipolar or multipolar nerve cell bodies are observed in vibratom sections
of the pyriform cortex (mainly layer II) as studied by immunocytochemistry using the PAP technique (see Köhler and Chan-
Palay, 1982). Normanski optics. 350X.

IBO LESIONED STRIATUM

☐ **INTACT CONTROL SIDE**

▨ **IBOTENATE LES. SIDE; 10 DAYS (4 x 0.5μg)**

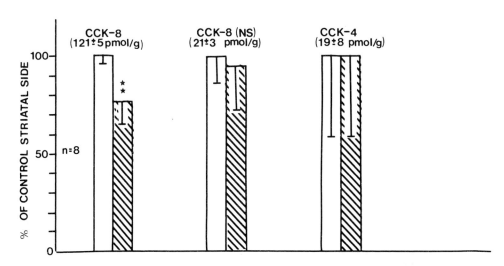

Fig. 4. Effects of unilateral striatal ibotenate lesions
on the contents of CCK-8, nonsulfated CCK-8 and CCK-4 in
the striatum. Means ± s.e.m. are shown out of 8 rats. The
values are expressed in per cent of the mean value of the
intact contralateral side. Mann-Whitney U-test. **= p<0.01.

As seen in fig. 3 the immunohistochemical analysis reveals the existence of bipolar or multipolar and medium sized CCK-8 immunoreactive cell bodies in the pyriform cortex located mainly in layer II. CCK immunoreactive terminals have also been observed, mainly in claustrum. These results support the existence of CCK immunoreactive interneurons in this area.

As seen in fig. 4 ibotenate striatal lesions induce differential changes among the striatal CCK peptides as evaluated 10 days following the lesion. Thus, the levels of CCK-4 and nonsulfated CCK-8 are not influenced by this lesion, while the striatal CCK-8 levels are significantly reduced by about 25 %. These results open up the possibility of the existence of a small population of striatal CCK-8 immunoreactive neurons, which are of the Golgi 2 type and which may contain only small amounts of nonsulfated CCK-8 and CCK-4.

Taken together, the results indicate that the CCK immunoreactive nerve cell bodies are highly sensitive to the neurotoxic action of ibotenic acid. Furthermore, the origin of the CCK-8 immunoreactive afferents to the striatum still remains to be determined.

3. Effects of pyriform ibotenate lesions on the ^{3}H-spiperone and ^{3}H-NPA binding sites in the striatum using receptor autoradiography

The receptor autoradiograms are shown in figs. 5,6,7 and 8 ^{3}H-spiperone binding is mainly observed in the striatum, nuc. accumbens and tuberculum olfactorium and especially in the lateral parts of the striatum (fig. 5). Following incubation in the presence of (+)butaclamol the labelling of these structures almost completely disappear. This is true also for the weakly labelled band seen in the cerebral hemispheres found in a layer of the cerebral cortex corresponding mainly to layer V. This band of grains is observed both in the medial cortex and in the dorsal and lateral cortex, but not within the pyriform cortex. The lesioned side is to the left in the figure. Computerized densitometry shows that the highest tones are mainly located in the lateral parts of the striatum (fig. 6). Furthermore, the analysis shows that specific ^{3}H-spiperone binding is increased on the lesioned side compared with the contralateral side when comparing the high tones in the striatum (fig. 9). This increase, however, is only observed at the two rostral levels analyzed.

As seen in fig. 6 also ^{3}H-NPA binding is mainly located in the lateral part of the striatum. When comparing by means of computerized densitometry the high tones in the striatum (fig. 8) an increase is found on the lesioned side at the intermediate rostrocaudal level analyzed (see fig. 9).

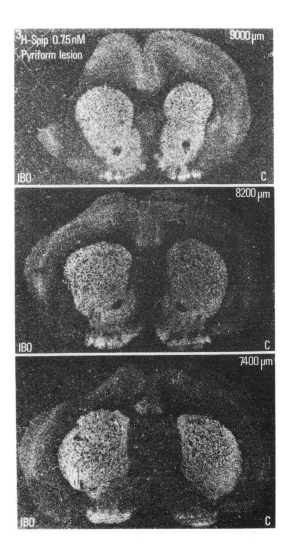

Fig. 5. Effects of unilateral ibotenate pyriform lesions on ³H-spiperone binding within the striatum, nuc. accumbens and tuberculum olfactorium at various rostrocaudal levels of the telencephalon. The König and Klippel level is indicated in the figure. For details on the experimental procedures, see text. ³H-spiperone binding is mainly located within the striatum, nuc. accumbens and tuberculum olfactorium and also within a band of the medial, dorsal and lateral cerebral cortex (which corresponds mainly to layer V). Following preincubation with (+)butaclamol (10⁻⁶ M) this labelling in the autoradiogram is markedly diminished.

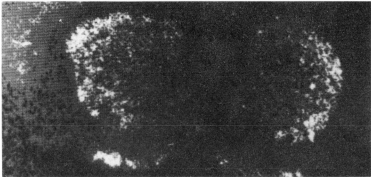

Fig. 6. This figure represent a computerized densitometric analysis of one of the figures shown in fig. 5. Only the high tones in the coronal section are shown. The high tones are mainly located in the lateral parts of the striatum.

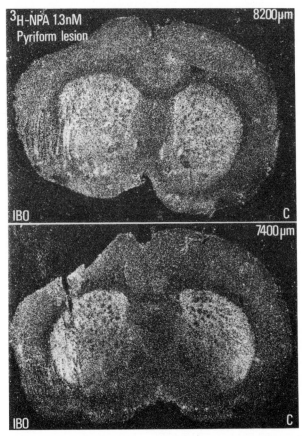

Fig. 7. The effects of unilateral ibotenate pyriform lesions on the ^{3}H-NPA binding in coronal sections of the forebrain. The ^{3}H-NPA binding is mainly located in the lateral part of the striatum. Signs of islands of grains are found within the tuberculum olfactorium and nuc. accumbens.

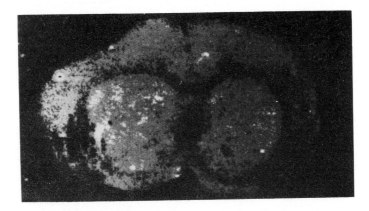

Fig. 8. Densitometric analysis of receptor autoradiograms
shown in the previous figure (upper part). Only the high
tones are demonstrated and shown to be located mainly within the lateral part of the lesioned striatum. The results
of the densitometric analysis are summarized in figure 9, showing
the increased binding of ^{3}H-NPA on the lesioned side (lateral part).

EFFECTS OF IB-A INDUCED LESION OF THE PYRIFORM CORTEX
ON ^{3}H-SPIPERONE(o) AND ^{3}H-NPA(•) BINDING SITES IN STRIATAL
CORONAL SECTIONS

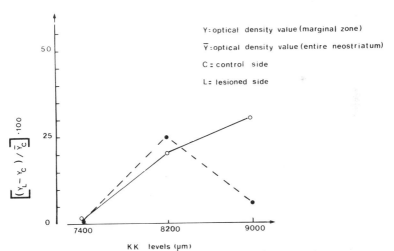

Y: optical density value (marginal zone)

$\overline{Y}$: optical density value (entire neostriatum)

C: control side

L: lesioned side

$\left[(Y_L - Y_C) / \overline{Y}_C \right] \cdot 100$

K K levels (μm)

Fig. 9. The effects of unilateral ibotenate pyriform lesions
on the ^{3}H-spiperone and ^{3}H-NPA binding sites in the lateral'
part of the striatum at various rostrocaudal levels. The difference in optical density between the two lateral zones on the
lesioned and unlesioned side is shown in per cent of the overall
optical density within the intact striatum. The ^{3}H-spiperone
and the ^{3}H-NPA binding are both increased at the intermediate
level analyzed, but at the most rostral level only the ^{3}H-
spiperone binding is increased in the lateral zone.

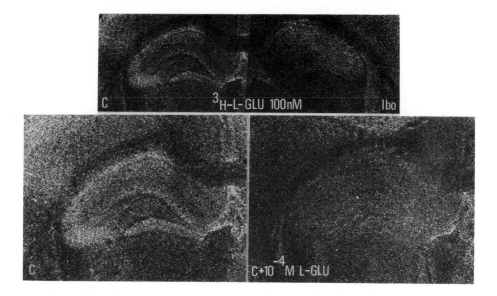

Fig. 10. The effects of hippocampal ibotenate lesions on
the ^{3}H-glutamate binding in the dorsal hippocampus seen
in studies on coronal sections of the dorsal hippocampus
using receptor autoradiography. For experimental details,
see text. As seen, ^{3}H-glutamate binding is mainly confined
to certain layers of the hippocampal formation (molecular
layer of the dentate gyrus (middle third) and the stratum
oriens of the CA-1 to CA-3 area. The ibotenate lesioned side is to the right in the upper part of the figure showing
the relative absence of grains. Unspecific binding in the
presence of 10^{-6} M l-glutamate is shown in the right lower
part of the figure. The left lower part of the figure shows
total binding. C= control side.

4. Effects of hippocampal ibotenate lesions on ^{3}H-gluta-mate binding using receptor autoradiography

As seen in fig. 10 certain layers of the dorsal hippocampus have been labeled
following incubation with ^{3}H-glutamate. The highest densities of grains are
found within the molecular layer (mainly middle third) of the dentate gyrus and
within the stratum oriens of subfields CA-3, CA-2 and CA-1. In the presence of
10^{-4} M l-glutamate the labelling disappears (fig. 10). Furthermore, following
ibotenate lesions this pattern of labeling following ^{3}H-glutamte incubation is
disrupted, and the specific label found is reduced and more evenly distributed
over the dorsal hippocampus.

It may be pointed out that the layers showing a high density of ^{3}H-glutamate
binding sites are richly innervated by presumed glutamate containing fibers of
the medial perforant pathway (middle third of the molecular layer of the dentate
gyrus) (Storm-Mathisen, 1981) and of the commissural pathway from the pyramidal
cells of the contralateral hippocampus (Storm-Mathisen, 1981). These results
imply that ^{3}H-glutamate binding sites shown by means of receptor autoradiography
at least to a large extent coincide with the distribution of glutamate termi-

nals. Ibotenate by destroying the granular and pyramidal cells of the hippocampal formation probably induces the demonstrated loss of ^{3}H-glutamate binding sites in the dorsal hippocampus. Thus, these receptors are probably mainly located on the dendrites of the granular cells and of the pyramidal cells.

GENERAL DISCUSSION

The present study has demonstrated that ibotenic acid in agreement with our previous papers represents a valuable tool in the analysis and characterization of transmitter-identified neurons, especially the monoaminergic and peptidergic neurons of the brain, both at the pre- and postsynaptic level. The following results were obtained:

1. Ibotenate striatal lesions lead to a prolonged increase of striatal DA turnover as seen 10 days following lesion.
2. Ibotenate pyriform lesions lead to a large reduction of CCK-8, nonsulfated CCK-8 and CCK-4 levels in the lesioned pyriform cortex, and striatal ibotenate lesions produce a small but significant reduction of striatal CCK-8, but not of CCK-4 levels on the lesioned side. These results indicate the existence of CCK-8 immunoreactive interneurons in the pyriform cortex containing also nonsulfated CCK-8 and CCK-4. The results also suggest the existence of a small population of striatal interneurons containing mainly CCK-8-like immunoreactivity.
3. Ibotenate pyriform lesions in combination with receptor autoradiography and computerized densitometry give evidence for the existence of plastic changes in postsynaptic DA mechanisms in the striatum on the lesioned side. Thus, in the lateral part of the striatum of the lesioned side an increase in ^{3}H-spiperone and ^{3}H-NPA binding is observed. These results indicate the existence of a striatal projection from the pyriform cortex, at least into the lateral area. Thus, when one afferent system is removed, the receptors belonging to another type of afferent systems (DA terminals) projecting into the same area, may change their affinity and/or density.
4. Studies on hippocampal ibotenate lesions in combination with receptor autoradiography of glutamate receptors in the dorsal hippocampus give evidence for a marked disappearance of glutamate receptors in the stratum oriens of the CA-1 – CA-3 area and of the molecular layers of the dentate gyrus following the ibotenic induced destruction of pyramidal and granular cells of this area.

ACKNOWLEDGEMENT

This work has been supported by a grant (04X-715) from the Swedish Medical Research Council, by a grant from Magnus Bergvalls Stiftelse, by a grant (MH 25504) from the National Institute of Health, Bethesda, Maryland, U.S.A., and by a grant from Knut & Alice Wallenberg's Foundation. We are grateful for the excellent technical assistance of mrs. Ulla Altamimi, miss Birgitta Johansson, miss Siv Nilsson, miss Barbro Tinner and mr. Giuseppe Mancinelli and for the excellent secreterial assistance of miss Elisabeth Sandqvist.

REFERENCES

Agnati, L.F., Andersson, K., Wiesel, F. and Fuxe, K (1979). Neurosci. Meth., 1, 365-373.

Andersson, K., Schwarcz, R. and Fuxe, K (1980). Nature 283(5742), 94-96.

Coyle, J.T. and Schwarcz, R (1976). Nature 263, 244-246.

Coyle, J.T., Zaczek, R., Slevin, J. and Collins, J (1981). Glutamate as a Neurotransmitter, (eds. G. Di Chiara and G.L. Gessa), pp. 337-346, Raven Press, New York.

Creese, I., Schneider, R. and Snyder, S.H (1977). Eur. J. Pharmacol., 46, 377-381.

Dockray, G.J., Gregory, R.A., Hutchison, J.B., Harris, I.J. and Runswick, M.J. (1978). Nature 711-713.

Fuxe, K., Hall, H. and Köhler, C (1979). Eur. J. Pharmacol., 58, 515-517.

Fuxe, K., Hökfelt, T., Jonsson, G. and Ungerstedt, U (1970). Contemporary Research Methods in Neuroanatomy, (eds. W.S.H. Wanta and S.O.E. Ebbesson), pp. 275-314,Springer-Verlag, Berlin.

Govoni, S., Olgiati, V.R., Trabucchi, L., Garau, E., Stefanini, E. and Spano, P.F. (1978). Neurosci. Lett., 8, 207-210.

Köhler, C. and Chan-Palay, V (1982). J. Comp. Neurol., 210, 136-146.

Köhler, C., Schwarcz, R. and Fuxe, K (1979a). Neurosci. Lett., 15, 223-228.

Köhler, C., Schwarcz, R. and Fuxe, K (1979b). Brain Res., 175, 366-371.

König, J. and Klippel, R (1963). The Rat Brain. A Stereotaxic Atlas, Robert E. Krieger Publishing Co. Inc., New York.

Löfström A., Jonsson, G., Wiesel, F.A. and Fuxe, K (1976). J. Histochem. Cytochem., 24, 430-442.

McGeer, E.G. and McGeer, P.L. (1976). Nature, (Lond.), 263, 517-519.

Rehfeld, J.F. (1978). J. Biol. Chem., 253, 4022-4030.

Roberts, P.J. and Sharif, N.A (1981). Glutamate as a neurotransmitter, (eds. G. Di Chiara and G.L. Gessa), pp. 295-305, Raven Press, New York.

Schwarcz, R., Creese, I., Coyle, J.T. and Snyder, S (1978). Nature 271, 766-768.

Schwarcz, R. and Fuxe, K (1979). Life Sci., 24, 1471-1480.

Schwarcz, R., Fuxe, K., Hökfelt, T., Andersson, K. and Coyle, J.T (1979c). Dopaminergic Ergot Derivatives and Motor Function, (eds, K. Fuxe and D.B. Calne), pp.115-126, Pergamon Press, Oxford and New York.

Schwarcz, R., Fuxe, K., Hökfelt, T., Terenius, L. and Goldstein, M (1979d). J. Neurochem., 34(4), 772-778.

Schwarcz, R., Hökfelt, T., Fuxe, K., Jonsson, G., Goldstein, M. and Terenius, L (1979a). Exp. Brain Res., 37, 199-216.

Schwarcz, R., Köhler, C., Fuxe, K., Hökfelt, T. adn Goldstein, M (1979b). Advances in Neurology, (eds. T.h. Chase, N.S. Wexler and A. Barbean), pp. 655-668,vol 23, Raven Press, New York.

Seeman, P (1980). Dopamine Receptors. Pharmacological Reviews, pp. 229-313, vol. 3, No. 3, William & Wilkins Comp., Baltimore.

Sternberger, L.A (1979). Immunocytochemistry (2nd Edition), John Wilney and Son, New York.

Storm-Mathisen, J (1981). Glutamate as a Neurotransmitter, (eds. G. Di Chiara and G.L. Gessa), pp. 43-55, Raven Press, New York.

CHARACTERIZATION OF STRIATAL IBOTENATE LESIONS AND OF 6-HYDROXYDOPAMINE INDUCED NIGRAL LESIONS BY MORPHOMETRIC AND DENSITOMETRIC APPROACHES

L. F. AGNATI*, K. FUXE**, L. CALZA*, F. BENFANATI*, N. BATTISTINI*,
I. ZINI*, L. FABBRI* and M. GOLDSTEIN***

*Departments of Human Physiology, Endochrinology and "Grandi Strumenti",
University of Modena, Modena, Italy
**Department of Psych., New York University Med. Center, New York, U.S.A.

ABSTRACT

The effects of the neurotoxins ibotenic acid and 6-hydroxydopamine (6OHDA) on the nigrostriatal dopamine (DA) system have been evaluated at the striatal level in the rat by means of a morphometrical and a densitometrical analysis using quantitative tyrosine hydroxylase immunocytochemistry and quantitative receptor autoradiography. 22 days following an ibotenic acid induced lesion a marked increase was observed in the contents of tyrosine hydroxylase immunoreactivity in the striatal DA nerve terminals as quantitatively evaluated from tone histograms in sagittal sections of the neostriatum. By means of the TESAK system to analyze images and suitable computer programs it has also for the first time been possible to quantitatively demonstrate supersensitivity development at DA receptors studying ^{3}H-spiperone binding by means of quantitative receptor autoradiography. Combined lesions with 6OHDA induced nigral lesions and controlateral striatal ibotenate lesions have also been analyzed by means of morphometrical and densitometrical methodologies. The results reveal a marked unbalance of ^{3}H-spiperone binding between the two striata of these animals. In line with these results it was shown that rotational behaviour induced by apomorphine was highest in animals with this type of combined lesions. It is suggested that synaptic plasticity in response to neurotoxin induced lesions at the pre- and postsynaptic level can be excellently studied by a morphometric and densitometric analysis of transmitter-identified neurons in the lesioned area. The usefulness of ibotenic acid as a neurotoxin, producing axon-sparing lesions in discrete areas of the mammallian brain without introducing distant lesions, is further documented in the present study.

KEYWORDS

Ibotenic acid; ^{3}H-spiperone; tyrosine hydroxylase; receptor autoradiography; immunohistochemistry; morphometry; densitometry.

INTRODUCTION

In recent years we have developed densitometric (Agnati et al., 1978, 1980) and morphometric methods (Agnati et al., 1982a,b,c,d) to study transmitter-identified neuronal systems. These methods were based on high contrast Kodalith plates and on the use of a semiautomatic image analyzer MOP AMO2 plugged into an Apple computer loaded with suitable programs, respectively. More recently we have expanded our techniques by performing such an analysis in a more rapid and reproducible fashion due to an automatic system to analyze and elaborate images: the TESAK system. By means of this new system and of suitable programs we can now quantitate immunocytochemically demonstrated antigens in terminals and cell bodies as well as characterize nerve cell bodies, processes and cell groups of transmitter-identified neurons.

The aim of the present paper is to evaluate by means of these morphometrical tools the effects of two neurotoxins, namely 6OHDA and ibotenic acid on the nigrostriatal DA system. The study has been carried out both at the presynaptic level (tyrosine hydroxylase (TH)-positive terminals and at the postsynaptic level (^{3}H-spiperone labeled DA receptors) on neuroanatomically defined areas in brain sagittal sections. A functional counterpart of this analysis has been obtained by studying the apomorphine induced rotational behaviour in these rats three weeks after lesion and two days before sacrifice.

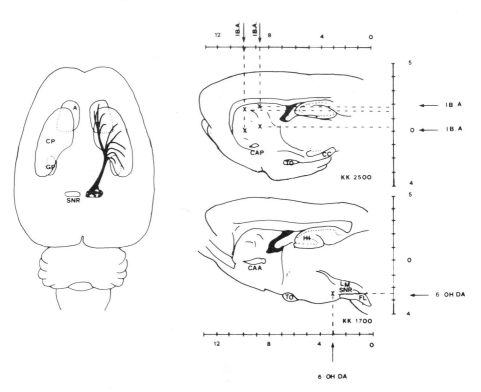

Fig. 1. The left panel shows a schematic drawing of the nigrostriatal DA pathway, while the right panels show the sites of ibotenic acid injection (upper panel) and of 6OH-DA injection (lower panel). The neuroanatomical landmarks and levels shown follow the König and Klippel (KK) atlas.

MATERIAL AND METHODS

Male Sprague-Dawley rats (about 200 gr b.wt.) have been used. The rats were lesioned with 6OHDA (2 μg/4μl, partial lesion) and with ibotenic acid (IB-A 4x5
μg/0.5 μl). The coordinates used (according to the König and Klippel atlas) (see
fig. 1) were for the 6OHDA injections as follows: anteroposterior (AP)= 3.1;
lateral (L)= 1.3; depth (D)= 7.8. For IB-A lesioned rats the L-coordinate was
always equal to 2.5. Two AP-coordinates (2.9; 1.9) were used, and at each of
these two AP-coordinates two D values were chosen. Thus, for AP= 2.9 the D-
coordinates were equal to 6.5 and 4.5; for AP= 1.9 the D-coordinates were equal
to 6.0 and 5.0.

By means of these two neurotoxins we have prepared four different animal models,
schematically shown in fig. 2. In the combined lesions (6OHDA+IB-A) the IB-A
lesion was performed three days after the 6OHDA lesion. Twenty days after lesion
the rats were tested for rotational behaviour induced by a subcutaneous injection
of apomorphine (1 mg/kg)

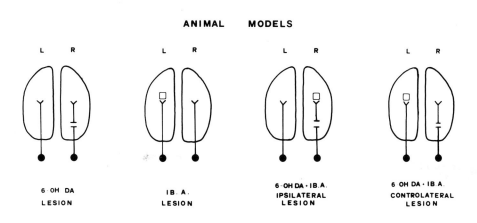

ANIMAL   MODELS

6-OH DA
LESION

IB. A.
LESION

6-OH DA · IB.A.
IPSILATERAL
LESION

6-OH DA · IB.A.
CONTROLATERAL
LESION

Fig. 2. Schematic representation of the four animal models
used in the present study.

Two days later the rats were sacrificed. Half of the rats were perfused for immunocytochemistry and half of them for receptor autoradiography using ^{3}H-spiperone
as a radioligand. The main difference between the two perfusions used is the
paraformaldehyde concentration which was 4% (W/V) for immunocytochemistry and
0.1% (W/V) for receptor autoradiography (see Hökfelt et al., 1975). Sagittal
sections (see fig. 1), 14 μm thick, have been obtained by cutting the brains in a
cryostat (see Hökfelt et al., 1975). The quantitation is principally based on
measurements of the optical density either in a negative taken from a certain
region (see fig. 1) of a section stained for TH-immunoreactivity (marker of DA
terminals) or in the LKB ^{3}H-Ultrofilm, which before development had been exposed

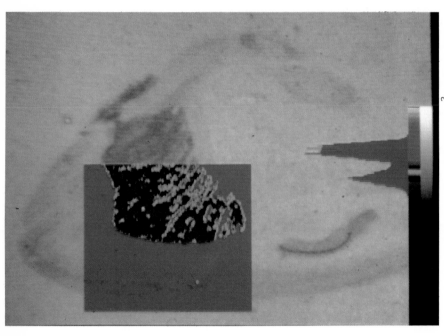

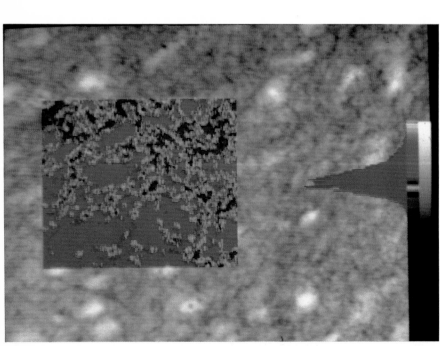

Fig. 3. Densitometric analysis of a TH-positive area in striatum made by the TESAK system. The different optical densities are coded with different colours. On the bottom of the fig. the tone histogram is shown (see text) of the optical densities present in the sampled window. Magnification of the original negative 62X. Final magnification 260X.

Fig. 4A. Densitometric analysis of ^{3}H-spiperone (27.5 Ci/mmol) binding in brain sagittal section (KK 1700). The different optical densities present in the window are coded with different colours (see also fig.3). On the right the tone histogram for the optical densities present in the window is shown. Magnification 15X.

to irradiation for four weeks at -70° C from sagittal sections labelled with
^{3}H-spiperone (1 nM). In the histochemical analysis a region such as the corpus
callosum was used as a tissue blank in view of its lack of TH-immunoreactivity.
As far as the autoradiographical analysis is concerned the blank was obtained by
preincubating an adjacent section with a buffer containing an excess of cold
(+)butaclamol (10^{-6} M) (see Creese et al., 1977). Thus, all the optical density
values presented are the differences between the total values observed in the
TH-positive areas or in the ^{3}H-spiperone labelled areas and the respective
blanks.

An example of these procedures is presented in figs. 3 and 4. In fig. 3 the TH-
positive terminals visualized in a striatal area are colour coded within a chosen
"window" and then a suitable computer program gives the tone histogram. The tone
histogram is obtained by considering the frequency (f_i value plotted on the Y-
axis) of a certain tone (t_i value plotted on the X-axis) in the window.

In this way we can obtain an overall evaluation of the intensity (I) of emission
(intensity of fluorescence) in the sampled area by considering the value $I = \sum_i f_i
t_i$, i.e. the overall intensity will be increased by an increase of the tone-his-
togram area or, coetiris paribus, by a displacement of the tone-histogram towards
the hot colours (red colours), thus moving away from the cold colours (blue colours).

Obviously as stated above we can obtain the specific overall fluorescence intensity by subtracting from the I_T value (fluorescence intensity measured in a TH-
positive area) the I_U value (fluorescence intensity measured in a TH-negative
area), where both I_T and I_U values have been obtained by using a window of the
same amplitude. We have also tested another possible measurement of I. Thus, the
modal value has been considered (i.e. the most frequent tone value in the sampled
region) of the histogram. By using this parameter similar results have been obtained to those obtained by the more complete parameter discussed above, which
gives an evaluation of the overall intensity of the sampled field.

Fig. 4A shows that for ^{3}H-spiperone binding in sections a slightly different
approach should be used, since the I_T value can be greatly affected by the background (note the two peaks in the tone histogram: one for the area labeled by
^{3}H-spiperone and the other one for the background). Obviously, however, we could
use the same window as shown in fig. 4A to measure the I_U value in the autoradiogram obtained by preincubation with a buffer containing (+)butaclamol (10^{-6} M) .
However, better results can be obtained if one considers only the area of interest in the autoradiogram. This can be achieved by comparing the autoradiogram
with the Nissl stained section. We can then use a window exactly equal to the
shape of the brain area of interest (fig. 4B). In this way we obtain a single
modal value in the tone-histogram.

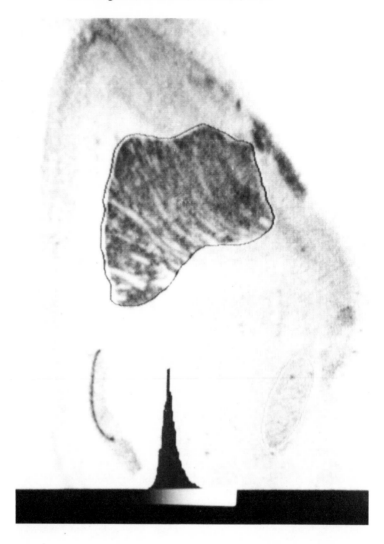

Fig. 4B. Densitometric analysis of ^{3}H-spiperone binding in the striatal area. The different optical densities are coded with different colours. Thus, in the black and white picture they will appear as different grey tones. Magnification 17X.

RESULTS

Before presenting a summing up table of the results obtained it is worthwhile to show three representative pictures of our data. The first one shows that at sites close to the IB-A injection there is an increase of TH-immunoreactivity (fig. 5). The second one demonstrates the increase of ^{3}H-spiperone binding in the partially denervated striatum after a nigral 6OHDA induced lesion (fig. 6). The third one shows that after a combined 6OHDA+IB-A induced lesion on the same

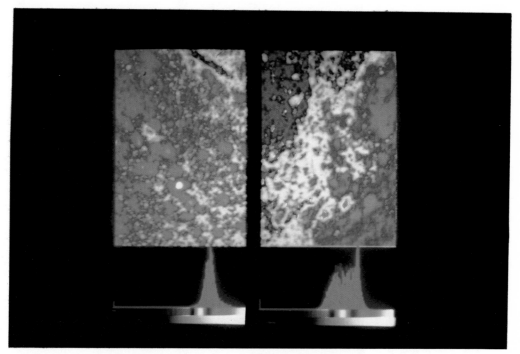

Fig. 5. Densitometric analysis of TH-immunoreactivity of corresponding striatal regions of the left striatum (i.e. ibotenic acid lesioned side) and of the controlateral intact side. Note the presence of hot tones on the lesioned side but not on the intact side. Note also the corresponding enlargment of the tone histogram and its displacement on the X-axis towards the hot tones for the lesioned side. Magnification of the original negative 16X.

side it is possible to detect the disappearance of the postsynaptic DA receptor due to the neurotoxic effects of IB-A (producing a disappearance of striatal nerve cells) and the postsynaptic increase in ^{3}H-spiperone linked DA receptors due to the presynaptic neurotoxic effects of 6-OHDA on the dopaminergic fibers (fig. 7). The experiments on rotational behaviour showed that it is possible to increase the apomorphine induced turning in 6OHDA lesioned rats by lesioning the contralateral side with IB-A (see fig. 8). In this animal model there exists on one side of the brain a striatum which is postsynaptically intact and presynaptically lesioned with regard to DA input, and on the other side a striatum which is postsynaptically lesioned and presynaptically intact.

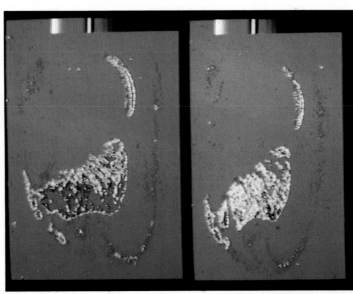

Fig. 6. Densitometric analysis of ³H-spiperone binding in the intact (upper panel) and on the 6-OHDA lesioned side (lower panel). Note the large amounts of hot tones present on the lesioned side. Magnification 7X.

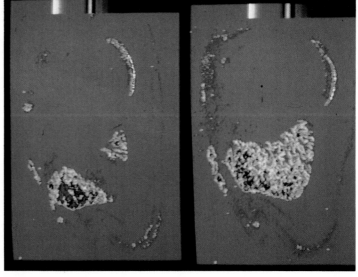

Fig. 7. Densitometric analysis of striata after a combined ipsilateral striatal lesion with 6-OHDA and IB-A. Note the loss of a large part of the nuc. caudatus on the lesioned side (lower panel) due to the IB-A lesion. However, large amounts of hot tones are present in the part of the striatum and nuc. accumbens spared from the neurotoxic action of IB-A. These hot tones demonstrate the supersensitivity in the DA receptors induced by the presynaptic destruction of the nigrostriatal DA system by 6-OHDA. Magnification 7X.

DISCUSSION

The increase in TH content produced by IB-A (see fig. 5) can be explained by the lack of striatal nerve cells which at the time interval studied leads to a compensatory increase in the TH-enzyme protein. The mechanism involved may be a disruption in the production of inhibitory factors by the striatal nerve cells. The factors may via the retrograde axoplasma flow be transported to the DA nerve cell bodies where they exert a restraining influence on TH protein synthesis via a possible action on the cell nucleus.

The increase in striatal ^{3}H-spiperone binding observed after a 6OHDA induced lesion of the nigrostriatal DA pathway (see fig. 6) is in line with the biochemical findings on development of supersensitivity in DA receptors after anatomical destruction or functional blockade of DA transmission (for a review, see Seeman, 1981). The present study is the first demonstration of DA receptor supersensitivity by quantitative receptor autoradiography and illustrates the powerful regional resolution of this analysis, which allows studies on the regulation of receptors in a morphologically intact brain. A quantitative receptor autoradiopgrahical technique has also been developed by Unnerstall et al., (1982).

It should be noted that the combined effect of ipsilateral treatment with 6OHDA, leading to an increase of ^{3}H-spiperone binding, and with IB-A, leading to a decrease of ^{3}H-spiperone binding (see fig. 7), can be appreciated only by means of these techniques, since with biochemistry the two opposite effects would tend to cancel each other.

Finally, these findings on TH contents and on ^{3}H-spiperone binding can explain the behavioural data (see fig. 8). In fact, if the per cent ratio of the value observed on the right side divided by the value observed on the left side is considered for each of the four animal models it is possible to observe that 1. the side partially lesioned with 6OHDA (right side) shows an increase in ^{3}H-spiperone binding and a decrease in TH contents, 2. the IB-A lesioned side (left side) shows a decrease in ^{3}H-spiperone binding and an increase in TH content, 3. the side lesioned with both 6OHDA+IB-A (right side) shows for ^{3}H-spiperone binding and TH contents the interaction of the two opposite neurotoxic effects and 4. animals with an ipsilateral 6OHDA induced lesion and an IB-A induced lesion of the contralateral side show above all the dramatic inbalance of ^{3}H-spiperone binding between the two striata. Hence, there is an inverse relationship between striatal TH-contents and striatal ^{3}H-spiperone binding.

L. F. Agnati, K. Fuxe, L. Calza, *et al.*

The highest degree of rotational behaviour was observed after an ipsilateral 6OHDA and a contralateral IB-A lesion. Therefore, rotational behaviour probably depends mainly on the imbalance of ^{3}H-spiperone binding between the two striata. However, as previously shown (Agnati et al., 1980, Fuxe et al., 1981, Schwarcz et al., 1979) supersensitive receptors probably have a higher intrinsic activity than normal receptors. Thus, even if the inbalance is more pronouced after IB-A than after a partial lesion with 6OHDA the rotational behaviour is higher in the latter animal model. In fact, the apomorphine-induced turning behaviour depends in the first case on the activation of the intact side (i.e. receptors with normal intrinsic activity), while in the second case it depends on the activation of the lesioned side (i.e. on receptors with higher intrinsic activity).

ANIMAL MODEL	^{3}H-SPIPERONE BINDING OPTICAL DENSITY OF CAUDATUS (L/R)·100	TH-POSITIVE TERMINALS OPTICAL DENSITY OF CAUDATUS (L/R)·100	ROTATIONAL BEHAVIOUR TOTAL ACTIVITY (turns/rat)
6OH-DA lesion 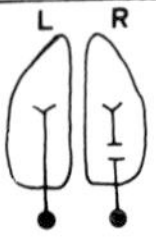	$(L/R^\uparrow) \cdot 100 = 79$	$(L/R^\downarrow) \cdot 100 = 155$	135
IB.-A. lesion 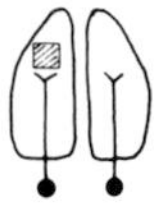	$(L^\downarrow/R) \cdot 100 = 62$	$(L^\downarrow/R) \cdot 100 = 115$	115
6OH-DA+IB.A. ipsilateral lesion 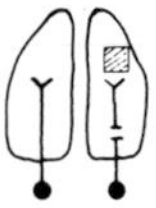	$(L/R) \cdot 100 = 92$	$(L/R) \cdot 100 = 109$	86
6OH-DA+IB.A. controlateral lesion 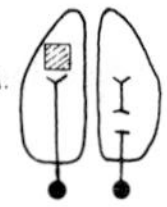	$(L^\downarrow/R^\uparrow) \cdot 100 = 40$	$(L^\downarrow/R^\downarrow) \cdot 100 = 118$	166

Fig. 8. Summing up table of the results observed in the four animal models at the postsynaptic level (^{3}H-spiperone binding) and at the presynaptic level (TH-immunoreactivity). The functional counterpart is studied by means of apomorphine induced rotational behaviour. The last column shows the mean value of the total number of turns (total activity) observed in each of the animal models.

From a more general standpoint the importance of morphomtrical and densitometric approaches in neurochemistry should be stressed (Fuxe et al., 1982a,b, Agnati et al., 1982e). In fact, it should be considered that by means of these techniques we cannot only provide direct evidence for structural changes in transmitter-identified neuronal systems, but also perform quantitative determinations of transmitter contents (Agnati et al., 1979) or more generally of antigen contents (Fuxe et al., 1982b).

It should be noted that special insights on terminal distribution can be obtained with the possibility to gather indirect evidence of axo-axonic contacts (Agnati et al., 1977) or to assess on a quantitative basis the existence of a particular pattern of innervation. Thus, we have e.g. demonstrated that it is possible to describe in quantitative terms islandic DA terminals in nuc. caudatus and discriminate between TH-contents and terminal density in these areas (Agnati et al., 1982f).

The importance of the above methods is clear if one remembers that all these techniques are carried out on an intact morphological substrate which is instead lost in biochemistry. Hence, coexistence can only be studied by means of these methods (Agnati et al., 1982g). In conclusion, we believe that new answers will be obtained in neuropsychopharmacology by matching the morphometrical and densitometric approaches with biochemical techniques.

ACKNOWLEDGEMENT

This work has been supported by a grant (04X-715) from the Swedish Medical Research Council, by a grant from Magnus Bergvalls Stiftelse, by a grant (MH 25504) from the National Institute of Health, Bethesda, Maryland, U.S.A., and by a grant from Knut & Alice Wallenberg's Foundation. We are grateful for the excellent technical assistance of mrs. Ulla Altamimi, miss Birgitta Johansson, miss Siv Nilsson, miss Barbro Tinner and mr. Giuseppe Mancinelli and for excellent secreterial assistance of miss Elisabeth Sandqvist.

REFERENCES

Agnati, L.F., Andersson, K., Wiesel, F. and Fuxe K (1979). J. Neurosci. Meth., 1, 365-373.
Agnati, L.F., Benfenati, F., Cortelli, P. and D'Alessandro, R. (1978). Neurosci. Lett., 9, 11-17.
Agnati, L.F. and Fuxe, K (1980). J. Neural Trans., 16, 69-81.
Agnati, L.F., Fuxe, K., Andersson, K., Benfenati, F., Cortelli, P. and D'Alessandro, R (1980). Neurosci. Lett., 18, 45-51.
Agnati, L.F., Fuxe, K., Andersson, K., Hökfelt, T., Skirboll, L., Benfenati, F., Battistini, N and Calza, L (1982a). Proc. of the 2nd Neurosci Meeting in Capoboj, Pergamon Press, New York, in press.
Agnati, L.F., Fuxe, K., Benfenati, F., Calza, L., Battistini, N. and Ögren, S.-O (1982e). In: Frontiers in Neuropsychiatric Research, CINP Satellite symposium, MacMillan Press, Corfu, Greece, June 28-30.
Agnati, L.F., Fuxe, K., Calza, L., Hökfelt, T., Johansson, O., Benfenati, F. and Goldstein, M (1982b). Brain Res. Bull., in press.
Agnati, L.F., Fuxe, K., Hökfelt, T., Benfenati, F., Calza, L., Johansson, O. and De Mey, J (1982c). Brain Res. Bull., in press.
Agnati, L.F., Fuxe, K., Hökfelt, T., Goldstein, M. and Jeffcoate, S.L (1977). J. Histochem. Cytochem., 25, 1222-1236.
Agnati, L.F., Fuxe, K., Locatelli, V., Benfenati, F., Zini, I., Panerai, A.E., El Etreby, M.F. and Hökfelt, T (1982g). J. Neurosci. Meth., 5, 203-214.
Agnati, L.F., Fuxe, K., Zini, I., Benfenati, F., Hökfelt, T. and De Mey, J (1982d). J. Neurosci. Meth., 6, 157-167.
Agnati, L.F., Fuxe, K., Zini, I., Calza, L., Benfenati, F., Zoli, M., Hökfelt, T. and Goldstein, M (1982f). Neurosci. Lett., in press.
Creese, I., Schneider, R. and Snyder, S.H (1977). Eur. J. Pharmacol., 46, 377-381.

Fuxe, K., Agnati, L.F., Hökfelt, T., Calza, L., Benfenati, F., Mascagni, F. and
Goldstein, M (1982a). WHO's study group on Neuroplasticity and Repair on the
CNS, Geneva, 28 June – 2 July.
Fuxe, K., Agnati, L.F., Köhler, C., Kuonen, D., Ögren, S.-O., Andersson, K. and
Hökfelt, T (1981). J. Neural Trans., 51, 3–37.
Fuxe, K., Agnati, L.F., Ögren, S.-O., Andersson, K. and Benfenati, F (1982b).
Symposium on Molecular Aspects on Nervous Stimulation, Transmission and Lear-
ning and Memory, Argentina, May 26–30.
Hökfelt, T., Fuxe, K. and Goldstein, M (1975). N.Y. Acad. Sci., 254, 407–432.
König, J. and Klippel, R (1963). The Rat Brain. A Stereotaxic Atlas, Robert E.
Krieger Publishing Co. Inc., New York.
Schwarcz, R., Fuxe, K., Hökfelt, T., Agnati, L.F. and Coyle, J.T (1979). Brain
Res., 170, 485–495.
Seeman, P. (1981). Pharmacol. Rev., 32, 229–313.
Unnerstall, J.R., Niehoff, D.L., Kuhar, M. and Palacios, J (1982). J. Neurosci.
Meth., 6, 59–73.

EFFECT OF IBOTENIC ACID STEREOTACTICALLY INJECTED INTO STRIATUM OR HIPPOCAMPUS ON LOCAL BLOOD FLOW AND GLUCOSE UTILIZATION IN RATS

Ch. OWMAN*, J. ANDERSSON*, N. H. DIEMER**, and K. FUXE***

*Department of Histology, University of Lund, Sweden
***Department of Histology, Karolinska Institutet, Sweden
**Department of Neuropathology, University of Copenhagen, Denmark

ABSTRACT

Local cerebral blood flow and glucose utilization were measured with an auto-radiographic, double-label technique (^{14}C-iodoantipyrine and ^{3}H-2-deoxyglucose, respectively) in rats following unilateral injection of 10 μg ibotenic acid into striatum or hippocampus. Five days after the injection there was a con-comitant reduction of flow and increase of glucose utilization in the injected regions, together with an enhanced metabolism in substantia nigra and probably also entorhinal cortex, which represent secondary projection sites.

KEYWORDS

Ibotenic acid; striatum; hippocampus; local cerebral blood flow; local cerebral glucose utilization.

INTRODUCTION

Injection of kainic acid into the brain of rats has been shown to produce selec-tive neuronal degeneration in several regions, including the striatum and the hippocampal formation (Schwarcz and Coyle, 1977; Schwarcz et al., 1978). Ibo-tenic acid, an isoxazole isolated from the mushroom Amanita muscaria also possesses neurotoxic properties when injected intracerebrally (Schwarcz et al., 1979). Transection of glutamate-containing afferent fibres have been found to reduce the kainic acid induced neuronal degeneration in both the striatum and the hippocampus (Biziere and Coyle, 1978; Köhler et al., 1978; Mc Geer et al., 1978). The neurotoxic action of ibotenic acid, however, does not appear to be dependent on the integrity of glutamate-containing afferents to the hippo-campus (Köhler et al., 1979b). Ibotenic acid may therefore exert its degenerative effects through some mechanism which is different from that underlying the de-generation caused by kainic acid.

The present study was undertaken to elucidate whether ibotenate-induced axonal degeneration in the striatum and hippocampus affects local cerebral blood flow, lCBF, and metabolism measured in terms of the cerebral metabolic rate of 2-deoxyglucose, lCMR(2DG), and to which extent remote effects can be detected in

251

secondary areas projecting to or receiving inputs from the two sites of injection.

MATERIAL AND METHODS

The experiments were carried out on 11 male Wistar albino rats weighing 200 g. The animals were anesthetized with pentobarbital (Mebumal, 60 mg/kg). Ten µg ibotenic acid was dissolved in phosphate buffer (pH 7.4), and 0.5 µl of the solution was slowly injected twice with a 3 min interval at the following coordinates in relationship to bregma: hippocampus, AP = 2.8; L = 1.8; V = 3.5 mm and striatum, AP = 7.9; L = 2.6; and V = 4.8 mm below the dura. Control animals received injections with the same volume of buffer solution alone.

At 5 days following the injections, the animals were taken for analysis of flow and metabolism in the brain.

A double autoradiographic technique was used, allowing in the same animal the determination of CBF and CMR(2DG). Approaches to such a double autoradiographic method have previously been made, but they involve procedures such as subtraction of autoradiograms or attenuation of one of the isotopes (Jones et al., 1979). In the present method, a double autoradiogram was made from two neighbour sections after extracting one of the isotopes with a solvent (Diemer and Rosenørn, 1981).

The non-anesthetized rats were injected i.v. with 500 µCi ^{3}H-2-deoxyglucose, and during the circulation period frequent samples of blood were taken for the determination of the plasma integral as described by Sokoloff et al. (1977). After the last 2DG-sample, the arterial catheter was connected to a constant velocity withdrawal pump (for mechanical integration of tracer concentration; Gjedde et al., 1980), and simultaneously 50 µCi ^{14}C-iodoantipyrine (Sakurada et al., 1978) was injected as an i.v. bolus, and the arterial tracer integral determined during a 20 sec circulation period. Twenty µm thick cryostat sections were used for autoradiography.

Experiments with extraction of the iodoantipyrine with different solvents have given various degrees of isotope retention in the sections. It was found (Diemer and Rosenørn, 1981) that 2,2-dimethoxypropane (DMP) removed all radioactive tracer. DMP reacts chemically with water, forming methanol and acetone, and this procedure was found not to influence the content or distribution of 2DG (and -phosphate) in the sections as measured by microdensitometry of the 2DG-autoradiograms on the ^{3}H sensitive film (LKB Ultrofilm). Microdensitometry was carried out with a computerized system (Leitz TAS PLUS).

RESULTS AND DISCUSSION

Intrahippocampal or intrastriatal injections of ibotenic acid causes a dose-dependent degeneration of cell bodies, with a threshold dose of approximately 1 µg (Köhler et al., 1979a). The pattern of neuronal degeneration in the hippocampus after injections of ibotenic acid differs in several respects from that described for kainic acid. Thus, the cell loss is more restricted to a region relatively close to the injection site, about 1.5 mm in diameter. Moreover, there is a sharp border separating intact and degenerated nerve cell bodies. Even after high doses of ibotenic acid there is no evidence of non-specific damage, such as that seen after kainic acid injections. No degeneration of cell bodies is observed in the contralateral or in any other brain region after injections of up to 10 µg of ibotenic acid.

The ^{3}H autoradiograms from the glucose metabolism experiments had the same high resolution in the present double-labelling approach as that described for single tracer experiments (Sokoloff et al., 1977; Faraco-Cantin et al., 1980). Although ^{3}H was present in the sections for CBF autoradiography, the irradiation from tritium was too weak to reach the emulsion on the X-ray film due to the thickness of the protective (gelatine) layer, and these autoradiograms thus reflected only the ^{14}C label.

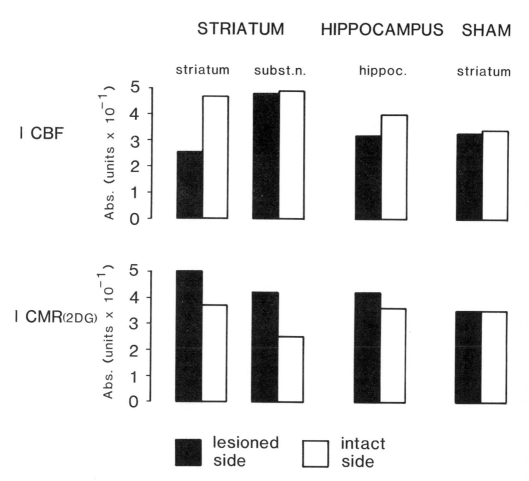

Fig. 1. Estimation of relative absorbance on autoradiograms, comparing lesioned with intact side, 5 days after unilateral injection of 10 μg ibotenic acid into striatum or hippocampus. There was a significant reduction in local blood flow, lCBF, in the injected regions, concomitant with a significant increase in local glucose utilization, lCMR(2DG). The metabolism was also significantly enhanced in substantia nigra.

The most prominent effects of ibotenic acid injections on the flow and glucose metabolism in the relevant regions of the brain are illustrated in Fig. 1, which expresses changes in terms of relative absorbance in the densitometric measurements, comparing the lesioned and intact sides.

Following striatal injections of the excitotoxin there was a highly significant local reduction in flow, with no discernible effect in substantia nigra. On the other hand, lCMR(2DG) was markedly increased in both regions. Control injections of the buffer solution alone had no significant local influence on either flow or metabolism. Corresponding findings were obtained after the hippocampal lesions, where lCBF was significantly reduced and lCMR(2DG) increased 5 days following the stereotaxic injection. There was also a tendency, though not statistically significant, for an elevated level of glucose utilization in the entorhinal cortex, directly connected with the hippocampus.

The results thus reveal a prominent reduction in the blood flow within the lesioned areas. This means that there was a disruption of the normally very close relationship between lCBF and lCMR(2DG) (Kuschinsky et al., 1982), the latter being enhanced in the respective lesioned regions. An observation that was unexpected in view of previous neuroanatomical and fluorescence histochemical studies following ibotenate injections is the increase in the local metabolism within substantia nigra and probably also the entorhinal cortex, both directly related to the lesioned brain regions.

The excitotoxic lesion provides an interesting model for studying mechanisms of CBF regulation through its ability to uncouple flow and metabolism. It also opens up possibilities to investigate more intricate mechanistic properties related to the neuron circuitry associating the lesioned brain area with more remote regions in a way not previously evident from the neuroanatomical and transmitter histochemical observations. The underlying mechanisms for the registered changes in flow and metabolism are presently being elucidated by evaluating effects on monoaminergic and peptidergic neuron systems in sections adjacent to those used for autoradiography following ibotenate lesions.

ACKNOWLEDGEMENT

Supported by grants from the Swedish (No. 14X-732 and 04X-715) and Danish (No. 12-3597) Medical Research Councils.

REFERENCES

Biziere, K., and J.T. Coyle (1978). Neurosci. Lett., 8, 303-310.
Diemer, N.H., and J. Rosenørn (1981). J. CBF Metab. 1, suppl. 1, S72-S73.
Faraco-Cantin, F., J. Courville and J.P. Lund (1980). Stain Tech. 55, 247-252.
Gjedde, A., A.J. Hansen and E. Siemkowicz (1980). Acta Physiol. Scand. 108, 321-330.
Jones, S.C., J.L. Lear, J.H. Greenberg and M. Reivich (1979). Acta Neurol. Scand. 60, suppl. 72, 202-203.
Köhler, C., R. Schwarcz and K. Fuxe (1978). Neurosci. Lett. 10, 241-246.
Köhler, C., R.Schwarcz and K. Fuxe (1979a). Neurosci. Lett. 15, 223-228.
Köhler, C., R. Schwarcz and K. Fuxe (1979b). Brain Res.175, 366-371.
Kuschinsky, W, S. Suda, R. Bünger and L. Sokoloff (1982). Developments in Neuroscience 14, 169-176.
McGeer, E.G., P.L. McGeer and K. Singh (1978). Brain Res. 139, 381-383.
Sakurada, O., C. Kennedy, J. Jehle, J.D. Brown, C.L. Carbin and L. Sokoloff (1978). Amer. J. Physiol. 234, H59-H66.
Schwarcz, R., and J.T. Coyle (1977). Brain Res. 127, 235-249.

Schwarcz, R., T. Hökfelt, K. Fuxe, G. Jonsson, M. Goldstein and L.Terenius
   (1979). Exp. Brain Res. 37, 199-216.
Schwarcz, R., R. Zaczek and J.T. Coyle (1978). Europ. J. Pharmacol. 50, 209-220.
Sokoloff, L., M. Reivich, C. Kennedy, M.H. Des Rosiers, C.S. Patlak,
   K.D. Pettigrew, O. Sakurada and M. Shinohara (1977). J. Neurochem. 28,
   897-916.

SYNAPTIC REARRANGEMENTS IN THE KAINIC ACID MODEL OF AMMON'S HORN SCLEROSIS

J. VICTOR NADLER, DAVID L. TAUCK, DEBRA A. EVENSON
and JAMES N. DAVIS

Departments of Pharmacology, Physiology and Medicine (Neurology), Duke University Medical Center, Durham, NC, USA 27710

ABSTRACT

Intraventricular and intravenous injections of kainic acid were used to create a model of Ammon's horn sclerosis in the rat. Anatomical studies demonstrated a number of synaptic rearrangements in the hippocampal formation. Neurons whose target cells were destroyed decreased the size of their terminal arborizations and numbers of synaptic contacts in the region of neuronal degeneration. Dentate granule cells rapidly shed a portion of their perforant path innervation by a mechanism that did not involve degeneration and later regained these connections. Finally, new connections were made to replace those which had formerly been provided by degenerated CA3-CA4 neurons. Most notably, the hippocampal mossy fibers sprouted recurrent collaterals that appeared to form electrophysiologically functional excitatory synapses with the dentate granule cell population. If sufficiently numerous, these recurrent collaterals could evidently mediate afterdischarge in the fascia dentata. We suggest that the formation of aberrant recurrent excitatory circuits in experimental or clinical Ammon's horn sclerosis could exacerbate or possibly even create an epileptic condition.

KEYWORDS

Kainic acid; hippocampus; Ammon's horn sclerosis; temporal lobe epilepsy; neuronal plasticity.

INTRODUCTION

In the nineteenth century, Sommer (1880) reported that about one-third of his epileptic patients were found at autopsy to have lost neurons from the hippocampal CA1 area (Sommer sector). Subsequent investigations extended and refined the description of this pathology, referred to as Ammon's horn sclerosis (AHS) or mesial temporal sclerosis (Corsellis and Meldrum, 1976). Classical AHS involves extensive loss of neurons from hippocampal area CA1, a less extensive neuronal deficit in the CA3-CA4 area (endblade, endfolium) and relative or complete sparing of neurons in the h_2 area of Rose (1927) ("resistant zone"; equivalent to area CA2 and the adjacent portion of area CA3a in Lorente de Nó's (1934) terminology) and in the fascia dentata. Loss of hippocampal neurons is followed by microglial overgrowth, atrophy and hardening (sclerosis). Some neuronal loss in certain other brain regions, particularly amygdala, thalamus and cerebral cortex, often accompanies the hippocampal lesion. AHS is a well recognized pathological finding in hippocampal tissue resected for intractable temporal lobe epilepsy. For example, in a review of 200 cases, Falconer (1971) reported that 47% of his surgical patients had such a lesion. The percentage was somewhat higher after excluding patients with malignant or benign glial tumors of the temporal lobe, vascular malformations, et cetera. Even the higher figures should be regarded as minimums, however, since a negative histopathological result may only mean that the necrotic portion of hippocampal tissue was not sampled. AHS is not confined exclusively to epileptics; similar lesions also characterize other neurological states, such as systemic anoxia (Brierley, 1976) and Alzheimer's disease (Corsellis, 1976), which are not necessarily associated with seizures. Thus AHS probably does not itself cause epilepsy. Rather, this lesion may result from repeated seizures or an episode of status epilepticus early in life (Falconer, 1974). It might then, in turn, exacerbate the epileptic condition.

Classical AHS is most commonly found upon histological examination of temporal lobes resected for pharmacologically intractable epilepsy. In a series of 55 autopsies on temporal lobe epileptics whose condition had not required surgery, Margerison and Corsellis (1966) reported that two-thirds of the patients who had hippocampal lesions had lost neurons only from the endblade. Endblade lesions usually were not associated with obvious damage to extrahippocampal brain regions. Occasionally, lesions confined to the endblade are present also in intractable cases selected for surgery (Brown, 1973), but they are far less common in such patients than is classical AHS. These observations suggest that endblade (or CA3-CA4) neurons are more readily destroyed by seizures than any others and that damage to area CA1 may possibly be associated with the transition to the intractable state. For convenience, the term AHS will be used in this chapter to designate all hippocampal lesions that are associated with temporal lobe epilepsy.

Although human neuropathological studies provide the framework for investigation of AHS, experimentation is required to define the relation between limbic seizures and hippocampal lesions and to explain these phenomena in terms of hippocampal anatomy and physiology. For these purposes, we need an animal model. Investigations over the last several years have shown that kainic acid (KA) injected parenterally, intraventricularly or into a region of brain remote from the hippocampal formation reproduces in the rat lesions remarkably similar to AHS in man (review: Nadler, 1981). Indeed intraventricular injections of KA at various doses reproduce the full range of brain lesions found in temporal lobe epileptics. Moreover, mounting evidence indicates that these lesions are, in fact, caused by the prolonged limbic status epilepticus that KA initiates. Accordingly, KA provides an appropriate animal model of AHS.

The hippocampal CA3-CA4 neurons, which are preferentially destroyed in AHS and by intraventricular KA, innervate and interconnect all parts of the hippocampal area (Gottlieb and Cowan, 1973; Swanson et al., 1978; Laurberg, 1979). One may therefore conclude that they play a central role in hippocampal function and that loss of their synaptic connections would severely disrupt these functions. However, the effect of AHS on hippocampus-dependent behaviors and on epileptogenesis depends not only on the loss of these neurons and their connections, but also on any synaptic rearrangements that result from this lesion. Such changes in connectivity have been demonstrated after a variety of brain lesions to the hippocampal area of experimental animals (review: Cotman and Nadler, 1978), and they are likely to occur also in man (DeLorenzo and Glaser, 1981). In this chapter we review the synaptic rearrangements that have been demonstrated in KA-induced experimental AHS and point out their possible significance for hippocampal pathophysiology.

REACTIVE AXONAL GROWTH AND SYNAPTOGENESIS

Slow infusion of KA (2.34-3.75 nmol) into each lateral ventricle of the rat brain destroys nearly all the CA3 hippocampal pyramidal cells and most neurons of the CA4 area, but spares the granule cells of the fascia dentata and usually the CA1 pyramidal cells (Nadler et al., 1978a,b). Bilateral destruction of the CA3 pyramidal cells extensively denervates the laminae of area CA1 to which axons of these cells project (stratum radiatum and stratum oriens). Similarly, bilateral destruction of CA4 neurons denervates the inner third of the molecular layer of the fascia dentata. Numerous instances of reinnervation or "reactive synaptogenesis" have been described in the mammalian CNS after a lesion of particular afferent fibers (review: Cotman et al., 1981). Quantitative electron microscopic studies have shown that the great majority of degenerated synaptic boutons are eventually replaced. Indeed, so regularly has reactive synaptogenesis been demonstrated, that it is considered by many an invariable result of denervation, provided that the denervated neurons survive. There is therefore every reason to think that such would be the case also in laminae denervated by experimental AHS.

Quantitative electron microscopic studies did, in fact, reveal an extensive reinnervation of the denervated hippocampal laminae (Nadler et al., 1980b). Bilateral destruction of the CA3-CA4 neurons reduced the synaptic density of the CA1 stratum radiatum by an average of 86% within three days. The synaptic density of the inner third of the dorsal dentate molecular layer declined by two-thirds and the corresponding zone of the ventral dentate molecular layer by about half. Within 6-8 weeks the synaptic density of these laminae had been largely restored to normal. After accounting for shrinkage of the tissue, the CA1 stratum radiatum regained about 72% of the synaptic contacts that had been destroyed. The inner third of the ventral dentate molecular layer recovered about 75% of its lost synapses and the inner third of the dorsal dentate molecular layer recovered essentially all of them. The newly formed synapses closely resembled those normally present.

Histochemical and autoradiographic techniques were employed to identify the projections responsible for the nascent synapses (Nadler et al., 1980a). The temporo-ammonic fibers did not sprout collaterals into stratum radiatum of area CA1 from their normal terminal zone in the adjacent stratum lacunosum-moleculare. Septohippocampal fibers, which are normally present in stratum radiatum and stratum oriens, were found not to proliferate in either lamina and mossy fibers did not grow from their normal terminus in area CA3 into area CA1. In addition, the density of synapses which featured a bouton that contained predominantly flattened vesicles did not change (Nadler et al., 1980b). These synapses are thought to be formed by axons of inhibitory interneurons. Thus inhibitory axons also failed to reinnervate synaptic sites made available by degeneration of afferent fibers from area CA3. It seems likely therefore that the nascent synapses were made predominantly by axons of the few surviving CA3 pyramidal cells. Some of these neurons in the temporal third of the hippocampal formation invariably escape destruction by intraventricular KA, and their axons have been shown to project a considerable distance rostrally (Swanson et al., 1978). In the remainder of the hippocampal formation, most of those CA3 pyramidal cells immediately adjacent to area CA2 survive the KA treatment. Surviving CA3 neurons evidently expand their synaptic territory in area CA1 about six-fold and thereby prevent heterologous projections from occupying the denervated synaptic sites.

In contrast, degeneration of projections from area CA4 readily elicited translaminar fiber growth in the fascia dentata. Collaterals of the mossy fibers, axons of the granule cells themselves, grew across the granular layer and formed a network whose density depended on the relative number of CA4 neurons that had been killed. Very few mossy fibers have recurrent collaterals in normal rats. Septohippocampal

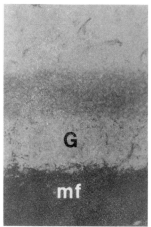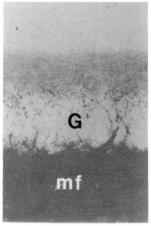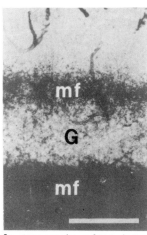

Fig. 1. Growth of recurrent mossy fiber (MF) collaterals two weeks after intravenous administration of KA. Left: Saline-injected rat. Center: 11 mg/kg KA
(small temporal CA4 lesion). Right: 11 mg/kg KA (large temporal CA4 lesion). G:
granule cell layer. Timm's sulfide silver stain. Scale bar = 0.05 mm.

fibers also grew into the denervated zone from adjacent laminae. Mossy fibers replaced the CA4 afferents more readily than did septohippocampal fibers. Even partial unilateral destruction of the CA4 projection provoked some mossy fiber
growth, but only extensive bilateral destruction of the CA4 projection elicited
the growth of septohippocampal fibers. Medial perforant path fibers did not grow
into the denervated zone, even when septohippocampal fibers were seen to do so in
the same animal (although complete isolation of the fascia dentata from area CA4
does elicit such growth (Stanfield and Cowan, 1979)). Thus heterologous projections reinnervate the CA4 terminal zone in a hierarchical manner, the mossy fibers
most readily replacing degenerated CA4 fibers and perforant path fibers replacing
them least readily. Evidently, either the degeneration preferentially evokes the
growth of mossy fibers or the denervated portion of the dendrite accepts alternative innervation most readily from the mossy fibers.

These results, in combination with previous reports (Nadler et al., 1977; Goldowitz et al., 1979), indicate that heterologous reinnervation occurs much more readily in the fascia dentata than in area CA1. The fascia dentata is likely to be
an important site for the processing of information communicated to the hippocampal formation. A miswired fascia dentata could therefore account for some of
the behavioral abnormalities in patients with AHS. To investigate this possibility, we have recently been studying the electrophysiological consequences of
mossy fiber collateral growth. At least some of these collaterals are likely to
form synapses with the dendrites of granule cells (Frotscher and Zimmer, 1982).
Thus, assuming these contacts are functional, experimental AHS creates an abnormally powerful pathway of direct communication among these cells.

To induce the formation of recurrent mossy fiber collaterals, adult male rats were
injected with KA either intraventricularly (2.34-3.75 nmol into each lateral ventricle over a 30-min period) or intravenously (11 mg/kg into a lateral tail vein).
In our hands, intravenous KA provides a rather poor model of AHS, since CA3 pyramidal cells appear relatively resistant, whereas CA1 pyramidal cells are relatively more sensitive to intravenous KA than to intraventricular KA, and since the
hippocampal formation is no more readily damaged than several other brain regions.
However, intravenous injections of KA usually destroy a larger percentage of the
temporal CA4 neurons than does bilateral intraventricular administration of KA,

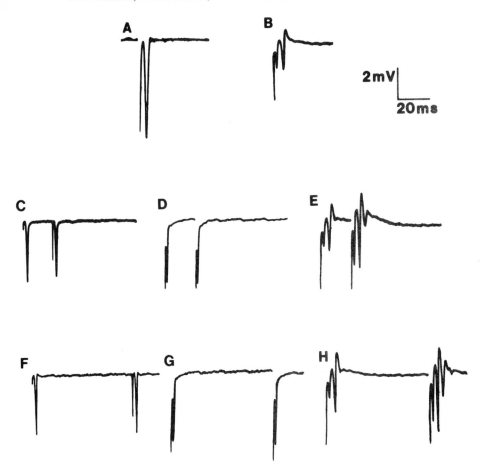

Fig. 2. Effects of KA-induced experimental AHS on responses of dentate granule
cells to antidromic stimulation of mossy fibers. Rats were given 11 mg/kg KA or
saline intravenously, and two weeks later hippocampal slices from these animals
were studied with extracellular recording techniques. Records shown are single
sweeps recorded AC. A: Antidromic population spike in slice from saline-injected
rat. B: Antidromic spike and afterdischarge in slice from KA-treated rat stimulated with the same current used in A (Expt. 4, TABLE 1). C-H: Responses to
paired stimuli, ISI of 20 ms (C-E) or 70 ms (F-H). C and F: Slice from vehicle-
injected rat; D and G: Slice from KA-treated rat - no afterdischarge; E and H:
Slice from KA-treated rat - afterdischarge present (Expt. 4, TABLE 1).

and it is mainly the temporal CA4 that projects to the fascia dentata (Swanson et
al., 1978). Presumably because the inner third of the dentate molecular layer is
more completely denervated by intravenous KA, extensive mossy fiber collateral
growth is more consistently provoked (Fig. 1). Thus intravenous injections have
an advantage for studies of this aberrant projection.

Transverse hippocampal slices were prepared from these rats about two weeks after
administration of KA or vehicle and were placed in a recording chamber for electrophysiological analysis. Adjacent slices were immersed in a solution of Na_2S
and subsequently stained for the presence of heavy metal cations by Timm's pro-

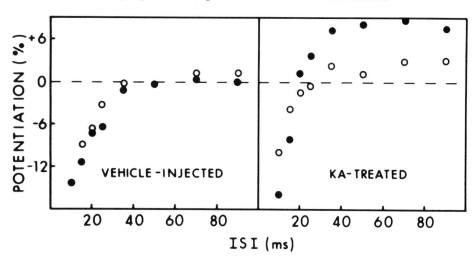

Fig. 3. Paired pulse potentiation of antidromic spike and the effect of Ca^{2+}-free medium. Left: Slice from rat injected with artificial CSF into each lateral ventricle. Right: Slice tested in the same experiment from rat injected with 3.75 nmol of KA into each lateral ventricle. Antidromic stimulation of mossy fibers did not elicit an afterdischarge. ●: Normal medium (1.3 mM Ca^{2+}, 1.2 mM Mg^{2+}). O: Ca^{2+}-free medium (no Ca^{2+}, 3.8 mM Mg^{2+}).

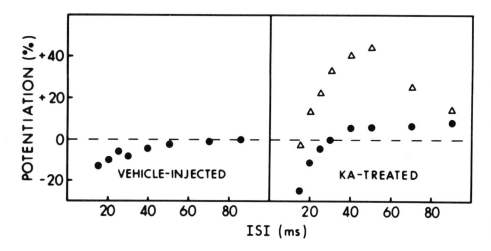

Fig. 4. Paired pulse potentiation of antidromic spike and afterdischarge. Left: Slice from rat injected with artificial CSF into each lateral ventricle. Right: Slice tested in the same experiment from rat injected with 3.75 nmol of KA into each lateral ventricle (Expt. 2, TABLE 1). ●: Antidromic spike; △: First spike of afterdischarge.

cedure (Danscher, 1981). The mossy fibers are easily demonstrated by this method, because they contain an extraordinarily high concentration of heavy metal, predominantly zinc. Other slices were fixed with formalin-saline, cut into sections and stained with cresyl violet to determine the extent of cell loss.

TABLE 1.   PAIRED PULSE POTENTIATION OF POPULATION SPIKE EVOKED BY
ANTIDROMIC STIMULATION OF MOSSY FIBERS

	Initial response (mV)		Test response (% change)	
	20 ms ISI	50-70 ms ISI	20 ms ISI	50-70 ms ISI
Vehicle-injected (N = 7)	4.6 ±0.6	4.6 ± 0.6	-9.7 ± 4.4	+0.4 ± 0.7
KA (no AD) (N = 5)	4.1 ± 0.4	4.2 ± 0.5	-5.0 ± 2.5	+9.5 ± 1.6
KA (AD)[*] Expt. 1	4.8, 3.3	4.4, 3.3	-9.6, +16	+19 , +47
2	5.3, 0.9	5.4, 0.8	-11 , +13	+5.9, +44
3[**]	4.8, 1.0	5.5, 1.3	-70 , +24	-8.2, +12
4	1.7, 2.9	1.5, 2.8	+85 , +46	+110 , +71

Pairs of identical stimuli were delivered to the mossy fibers with various ISI's,
each pair separated from the next by 30-45 s.   Population spikes were recorded in
the granular layer at the center of the dorsal leaf of the fascia dentata.   The
mossy fibers were stimulated with 5-10 pairs of pulses at each ISI and the peak
amplitudes of all responses were averaged.   See Fig. 2 for sample records.   Values are means ± S.E.M. for the number of experiments given in parentheses (each
experiment on slices from a different animal) or results of single experiments.

[*]First value in each set is amplitude or potentiation of the antidromic spike and
second value is amplitude or potentiation of first spike of afterdischarge.

[**]For technical reasons, stimulus intensities required to evoke a larger antidromic spike made accurate measurements impossible.   Small amplitude of the initial
antidromic spike may partially account for large paired pulse potentiation in this
experiment.

In slices from vehicle-injected rats, antidromic stimulation of the mossy fibers
elicited only a single population spike in the granular layer of the fascia dentata (Fig. 2A).   In contrast, antidromic stimulation of the mossy fibers in slices from 8 of 12 KA-treated rats also evoked an afterdischarge (Fig. 2B).   The
afterdischarge consisted of one or more population spikes that were superimposed
on a positive wave and separated from the antidromic spike and from each other by
about 4 ms.   Although large stimulus currents were often required to elicit this
response, it was never observed in control slices, however large the input current.
The afterdischarge did not appear to result from any reduction of GABAergic inhibition, since it was not reproduced by superfusion of control slices with 100 μM
bicuculline methiodide.   Superfusion with Ca^{2+}-free medium (with 3.8 mM Mg^{2+}) abolished the afterdischarge without affecting the antidromic spike, suggesting a
dependence on synaptic transmission.   Moreover, the Timm's sulfide silver stain
revealed that the propensity for generating afterdischarge at low or moderate stimulus currents characterized slices from animals with the densest network of recurrent mossy fiber collaterals.   These results are consistent with the lesion-
induced formation of a recurrent excitatory circuit.

In some of these experiments we applied a second test of excitatory function.
Subthreshold recurrent excitation would be expected to increase the excitability
of granule cells, thus bringing more of these cells to threshold with a submaximal
stimulus.   Consequently, an initial submaximal antidromic stimulus should increase

the amplitude of an antidromic spike fired in response to an identical test stimulus delivered during the recurrent EPSP. To detect such potentiation, pairs of antidromic stimuli were delivered to the mossy fibers with various interstimulus intervals (ISI). The intensity and duration of stimulus pulses were adjusted to produce an initial submaximal antidromic spike of 3-6 mV. In all but one case, slices from KA-treated and vehicle-injected rats were studied in the same experiment.

In slices from vehicle-injected rats the amplitude of the second antidromic spike was less than that of the first of the pair, when short ISI's were used (Fig. 2C, 3,4; TABLE 1). At an ISI of 35 ms or more, the two responses were of approximately equal magnitude (Fig. 2F,3; TABLE 1). The reduction of the second antidromic spike obtained with a relatively brief ISI appears not to have resulted from activation of the recurrent GABAergic inhibitory circuit, because it was little affected by replacing all Ca^{2+} in the medium with twice the concentration of Mg^{2+} and was unaffected by addition of 100 μM bicuculline methiodide to the medium.

Slices from three KA-treated rats which did not fire an afterdischarge and from two rats tested at a stimulus intensity below that required to elicit an afterdischarge exhibited paired pulse potentiation of the antidromic population spike at ISI's of 30-90 ms (Fig. 2G,3). Assuming that the amplitude of individual action potentials was unchanged, this result implies that the second stimulus brought more granule cells to threshold than the first. The amplitude of the second antidromic spike of the pair exceeded that of the first by an average of 9.5% at the optimal ISI of 50-70 ms, but usually was still less than that of the first spike at an ISI of 20 ms (TABLE 1). Although the antidromic spike potentiated only modestly under our experimental conditions, any plasticity of this response is likely to be meaningful, since the safety factor for antidromically-induced firing is very high. When antidromic stimulation evoked an afterdischarge, the antidromic spike potentiated in three of four cases studied at an ISI of 50-70 ms (Fig. 2H,4; TABLE 1), but in only one case at an ISI of 20 ms (Fig. 2E, 4; TABLE 1). However, the second, presumably synaptically-generated, population spike always potentiated at both ISI's. In addition, a conditioning volley often unmasked one or two more population spikes, thus prolonging the afterdischarge. Paired pulse potentiation was markedly reduced by replacing all Ca^{2+} in the medium with twice the concentration of Mg^{2+}.

All these preliminary data could be explained by the creation of an aberrant recurrent mossy fiber circuit in response to destruction of the CA4 projection. However, further experiments are required to establish this hypothesis. We are presently attempting to repeat these studies with an inhibitor of mossy fiber transmission and with intracellular recordings. One would expect an antidromic spike to evoke a long-lasting EPSP that was selectively blocked by an inhibitor of mossy fiber transmission.

Assuming that the recurrent mossy fiber collaterals which form in the KA model of AHS are indeed responsible for the excitability changes we have demonstrated, our results have important implications for the relation between AHS and limbic seizures. If these collaterals innervate the dentate granule cells densely enough, they can evidently mediate afterdischarge. It seems likely that multiple firing of dentate granule cells in response to stimuli that normally elicit only a single discharge would further compromise hippocampal function that had already been disrupted by destruction of CA3-CA4 cells. In fact, these aberrant recurrent connections might well create an epileptogenic focus in the fascia dentata. Afterdischarge in the fascia dentata would be conveyed to the surviving pyramidal cells of the h_2 area via the mossy fibers. These neurons are easily induced to burst and thus to cause afterdischarge in area CA1 (Traub and Wong, 1982). If the initial activation of the dentate granule cells were sufficiently intense, a full-blown limbic seizure could result. Thus synaptic reorganization in KA-induced experimental AHS, and potentially in clinical AHS as well, could exacerbate or possibly even initiate an epileptic condition. The development of aberrant recurrent excitatory circuitry might well explain the spontaneous behavioral seizures we have observed in rats with extensive bilateral KA lesions even months after treatment with the convulsant.

RESPONSES OF CNS NEURONS TO LOSS OF TARGET CELLS

The hippocampal mossy fibers exclusively innervate the neurons of the CA3-CA4 area. When the latter are destroyed with KA or in AHS, the dentate granule cells are deprived of their postsynaptic targets. Studies on various peripheral and central neurons suggest that connections between neurons and their target cells are required to maintain several of their differentiated properties (review: Purves and Njå, 1978). Among these are the ability to maintain afferent synapses and to respond to application of neurotransmitters. Thus neurons that have been axotomized or in which retrograde axoplasmic transport has been blocked with colchicine or other toxins suffer a loss of afferent synaptic connections and are not readily depolarized by excitatory transmitters like acetylcholine. In axotomized neurons these effects reverse once the axon regenerates and forms new synaptic connections with its target cells. In the CNS functional regeneration does not occur, but collateral branches of the transected axon can form new connections to make up for those which were lost (e.g., Schneider and Jhaveri, 1974; Pickel et al., 1974). Perhaps in the CNS axon sprouting takes the place of regeneration. Shedding excitatory synapses and reducing their population of neurotransmitter receptors may be adaptive mechanisms which allow neurons to focus their metabolic machinery on growth, instead of on electrical activity.

In light of the foregoing considerations, it is of interest that bilateral intraventricular administration of KA reduced the synaptic density of the outer two-thirds of the dentate molecular layer by about 30% within 3-5 days (TABLE 2). A definite reduction could be seen in one day, but not in four hours. Evidence of presynaptic degeneration was very rarely observed in this zone (0.1% of all synapses). Since perforant path fibers contribute at least 86% of the synapses identified there (Matthews et al., 1976), these observations imply a substantial non-degenerative loss of perforant path innervation. Postsynaptic specializations associated with these synapses disappeared concurrently and small dendritic spines, on which most perforant path synapses are normally found, were less frequently encountered. This loss of synapses was completely reversible; in 6-8 week survivors the synaptic density of the perforant path terminal zone was normal.

In many respects these observations resemble those reported in electron microscopic studies of axotomized neurons, and thus the synaptic deficit may have arisen from the destruction of neurons to which the granule cells had projected. However, alternative explanations must be considered. The loss of perforant path synapses does not appear attributable to a direct action of KA, since this effect was not seen until hours after the CA3-CA4 neurons had already shown advanced signs of degeneration (Nadler et al., 1980c). It also did not correlate in time with KA-induced seizure activity. The density of perforant path synapses declined equally in both dorsal and ventral dentate molecular layers, whereas the loss of CA4-derived innervation was much greater in the dorsal molecular layer. On this basis, the disappearance of perforant path synapses seemed independent of the degeneration of CA4-derived fibers. However, after a perforant path lesion the synaptic density of every dentate lamina reportedly declines at some survival time, even the density of laminae not innervated by perforant path fibers (Hoff et al., 1981). Therefore the effect of denervation per se must be seriously considered.

TABLE 2. SYNAPTIC DENSITY OF PERFORANT PATH TERMINAL ZONE
AFTER BILATERAL CA3-CA4 LESION

Survival time	N	Synapses/100 μm^2	
		Dorsal leaf	Ventral leaf
Control	4	36 ± 1	44 ± 2
4h	2	34 ± 1	47 ± 3
1d	2	30 ± 1	32 ± 1
3-5d	5	24 ± 2	31 ± 2
6-8 wk	5	36 ± 2	41 ± 2

Values are means ± S.E.M. for N = number of animals. Data recalculated from Nadler et al. (1980b).

An important reason for favoring the view that the density of perforant path innervation depends on the maintenance of mossy fiber contacts is that it varied temporally and quantitatively with the number of mossy fiber boutons remaining in area CA3 (see below). One could speculate that the granule cells can accept innervation only in proportion to the quantity of trophic material accumulated by mossy fiber boutons. The most definitive evidence favoring a relation of these results to axotomy, however, is the preliminary finding of Tarrant and Routtenberg (presentation to Society for Neuroscience, 1978) that transection of the mossy fibers similarly reduces the density of perforant path innervation. In contrast to axotomized peripheral neurons, dentate granule cells could not have reacquired a normal synaptic complement through axonal regeneration and reformation of the original contacts. However, the development of recurrent axon collaterals and nascent synapses by the mossy fibers might substitute for regeneration. Some new mossy fiber synapses may be formed in the CA3-CA4 area as well (Nadler et al., 1981b).

These issues are currently the subjects of more thorough investigation. We are also attempting to determine whether destruction of CA3-CA4 neurons reduces the responsiveness of dentate granule cells to the transmitters used by their afferent fibers. It should be noted that Scarnati and Pacitti (1982) found that dopaminergic neurons of the substantia nigra lost sensitivity to three neurotransmitters after destruction of striatal neurons with KA. These workers did not consider disconnection of these cells from their postsynaptic targets as an explanation for their finding, however.

RESPONSES OF AFFERENT FIBERS TO LOSS OF TARGET CELLS

Although selective neuronal cell death, such as occurs in AHS, is a common occurrence in the mammalian CNS, little attention has been paid to the fate of afferents that projected to those cells. In KA-induced and clinical AHS the hippocampal mossy fibers lose many of their postsynaptic targets, but their cell bodies of origin survive. One wonders how long their boutons can survive in the absence of a postsynaptic element. To answer this question, the fate of these afferent fibers was studied by light and electron microscopy after destruction of CA3-CA4 neurons with intraventricular KA (Nadler et al., 1981b).

Histochemical staining for heavy metal showed a substantial bleaching of the mossy fiber terminal zone within one day, which suggested a loss of mossy fiber boutons. This visual impression was confirmed by microdensitometric analysis. A quantitative electron microscopic study revealed about a 50% decrease in the incidence of mossy fiber boutons in area CA3 1-7 days after KA treatment. Electron dense degeneration accounted for a portion of this reduction. At a 4-hour survival time, about 10-20% of the total population of mossy fiber boutons was already electron dense and in one day large degeneration products could be demonstrated by the Fink-Heimer procedure in the mossy fiber terminal zone. However, frank electron dense degeneration did not appear to account for the entire loss of boutons. Some mossy fiber boutons may have been resorbed into the parent axon.

Mossy fiber boutons were lost about as rapidly after KA administration as after lesions of the fascia dentata (Haug et al., 1971). This surprisingly rapid presynaptic response to the toxin differed markedly from the apparent retraction of cholinergic septohippocampal (Nadler et al., 1981a) and catecholaminergic (CA) (Fig. 5C) fibers from the region of neuronal cell death. The latter effects occur over a time course of weeks, not hours. Similarly, extrinsic afferents to the lateral geniculate nucleus die back slowly after retrograde degeneration of geniculate neurons (Stenevi et al., 1972), as do striatal afferents after focal injections of KA (Zaczek et al., 1978). The apparently unique vulnerability of mossy fiber boutons to destruction of their postsynaptic targets may be explained by their unusual structure. These extremely large boutons are extensively invaginated by the thorny dendritic excrescences with which they make synaptic contact. The rapid loss of mossy fiber boutons may be attributable to the unusual fragility of such a structure when it is deprived of the mechanical support normally provided by the postsynaptic cell. However, a direct toxic effect of KA on the mossy fiber boutons themselves has not been excluded.

Studies on the mossy fiber projection established that synapses lost by destruction of target cells can be compensated, at least in part, by axon sprouting in other regions innervated by the same projection, if unoccupied postsynaptic sites are available there. Recently, however, we have obtained evidence which suggests the sprouting of hippocampal CA fibers into even normally innervated regions.

Rats were injected with 2.81 nmol of KA into each lateral ventricle and sacrificed about one month later. Fluorescence microscopy demonstrated, as expected, a relative paucity of CA fibers in regions of hippocampal cell loss (Fig. 5A,C). In five animals with relatively complete CA3-CA4 lesions we also found a compensatory increase of CA fibers in other hippocampal regions. Surprisingly, there was no clear relationship to the pattern of terminal degeneration. This apparent proliferation could be seen most clearly in the molecular layer of the fascia dentata (Fig. 5 B,D). Normally, this layer receives only a very sparse CA innervation; only scattered fluorescent varicosities are present and few fibers are visible. After KA treatment, however, the number of fluorescent varicosities increased and numerous beaded fibers could be seen oriented perpendicularly to the granular layer. The density of CA elements was no greater in the denervated CA4 terminal zone than in the rest of the molecular layer. All these fibers had the appearance of central noradrenergic fibers that originate in the nucleus locus coeruleus rather than of peripheral sympathetic axons.

One possible explanation for increased CA fluorescence throughout the dentate molecular layer is that CA fibers replaced synapses lost by degeneration of CA4-derived fibers as well as some of the perforant path synapses that were shed in response to destruction of CA3-CA4 neurons. This explanation seems unlikely, however, since septohippocampal fibers did not proliferate in the perforant path terminal zone, even though they replace degenerated perforant path fibers much more readily than do CA fibers (Cotman and Nadler, 1978). Another possibility is that little or no growth of CA fibers actually took place, but instead the KA treatment increased the CA content, and hence the demonstrability, of varicosities that normally are undetected by fluorescence microscopy. Biochemical data suggest that this explanation may be at least partially correct. KA treatment did not significantly alter the norepinephrine content of the hippocampal formation (KA-treated: 0.52 ± 0.07 µg/g wet wt.; vehicle-injected: 0.56 ± 0.08 µg/g wet wt.; N = 3

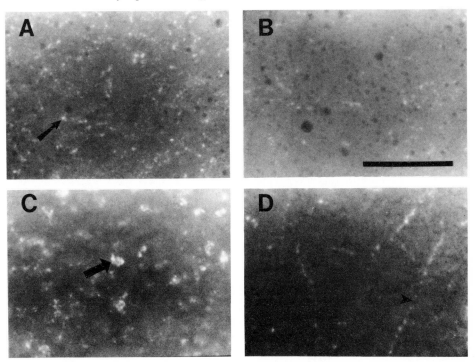

Fig. 5. Glyoxylic acid-induced CA fluorescence one month after bilateral intra-ventricular administration of KA. A: Area CA3 pyramidal cell layer from vehicle-injected rat. Numerous fluorescent varicosities (small arrow) can be seen. B: Dentate molecular layer from vehicle-injected rat. A few scattered fluorescent varicosities are present. C: Area CA3 pyramidal cell layer from KA-treated rat. Many autofluorescent phagocytes (large arrow) are present, but relatively few of the smaller CA varicosities remain. D: Dentate molecular layer from KA-treated rat. More CA structures than normal are present. Beaded fluorescent fibers (arrowhead) radiate outward from the granular layer (at top). Scale bar = 0.1 mm.

in each group), but reduced the high affinity uptake of [^{3}H]norepinephrine by hippocampal particulate fractions (KA-treated: 1.39 ± 0.19 pmol in 7 min/mg protein; vehicle-injected: 1.96 ± 0.12 pmol in 7 min/mg protein; N = 3 in each group; P < 0.03, Student's t-test). These results could be interpreted to signify a net decrease in the total number of CA terminals, but an increase in the norepinephrine content of each terminal. It is unclear, however, whether a 40% increase in average CA content would be sufficient to reveal so many latent structures, especially to induce the appearance of so many more fibers. Finally, CA fibers may proliferate in some terminal regions to compensate for the contraction of their terminal arborization in regions where postsynaptic cells degenerate. Such compensatory proliferation of central CA fibers has been documented previously (Pickel et al., 1974; Reis et al., 1978), although those studies involved actually cutting one branch of the CA axon. Here we are suggesting that degeneration of neurons contacted by central CA fibers may trigger the same compensatory growth as axotomy. The abnormal growth of surviving axonal branches after damage to another branch has been referred to as the "pruning" effect (Devor and Schneider, 1975). Such growth may be expected to have behavioral consequences.

DISCUSSION

AHS was first described in human temporal lobe epileptics more than a century ago, yet even today the relationship between the seizures, brain lesions and deteriorating mental function in these patients is a matter of controversy. The KA model promises to provide some insights into these relationships. Already it is clear that not only do specific neuronal populations degenerate in KA-induced experimental AHS, but, in addition, synaptic relationships are permanently altered. Neurons reduce the size of their terminal arborizations to accomodate a reduction in the target cell population. During this period these neurons may also shed and then regain afferent innervation. Finally, new connections are made to replace those which were lost, sometimes possibly even in regions that were not denervated. Each of these synaptic rearrangements could either ameliorate or exacerbate the behavioral disorder initially caused by neuronal cell death.

Perhaps the most important finding to date is that collateral branches of the hippocampal mossy fibers form a recurrent circuit that appears to increase the excitability of dentate granule cells and even to generate afterdischarge. Recurrent excitatory circuits might also be created in other regions that are deprived of afferent fibers in AHS. Creation of such aberrant circuits may explain how AHS, once established, can sustain or exacerbate the underlying epileptic condition. This hypothesis must be tentative, however, for two reasons. First, it is not yet clear whether KA-induced AHS reproduces the spontaneous and repetitive seizures that are the hallmarks of clinical epilepsy. Second, it has not been determined whether recurrent excitatory circuits are created in the brains of patients with AHS. On the other hand, we are encouraged by recent brief reports of spontaneous seizures weeks after destruction of limbic neurons by focal injections of KA (Cavalheiro et al., 1982) and of synaptic rearrangements in the brains of temporal lobe epileptics (DeLorenzo and Glaser, 1981; DeLorenzo et al., 1982).

In addition to their clinical implications, the changes in synaptic organization reviewed here suggest caution in the use of KA or other excitotoxins as lesioning agents. In most cases, use of these compounds has the advantage over other available methods of destroying neurons exposed to them while sparing fibers that pass to or through the target zone. Studies of the hippocampal mossy fibers suggest that this is not always so, however. Furthermore, if one wishes to relate results of biochemical, physiological or behavioral studies to the destruction of specific neurons, the use of survival times long enough to permit reinnervation or other anatomical adjustments may lead to misinterpretation. Unfortunately, membrane-bound constituents, such as neurotransmitter and drug receptors, may persist on degenerating bits of membrane for weeks. Thus the use of long survival times in receptor localization studies is sometimes unavoidable. Even when short survival times can be used, this difficulty may not be obviated, since some changes in connectivity other than those involving direct neurotoxin-induced degeneration have been observed within a few days. These considerations emphasize the need for comprehensive anatomical monitoring of all excitotoxin lesions. Valid conclusions can be drawn only when the possible contributions of synaptic reorganization to the observed result have been evaluated.

ACKNOWLEDGMENTS

We thank Ms. Patterson McKinnon and Ms. Jamila Tayeb for technical assistance. Some of these studies were supported by research grants NS 06233 and NS 17771 and Research Career Development Award NS 00447 from the National Institutes of Health.

REFERENCES

Brierley, J.B. (1976). Greenfield's Neuropathology, pp. 43-85, Edward Arnold,

London.
Brown, W.J. (1973). Epilepsy: Its Phenomena in Man, pp. 339-374, Academic Press, New York.
Cavalheiro, E.A., D.A. Riche and G. Le Gal La Salle (1982). Electroenceph. Clin. Neurophysiol., 53, 581-589.
Corsellis, J.A.N. (1976). Greenfield's Neuropathology, pp. 796-848, Edward Arnold, London.
Corsellis, J.A.N. and B.S. Meldrum (1976). Greenfield's Neuropathology, pp. 771-795, Edward Arnold, London.
Cotman, C.W. and J.V. Nadler (1978). Neuronal Plasticity, pp. 227-271, Raven Press, New York.
Cotman, C.W., M. Nieto-Sampedro, and E.W. Harris (1981). Physiol. Rev., 61, 684-784.
Danscher, G. (1981). Histochemistry, 71, 1-16.
DeLorenzo, R.J. and G.H. Glaser (1981). Neurology, 31, 114.
DeLorenzo, R.J., G.H. Glaser, P. DeLucia, and D. Schwartz (1982). Neurology, 32, A92.
Devor, M. and G.E. Schneider (1975). Aspects of Neural Plasticity, pp. 191-201, INSERM, Paris.
Falconer, M.A. (1971). Epilepsia, 12, 13-31.
Falconer, M.A. (1974). Lancet, 2, 767-770.
Frotscher, M. and J. Zimmer (1982). Neuroscience, 7, S73.
Goldowitz, D., S.W. Scheff and C.W. Cotman (1979). Brain Res., 170, 427-447.
Gottlieb, D.I. and W.M. Cowan (1973). J. Comp. Neurol., 149, 393-422.
Haug, F.-M.S., T.W. Blackstad, A. Hjorth-Simonsen and J. Zimmer (1971). J. Comp. Neurol., 142, 23-32.
Hoff, S.F., S.W. Scheff, A.Y. Kwan and C.W. Cotman (1981). Brain Res., 222, 1-13.
Laurberg, S. (1979). J. Comp. Neurol., 184, 685-708.
Lorente de Nó, R. (1934). J. Psychol. Neurol. (Leipzig), 46, 113-177.
Margerison, J.H. and J.A.N. Corsellis (1966). Brain, 89, 499-530.
Matthews, D.A., C. Cotman and G. Lynch (1976). Brain Res., 115, 1-21.
Nadler, J.V. (1981). Life Sci., 29, 2031-2042.
Nadler, J.V., C.W. Cotman and G.S. Lynch (1977). J. Comp. Neurol., 171, 561-588.
Nadler, J.V., D.A. Evenson and G.J. Cuthbertson (1981a). Neuroscience, 6, 2505-2517.
Nadler, J.V., B.W. Perry and C.W. Cotman (1978a). Nature, 271, 676-677.
Nadler, J.V., B.W. Perry and C.W. Cotman (1978b). Kainic Acid As a Tool in Neurobiology, pp. 219-237, Raven Press, New York.
Nadler, J.V., B.W. Perry and C.W. Cotman (1980a). Brain Res., 182, 1-9.
Nadler, J.V., B.W. Perry, C. Gentry and C.W. Cotman (1980b). Brain Res., 191, 387-403.
Nadler, J.V., B.W. Perry, C. Gentry and C.W. Cotman (1980c). J. Comp. Neurol., 192, 333-359.
Nadler, J.V., B.W. Perry, C. Gentry and C.W. Cotman (1981b). J. Comp. Neurol., 196, 549-569.
Pickel, V.M., M. Segal and F.E. Bloom (1974). J. Comp. Neurol., 155, 43-50.
Purves, D. and A. Njå (1978). Neuronal Plasticity, pp. 27-47, Raven Press, New York.
Reis, D.J., R.A. Ross, G. Gilad and T.H. Joh (1978). Neuronal Plasticity, pp. 197-226, Raven Press, New York.
Rose, M. (1927). J. Psychol. Neurol. (Leipzig), 34, 1-111.
Scarnati. E. and C. Pacitti (1982). Exp. Brain Res., 46, 377-382.
Schneider, G.E. and S.R. Jhaveri (1974). Plasticity and Recovery of Function in the Central Nervous System, pp. 65-109, Academic Press, New York.
Sommer, W. (1880). Arch. Psychiatr. Nervenkr., 10, 631-675.
Stanfield, B. and W.M. Cowan (1979). Anat. Embryol., 156, 37-52.
Stenevi, U., A. Björklund, and R.Y. Moore (1972). Exp. Neurol., 35, 290-299.
Swanson, L.W., J.M. Wyss and W.M. Cowan (1978). J. Comp. Neurol., 181, 681-715.

Traub, R.D. and R.K.S. Wong (1982). Science, 216, 745-747.
Zaczek, R., R. Schwarcz and J.T. Coyle (1978). Brain Res., 152, 626-632.

ON THE PROBLEM OF DISTANT LESIONS IN BEHAVIOUAL STUDIES UTILIZING KAINIC ACID

H. C. FIBIGER and S. ATMADJA

Department of Psychiatry, University of British Columbia, Vancouver, B.C. V6T 1W5, Canada

ABSTRACT

This role of the dorsal striatum in d-amphetamine-induced motor responses has been re-investigated using kainic and ibotenic acid lesions. In accordance with previous observations, bilateral stereotaxic injections of kainic acid into the striatum resulted in large increases in d-amphetamine-induced locomotor activity. Intraventricular injections of kainic acid, which cause insignificant damage to the striatum, while producing a pattern of distant lesions that are similar to those found after intrastriatal injections, also enhanced the locomotor stimulant effects of amphetamine but to a smaller extent. These results indicate that the distant, extrastriatal lesions that are found after intrastriatal injections of kainic acid contribute to the enhanced locomotor stimulant effects of d-amphetamine. However, damage to the striatum itself is also partly responsible for the potentiation of amphetamine-induced locomotor activity because bilateral ibotenic acid lesions of the striatum, which do not cause distant, extrastriatal lesions, also enhanced this effect of amphetamine. Unilateral intrastriatal injections of kainic acid resulted in ipsilateral turning after d-amphetamine. This observation is not compatible with the hypothesis that kainic acid lesions of the striatum interrupt a striato-nigral negative feedback loop. The discrepancies obtained using unilateral and bilateral excitotoxic lesions of the striatum indicate that at present it is not possible to provide a unified theoretical framework within which to account for the effect of striatal lesions on amphetamine-induced motor behaviors. In contrast to previous findings with kainic acid, bilateral ibotenic acid lesions of the dorsal striatum did not enhance spontaneous locomotor activity during the dark phase of the day-night cycle. This result indicates that the previous finding of increased nocturnal activity after intrastriatal injections of kainic acid is best attributed to the non-striatal, distant lesions produced by this toxin. Some advantages of ibotenic acid over kainic acid in behavioral studies are discussed.

KEYWORDS

Kainic acid - Ibotenic acid - Striatum - Amphetamine - Locomotor activity - Stereotypy - Rotation

INTRODUCTION

The introduction of kainic acid as a tool for producing relatively selective damage to neuronal perikarya while sparing fibers of passage has proven to be of considerable value in many branches of neuroscience, including physiological psychology and behavioral pharmacology. With respect to behavioral studies, this compound has been employed in attempts to determine if local neurons in the vicinity of an intracerebral kainic acid injection site participate in specified behavioral functions or whether the behavioral changes that occur after non-specific (e.g. electrolytic or mechanical) lesions of the same site should be attributed to damage to fibres that pass through the lesioned site. This approach has been used to explore specific behavioral functions of the striatum (Fibiger, 1978; Divac, et al, 1978; Sanberg, et al,1979; Pisa, et al,1980; 1981; Rieke,1980),the lateral hypothalamus (Grossman, et al, 1978), and the hippocampus (Munoz and Grossman,1981).

In the course of studies with intracerebral injections of kainic acid it became evident that its use has a major limitation that is of particular importance in studies concerned with brain-behavior relationships. This concerns the now extensively documented finding that neuronal damage produced by this compound is rarely confined to the area in the injection but typically also includes regions that are remote from this site (Schwob, et al, 1980; Ben-Ari, et al, 1979). This, of course, introduces considerable interpretative difficulties for functional studies because when behavioral changes occur as a result of intracerebral injections of kainic acid, the attribution of these effects to local or distant lesions, or a combination of both, can be uncertain and difficult.

An example of this problem concerns a report from this laboratory that kainic acid injections aimed at the striatum in the rat enhance the locomotor stimulant and stereotypy-inducing properties of d-amphetamine (Mason and Fibiger, 1978). Although these findings were interpreted as being due to a lesion-induced disruption of a striato-nigral negative feedback mechanism that normally controls the activity of dopaminergic neurons in the substantia nigra, a substantially different interpretation of these findings is possible. Specifically, it is known that lesions of the hippocampus can potentiate the motor stimulant effects of amphetamine (Campbell, et al, 1971), and inasmuch as striatal injections of kainic acid typically also cause damage to pyramidal neurons in the CA3 field of the hippocampus (Pisa, et al, 1981), it is possible that damage to the hippocampus rather than the dorsal striatum was the basis for these observations.

The experiments reported here were designed to discriminate between these two alternatives. The first experiment employed animals with intraventricular injections of kainic acid, a procedure that produces many of the distant lesions produced by intrastriatal injections of kainic acid but causes relatively little damage to the striatum itself (Nadler, et al, 1978). The second experiment studied the effects of ibotenic acid, a neurotoxin that is also selective for neuronal perikarya while leaving fibers of passage intact, but which does not cause detectable distant lesions (Schwarcz, et al, 1979; Guldin and Markowitsch, 1981;1982).

METHODS

Male Wistar rats weighing 290-310 gm. at the time of surgery were used in all experiments. The animals were anaesthetized with halothane and placed in a stereotaxic instrument. Some animals received either unilateral or bilateral intrastriatal injections of kainic acid (3 nmol in 0.5µL) or vehicle as described previously (Mason and Fibiger, 1978). Others received identical bilateral injections of kainic acid (3nmol in 0.5 µL) or vehicle, except that the injections were aimed at the lateral ventricles (coordinates AP + 9.6 mm, L±1.3 and DV + 4.5 from stereotaxic zero, with the animal's head held in the horizontal plane). Other groups of animals received bilateral intrastriatal injections of ibotenic acid 28 nmol in 1.0 µL) at the same coordinates as were used for the intrastriatal kainic acid injections (Mason and Fibiger, 1978).

After a recovery period of 30 days (kainic acid) or 15 days (ibotenic acid), during which they were housed singly and maintained on ad libitum food and water, the rats were tested for spontaneous locomotor activity during the day and night, d-amphetamine sulphate (1.0 mg/kg) induced locomotor activity, apomorphine hydrochloride (2.0 mg/kg) induced stereotypy, or d-amphetamine sulphate (1.0 and 2.0 mg /kg) induced rotation. All injections were intraperitoneal. At the end of the behavioral tests the animals were killed and the brains were examined histologically to determine the extent of the lesions.

RESULTS

1. The effect of intrastriatal injections of kainic acid on d-amphetamine-induced locomotor activity. The results of this experiment are given in Fig. 1 and confirm the previous observation that these lesions result in a large enhancement of the locomotor stimulant effects of d-amphetamine (Mason and Fibiger, 1978). As expected the kainic acid injections caused considerable neuronal loss in the dorsal two-thirds of the striatum. In addition, distant lesions were observed in the hippocampus, in some thalamic nuclei, and in the pyriform cortex (Pisa et al, 1981).

2. The effect of intrastriatal injections of ibotenic acid on d-amphetamine-induced locomotor activity and apomorphine-induced stereotypy. As is evident in Fig. 2, ibotenic acid-induced lesions of the striatum resulted in a significant (p <.01) potentiation of the locomotor stimulant effects of d-amphetamine. It is evident, however, that the magnitude of this increase was less than that observed after injection of kainic acid into the same striatal coordinates (Fig. 1). In accordance with earlier results obtained after kainic acid lesions of the striatum (Mason and Fibiger, 1978), intrastriatal injections of ibotenic acid did not affect apomorphine-induced stereotypy (Fig. 3). Histological analysis of the brains of animals receiving the ibotenic acid lesions indicated that the extent of the striatal damage was similar to that in the kainic acid group. In contrast to the latter group, however, extrastriatal damage was not observed in the ibotenic acid lesioned animals except occasionally in the neocortex overlying the striatal injection.

3. The effect of intraventricular injections of kainic acid on d-amphetamine-induced locomotor activity. Intraventricular injections of kainic acid resulted in a small, but statistically significant (p <.01) increase in the locomotor stimulant of amphetamine (Fig. 4). Histological analysis indicated that while the intraventricular injections produced little, if any,loss of neurons in the striatum, the patterns of degeneration in the CA3 and CA4 regions of the hippocampus, in the thalamus,and in the pyriform cortex, were similar to the distant lesions observed after the intrastriatal injections of kainic acid.

4. The effect of unilateral injections of kainic acid on rotation produced by d-amphetamine. Unilateral intrastriatal injections of kainic acid resulted in significant, dose-related ipsilateral rotation (i.e. towards the lesioned side) in response to d-amphetamine (Fig. 5). Histological examintion indicated that the lesion was restricted to the striatum, except for occasional damage to the overyling deep layers of neocortex around the track of the injection cannula.

5. The effect of bilateral intrastriatal injections of ibotenic acid on spontaneouss locomotor activity measured during the night. As is seen in Fig. 6, bilateral ibotenic acid lesions of the striatum failed to affect spontaneous locomotor activity during the dark phase of the day-night cycle.

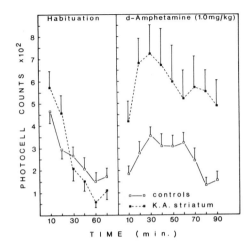

Fig. 1.   The effect of bilateral injections of kainic acid (3 nmol in 0.5 µL) aimed at the dorsal half of the striatum (see Mason and Fibiger, 1978) on spontaneous (habituation) and d-amphetamine sulphate induced loco- motor activity.   Data represent means and S.E.M.'s of 10 animals   in each group, and were obtained approximately 30 days after the kainic acid lesions.

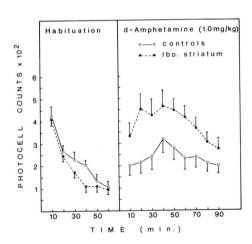

Fig. 2.   The effect of bilateral ibotenic acid lesions (28 nmol in 1 µL) of the dorsal half of the striatum on spontaneous (habituation) and d-ampheta- mine sulphate induced locomotor activity.   Data represent means   and S.E.M.'s of 12 animals in each group, and were obtained about 15 days after the ibotenic acid lesions.

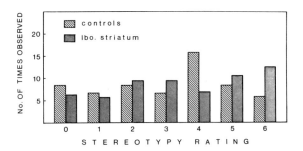

Fig. 3.   The effect of bilateral ibotenic acid lesions of the dorsal striatum
         (28 nmol in 1 μL) on apomorphine hydrochloride (2.0 mg/kg) induced
         stereotypy. Stereotypy scores were recorded every 10 min for 1 hour
         after the injection according to Creese and Iversen's (1975) rating
         scale. There were no statistically significant differences between
         the control (n=12) and ibotenic acid lesioned (n=12) groups.

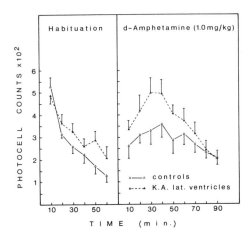

Fig. 4.   The effect of bilateral injections of kainic acid (3 nmol in 0.5 μL)
         into the lateral ventricles on spontaneous (habituation) and d-
         amphetamine induced locomotor activity. Data represent means and
         S.E.M.'s of 10 animals in each group, and were obtained about 30
         days after the kainic acid injections.

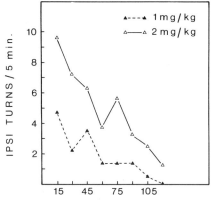

Fig. 5.   The effect of unilateral injections of kainic acid (3 nmol in 0.5 μL)
          aimed at the dorsal striatum on d-amphetamine sulphate induced rotation.
          Data represent mean number of turns towards the lesioned side in 10
          animals, and were obtained 30-35 days after the kainic acid lesions.

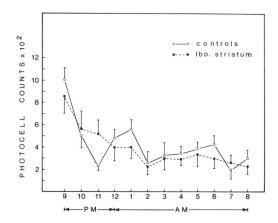

Fig. 6.   The effect of bilateral ibotenic acid lesions (28 nmol in 1 μL) of the
          dorsal half of the striatum on spontaneous locomotor activity during
          the dark phase of the day (12 hr) -night (12 hr) cycle. The animals
          were placed in the photocell activity cages at the beginning of the dark
          phase (8 p.m.). Data represent means and S.E.M.'s of 12 animals in
          each group, and were obtained about 25 days after the ibotenic acid
          lesions. There were no statistically significant group differences.

DISCUSSION

Mason and Fibiger (1978) reported that kainic acid lesions of the dorsal striatum enhanced the locomotor stimulant effects of d-amphetamine. The present results suggest that two neuropathological effects of striatal injections of kainic acid contributed to this effect. First, intraventricular injections of kainic acid were found to result in a modest, although statistically significant potentiation of amphetamine-induced locomotor activity. Because this procedure spares the striatum but damages many of the same extrastriatal regions that undergo neuropathological changes after intrastriatal injections of kainic acid, a contribution of these distant lesions to the enhanced locomotor stimulant effects of d-amphetamine is indicated. It should be noted, however, that the magnitude of facilitation of amphetamine motor stimulation was considerably greater in rats with intrastriatal injections of kainic acid than it was in rats with intraventricular injections (compare Figs. 1 and 4). Thus, it is unlikely that extrastriatal damage can account completely for the potentiation of the amphetamine effect. This conclusion is supported by the observation that bilateral injections of ibotenic acid into the striatum, which caused striatal damage that was qualitatively and quantitatively similar to that produced by intrastriatal injections of kainic acid, also significantly facilitated amphetamine-induced locomotor activity. Again, however, the magnitude of this effect was less than that observed in rats that had received bilateral kainic acid injections into the striatum. Thus while Mason and Fibiger's (1978) hypothesis concerning damage to a striato-nigral negative feedback loop receives a degree of support from the present observations in the ibotenate lesioned rats,it appears that striatal damage accounts for only part of the potentiation of the amphetamine effect in rats with bilateral kainic acid lesions of the striatum, and that extrastriatal damage is also a significant contributing factor.

Although damage to a striato-nigral negative feedback loop appears to account for at least part the increased motor stimulant effects of amphetamine in rats with bilateral kainic acid lesions of the striatum, the observations on rats with identical unilateral lesions indicate that complexities remain and that it is not possible to explain the effects of these lesions on amphetamine-induced behaviors in terms of a single striatal mechanism. Specifically, amphetamine was found to cause ipsilateral rotation in rats with unilateral kainic acid lesions of the striatum. The most parsimonious explanation for this observation is that the lesions damaged a striatal mechanism that is normally involved in the expression of amphetamine-induced motor output. If, as data obtained in animals with bilateral lesions would suggest, the unilateral kainic acid lesions had damaged a negative striato-nigral feedback mechanism (Mason and Fibiger, 1978), then amphetamine should have caused contralateral rather than ipsilateral rotation due to the enhanced dopaminergic function on the lesioned side (Ungerstedt, 1971). Clearly, opposite results were obtained and at present the basis of these discrepancies remain to be determined. One possibility is that the neural mechanisms underlying amphetamine-induced rotation differ from those that mediate locomotor activity, and are perhaps more similar to those involved in amphetamine-induced stereotypy. In this regard, it is noteworthy that the doses of amphetamine required to elicit maximal rotational behavior are "stereotypic" doses in intact animals (Ungerstedt, 1971). According to this hypothesis bilateral kainic acid-induced lesions of the striatum would be expected to decrease amphetamine-induced stereotypy. However, rats with these lesions have been found to display enhanced stereotyped behaviors in response to high doses of d-amphetamine (Mason et al, 1978). At present, therefore, it does not appear possible to offer a unified framework within which to account for the effects of kainic acid lesions of the striatum on amphetamine-induced motor behaviors.

Mason and Fibiger (1979) reported that kainic acid lesions of the striatum in-

creased the spontaneous nocturnal locomotor activity of rats. In the present experiments, we were unable to demonstrate a similar effect in rats with striatal
ibotenic acid lesions. The major histopathological difference between the kainic
and ibotenic acid lesioned groups is that the former also possess extrastriatal
lesions. We conclude therefore, that the enhanced nocturnal locomotor activity of
the kainic acid lesioned rats is most likely due to damage to neuronal structures
lying outside the striatum. In this regard, it is interesting to note that lesions of the hippocampus have been reported to result in large increases in spontaneous locomotor activity (Campbell et al, 1971). The hippocampal damage produced by intrastriatal injections of kainic acid seems, therefore, to be a likely
candidate for neural basis of this behavioral observation.

The present experiments point to certain advantages of using ibotenic acid in behavioral studies. The most marked benefit is that this compound does not produce
the distant lesions that occur regularly after local intracerebral injections of
kainic acid. The absence of distant lesions obviously greatly simplifies the interpretation of functional changes that occur after local injections of ibotenic
acid. Another significant advantage of ibotenic acid is that we have found that
the lesions produced by this compound are much more reproducible from one animal
to the next both in terms of size and shape. In addition, compared to kainic
acid, the size of the lesion produced by ibotenic acid is more consistently and
predictably related to the dose employed. The introduction of ibotenic acid
seems to leave little justification for the continued use of kainic acid in studies concerned with the role of specific neuronal systems in behavior.

The above considerations indicate that ibotenic acid has a number of distinct ad-
advantages over kainic acid in programs of research that are concerned with the
role of specific neuronal systems in behavior.

ACKNOWLEDGEMENT

Supported by the Medical Research Council. The generous supply of ibotenic acid
provided by Dr. C.H. Eugster is most gratefully acknowledged.

REFERENCES

Ben-Ari, Y., E. Tremblay, O.P. Ottersen and R. Naquet (1979). Brain Res. 165, 362-
    365.
Campbell, B.A., P. Ballantine and G. Lynch (1971). Exp. Neurol., 33, 159-170.
Divac, I., H.J. Markowitsch and M. Pritzel (1978). Brain Res., 151,523-532.
Fibiger, H.C. (1978). Kainic Acid As a Tool in Neurobiology, 161-176, ed. E.G.
    McGeer, Raven Press, New York.
Grossman, S.P., D. Dacey, A.E. Halaris, T. Collier and A. Routtenberg (1978).
    Science, 202, 537-539.
Guldin, W.O., and H.J. Markowitsch (1982). J. Neurosci. Meth., 5, 83-93.
Guldin, W.O., and H.J. Markowitsch (1981). Brain Res., 225, 446-451.
Mason, S.T., and H.C. Fibiger (1979). Neuropharmacol., 18, 403-407.
Mason, S.T., and H.C. Fibiger (1978). Brain Res., 155, 313-329.
Mason, S.T., P.R. Sanberg and H.C. Fibiger (1978). Science, 201, 352-355.
Munoz, C., and S.P. Grossman (1981). Brain Res. Bull., 6, 399-406.
Nadler, J.V., B.W. Perry and C.W. Cotman (1978). Nature, 271, 676-677.
Pisa, M., P.R. Sanberg and H.C. Fibiger (1981). Exp. Neurol., 74, 633-653.
Pisa, M., P.R. Sanberg and H.C. Fibiger (1980). Physiol. Behav., 24, 11-19.
Rieke, G.K. (1980). Physiol. & Behav., 24, 683-687.
Sanberg, P.R., M. Pisa and H.C. Fibiger (1979). Pharmacol. Biochem. Behav., 10,
    10, 137-144.

Schwarcz, R., C. Kohler, K. Fuxe, T. Hokfelt and M. Goldstein (1979). In <u>Advances in Neurology, Vol. 23,</u> ed. T.N. Chase et al, Raven Press, New York.
Schwob, J.E., T. Fuller, J.L. Price and J.W. Olney (1980). <u>Neurosci.,</u> 5, 991-1014.
Ungerstedt, U. (1971). <u>Acta Physiol. Scand. Suppl.,</u> 367, 49-68.

KAINIC ACID INJECTIONS INTO THE RAT NEOSTRATUM:
EFFECTS ON LEARNING AND EXPLORATION

MICHELE PISA

Department of Neurosciences, McMaster University, Hamilton, Ontario, Canada, L8N 3Z5

Hamilton, Ontario, Canada, L8N 3Z5

ABSTRACT

Rats with bilateral injections of kainic acid (KA) in the neostriatum showed alterations of locomotor, exploratory, and learning and memory performance. Thus, compared with vehicle-injected rats, the KA-treated rats ran more slowly, were resistant to extinction of appetitive bar pressing, showed greater hesitation to explore novel environments and to eat novel food, and were impaired in performance of spatial and hedonic memory tasks, and in learning and extinction of aversive locomotor responses. The KA injections induced massive neuronal loss in the dorsal-central region of the neostriata. Neuronal loss was also detected in the rostral globus pallidus, frontal cortex, hippocampus and olfactory tubercle. Both the multifocal neuronal loss and the complex pattern of locomotor, affective and cognitive alterations resembled those of patients with Huntington's Disease (HD), thus supporting the view that the KA striatal preparation may be a useful anatomical, biochemical and behavioral model of the human disease. On the other hand, the multifocality of the KA-induced pathology counterindicates the use of KA striatal injections for investigations of the behavioral effects of selective loss of neostriatal neurons.

KEYWORDS

Kainic acid; striatum; learning; memory; exploration; neophobia.

INTRODUCTION

On the basis of behavioral studies of animals with coagulative lesions of the neostriatum, a role has been proposed for this brain nucleus in cognition (Oberg and Divac, 1978), and inhibitory control of arousal reactions (Kirkby, 1973). Unfortunately, coagulative lesions indiscriminately destroy all neural elements, including the corticofugal fibers traversing the neostriatum, thus preventing a convincing attribution of the resulting behavioral disorders specifically to loss of striatal neurons. Furthermore, the mechanisms by which thermal or electrolytic coagulations cause neural destruction are unlikely to bear any resemblance to those responsible for striatal neurodegeneration in human diseases, thus limiting the usefulness of these methods in experimental neurophysiopathology.

In recent years, it was found that injections of the neurotoxin kainic acid (KA) into the rat neostriatum induced degenerative loss of neurons and reactive glial proliferation in the neostriatum, with sparing of both the afferent fibers and the fibers of passage (Divac et al., 1978; Mason and Fibiger, 1978; Schwarcz and Coyle, 1977). Both these morphological alterations and the attendant biochemical changes (Coyle and Schwarcz, 1976; McGeer and McGeer, 1976) resembled those found in the caudate-putamen of patients with Huntington's disease (HD), suggesting that the mechanisms of HD and KA-induced neurodegenerations may have some basic features in common.

The degenerative process of HD, although especially conspicuous in the caudate-putamen, also affects the cortex and other subcortical structures (Bruyn et al., 1979; Forno and Jose, 1973; Lange et al., 1974). In spite of the traditional wisdom attributing the motor disorders (chorea) to caudate-putamen pathology and the cognitive and affective disorders to cortical pathology, there is in fact no conclusive evidence on the specific anatomical correlates of the behavioral impairments of HD patients.

The objective of the studies reviewed here was to determine whether alterations of learning and memory performance and of reactivity to novel stimuli attended the KA-induced loss of striatal neurons in the rat, and whether the observed behavioral alterations resembled those found in patients with HD. Some of the results have already been published elsewhere (Pisa et al., 1980; Pisa et al., 1981; Sanberg et al., 1979).

GENERAL METHOD

Male Wistar rats (275-300 gm), were anaesthetized with 50 mg/kg sodium pentobarbital ip, and positioned on a rodent stereotaxic instrument. A solution of 3 nmol KA dissolved in 0.5 µl phosphate buffer, pH 7.2, was infused into the brains of the rats assigned to KA treatment, at the following coordinates: 9.6 mm rostral and 4.5 dorsal to the interaural line, and 2.8 mm lateral to the sagittal suture. The infusions were made bilaterally with a 34 gauge cannula over a 3-min period. The control rats received infusions of the vehicle solution, with no KA, at the same coordinates. Postoperatively, the rats were individually housed in stainless steel cages in a colony room with 12-h light: 12-h dark cycle, and maintained on ad-lib Rat Purina Chow and tap water. Rats that showed a transient post-operative aphagia and adipsia were tube-fed with 10 ml Soyalac® twice daily, until they resumed spontaneous feeding. The behavioral tests began at least three weeks after surgery. The rats trained in the appetitive tasks were subjected to a food restricted diet that reduced their body weights to 85% of the free-feeding values. Before training, these rats were given adaptation sessions to both the test environments and the 45-mg food pellets (Noyes, Inc.) used as reward. After completion of behavioral testing, the rats were deeply anaesthetized with either ether or an overdose of pentobarbital, and perfused intracardially with isotonic saline solution followed by a 10% formol-saline solution. The brains were extracted, stored for two weeks in the fixative, frozen, and cut in coronal sections 40 µm thick. The sections were stained with cresyl violet and luxol fast blue (Kluver and Barrera, 1953), and examined by light microscopy.

PROCEDURE AND RESULTS

Acquisition and extinction of continuously reinforced appetitive responses. Two experiments were conducted to examine the effects of KA treatment on acquisition and extinction of appetitively reinforced behaviors.

In the first experiment, groups (N=10) of control and KA-injected rats were trained to press a bar on a schedule of continuous food (one pellet) reinforcement (CRF) in standard operant boxes (BRS, Foringer), for 12, 30-min daily sessions. On sessions 13 to 17 reinforcement was discontinued, and each session lasted until the rats reached the extinction criterion of no bar presses for 3 consecutive minutes.

Analysis of the number of responses in acquisition showed a significant effect of sessions, $F(11, 98) = 342$, $p < .001$, reflecting the increase of bar pressing with practice, with no reliable lesion effect, $F(1, 18) = 2.5$, or lesion x sessions interaction effect, $F(11, 98) = 1.0$, $p_s > .1$, indicating no differences between groups in either overall number of bar presses or rate of learning. In extinction, however, there was a significant lesion x sessions interaction, $F(4, 72) = 3.7$, $p < .05$. Tests of simple main effects of lesion ($p < .05$) revealed that the KA-treated rats bar pressed significantly more, and took significantly longer to reach the extinction criterion than the controls in both the first and the second session (Fig. 1).

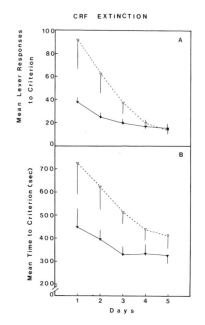

CRF EXTINCTION

Fig. 1.   Mean ± SE bar presses (A) and latencies (B) of control (open) triangles) and KA-treated (filled triangles) rats to reach the criterion of bar press extinction (from Sanberg et al., 1979).

In the second experiment, groups (N=20) of control and KA-injected rats were trained to run on a CRF schedule in a wooden, L-shape runway, 12 cm wide and 30 cm high, and with start box, alley, and goal box 35 cm, 132 cm, and 35 cm long, respectively. The goal box was entered with a 90° right turn from the alley. Each daily session consisted of 5 run trials. In the trials of the 5 acquisition sessions, running was rewarded with 5 food pellets in a cup at the rear end of the goal box. In the trials of the 5 extinction sessions running was not rewarded.

Analysis of the logarithmically transformed running times (log times) in the alley during acquisition (Fig. 2) revealed a significant effect of sessions, $F(5, 180) = 50.2$, $p < .001$, reflecting the increase of running speed with practice, with no significant lesion x sessions interaction, $F < 1$, indicating that the two groups did not reliably differ in learning of the running response. However, the lesion x trials interaction was significant, $F(4, 864) = 3.7$, $p < .01$, with Neumann-Keuls post-hoc comparisons ($p < .05$) showing that the KA-treated rats ran

significantly more slowly than the controls in the first trial of the daily
sessions, although not in the subsequent trials.

Analysis of the logtimes in extinction revealed a significant lesion x sessions
interaction, $F(4, 144) = 2.8$, $p < .05$. The KA-treated rats ran significantly
more slowly than the controls in session 5 ($p < .05$), although not in the previous
sessions. As in acquisition, the lesion x trials interaction was significant,
$F(4, 720) = 5.3$, $p < .005$, with Neumann-Keuls post-hoc comparisons ($p < .05$)
showing that the KA-treated rats ran more slowly than the controls in the first
daily trial although not in the subsequent trials.

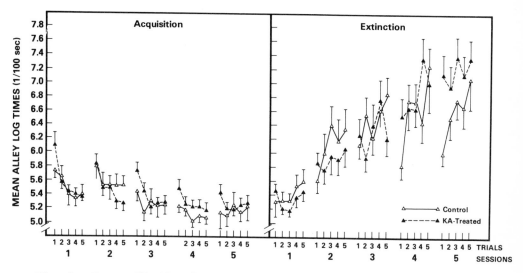

Fig. 2.   Mean ± SE alley logtimes of control and KA-treated rats in acquisition and extinction of continuously reinforced running (from
Pisa et al., 1981, modified).

Thus, striatal injections of KA did not appreciably alter learning of continuously reinforced appetitive responses. However, they appeared to produce both a
releasing effect on performance of manipulative responses, as indicated by the
resistance to extinction of bar pressing, and an impairment in performance of
fast locomotor responses, as indicated by the relatively slow running speed both
in the last session of extinction and in the first daily trial of both the acquisition and the extinction sessions.

Learning of spatial alternation and speed alternation.   To examine the effects of
KA striatal injection on working memory (Honig, 1978) for past places and past
reward events, two experiments were conducted.

In the first experiment, groups (N = 10) of control and KA-treated rats were
trained on a schedule of contingent food reinforcement (five pellets) for left-
right alternation in a wooden, grey-painted T-maze, 17 cm high, 8 cm wide, and
with start box, stem and goal arms 27 cm, 66 cm, and 39 cm long, respectively.
The rats were given 5 daily trials (four alternation opportunities), with inter-
trial interval (ITI) of 20 sec spent in a waiting box, until they reached the
learning criterion of 18 alternations in 4 consecutive sessions, or up to a
maximum of 25 sessions.

The results were clearcut. All control rats but one reached the learning criterion, taking an average of 16.3 sessions. In contrast, none of the KA-treated

rats met the learning criterion before the end of training (one KA-treated rat
was discontinued from training after four sessions because it did not run in the
maze). Mean errors (nonalternated responses) before the end of training were
23.1 and 84.0 for the control and the KA-treated rats, respectively, $U=5$, $n_1/n_2=$
9/10, $p < .01$.

Normal rats trained to run on a schedule of alternated food reinforcement, learn
to run more slowly in the nonrewarded than in the rewarded trials. This behavior
has been interpreted to reflect hedonic memory, or memory of past reward events
(Capaldi, 1971). In the second experiment, groups (N=9) of control and KA-treated rats were trained to run from the start box to the goal box of the runway on
a schedule of alternated food reinforcement. Each daily session consisted of
12 run trials. In the 32 acquisition sessions, five pellets of food reward were
placed in a food cup at the rear end of the goal box in the even, but not in the
odd trials. In the subsequent 5 extinction sessions, no reward was available in
any trials. In the first 22 sessions of acquisition, the ITI was 1 min. To
challenge hedonic memory more severely, the ITI was increased to 5 min in the
last 10 acquisition sessions.

Acquisition performance is shown in Figure 3. The first result to be noted is
that, independent of trial outcome, the KA-treated rats ran significantly more
slowly than the controls both in the sessions with 1-min ITI and those with 5-min
ITI (in the ANOVA of the logtimes in the alley, $p < .01$ for all values of the
main lesion effect).

It has been shown that, once normal rats learn to alternate speed, they display
less marked speed alternation in the late than in the early trials of the daily
sessions, presumably on account of proactive interference (Flaherty and Davenport, 1972). Thus, if the KA-induced brain lesions impaired hedonic memory,
differences between groups in alternation performance would be especially expected in the late daily trials. Planned orthogonal contrasts were therefore set up,
independently testing the effect of reward alternation on the logtimes of the
first 2 daily trials and on the logtimes of the last 10 daily trials, in the
blocks of initial 5 sessions, last five sessions with 1-min ITI, and last 5
sessions with 5-min ITI.

Analyses of the alley logtimes in the first 2 daily trials showed that both the
control and the KA-treated rats ran significantly faster in Trial 2 than in Trial
1 at the end of training with either 1 or 5-min ITI ($p < .01$). For the control
rats, this speed difference clearly resulted from learning of the reinforcement-
alternation contingency, as indicated by the nonsignificant ($p > .1$) speed difference between first and second trials in the initial 5 sessions of training. On
the other hand, the KA-treated rats showed significant ($p < .05$) speed differentiation not only in the late sessions, but also in the initial 5 sessions, indicating that a bradykinetic disorder contributed to the relatively low running speed
in the first daily trial. With practice, however, the KA-treated rats showed an
increase of the speed difference between first and second trial, indicating learning of the alternation contingency.

Analysis of the alley logtimes in the last 10 daily trials showed that in the
initial five sessions neither the control rats nor the KA-treated rats alternated
speed significantly ($p_s > .1$). However, in the last 5 sessions with either
1-min or 5-min ITI, the control rats showed a significantly lower speed in the
nonrewarded than in the rewarded trials ($p_s < .05$), the KA-treated rats did not
($p_s > .05$).

Analysis of the alley logtimes in extinction showed that the KA-treated rats ran
more slowly than the controls in session 5 (Neumann-Keuls post-comparisons,

p < .05), although not in the earlier extinction sessions.

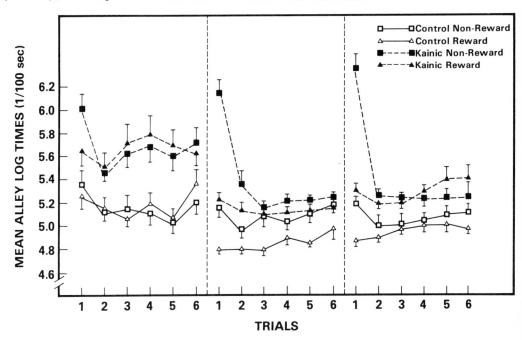

Fig. 3.   Mean ± SE alley logtimes of control and KA-treated rats in the
rewarded and nonrewarded trials of the first 5 sessions with
1-min ITI (left panel), last 5 sessions with 1-min ITI (central
panel), and last 5 sessions with 5-min ITI (right panel) of
alternately reinforced running (from Pisa et al., 1981,
modified).

The results thus indicated an impairment of the KA-treated rats in performance
of spatial and hedonic memory tasks. Furthermore, the bradykinesia of the KA-
treated rats in the task of CRF running was confirmed in the task of alternately
reinforced running.

<u>Learning of aversively motivated responses</u>. Two experiments were conducted to
investigate the effects of KA striatal injections on learning performance of
aversively motivated responses.

In the first experiment, acquisition and retention of passive avoidance were
examined. The rats, which had previously participated to the experiment of appetitive bar pressing, were trained in a 27x27x30 cm box with Plexiglas walls, a
grid floor connected to an AC current generator and scrambler (Layfayette, mod.
82404), and a 26.7x7.5 cm wooden platform hinged on a microswitch 9.4 cm above
the floor. In the first session, the rats were placed on the platform. Upon
releasing the microswitch and stepping down on the grid, the rats received a 2 mA
footshock, which lasted until the rats climbed on the platform. The session
continued until the rats reached the learning criterion of 3 consecutive minutes
spent on the platform. The next day, retention was tested: the rats were placed
on the platform, and their step down latencies, up to a maximum of 3 min, recorded. To determine whether the KA-induced brain lesions altered sensitivity to
footshock, 3 days after the retention test the platform was removed from the box,
the rats placed on the grid floor, and a series of inescapable 0.5 sec footshocks

of ascending intensities delivered with an intershock interval of 15 sec. Threshold shock intensities for flinch, jump and vocalization were determined as the
occurrence of these behaviors at least in 3 out of 5 shock presentations at that
intensity.

Acquisition and retention data are shown in Table 1. In session 1, control and
KA-treated rats did not significantly differ in latency to the first step-down
response, t < .1. After the first footshock, however, the KA-treated rats took
significantly longer, and made significantly more step-down responses to reach
the learning criterion than the controls, indicating an impairment of learning
performance. In the retention test, the rats of both groups showed much longer
step-down latencies than in Session 1, indicating memory of the footshock experience. However, the latencies of the KA-treated rats were significantly shorter
than those of the controls, indicating an impairment of retention performance.
The two groups did not significantly differ in shock-detection thresholds, as
measured by either flinch, jump, or vocalization reactions, t_s < 1.

TABLE I

Acquisition and retention of passive avoidance

Group	N	Latency to first step down	Time to criterion	Responses to criterion	Retention step down latency
Control	10	3.58 ± 1.0	298.7 ± 28.7	3.1 ± 0.2	148.2 ± 16.7
Striatal kainic	11	3.78 ± 1.4	502.6 ± 42.8[*]	6.1 ± 0.6[**]	83.5 ± 23.1[§]

Note. Data are means ± SE. Time data are expressed in seconds.

[*] t(19) = 3.64, p < .005; [**] t(19) = 4.62, p < .0005 (two-tailed test).

[§] U(10/11) = 25.5, p < .05 (Mann-Whitney test, two-tailed).

In the second experiment, acquisition, extinction and reversal of active avoidance
were examined. Groups (N = 9) of control and KA-treated rats were trained in a
wooden box 29 cm high and 30 cm wide, with a guillotine door dividing the 70 cm
length of the box into equal halves, and with a grid floor connected to a generator of scrambled AC current. On each trial, the rat was placed in the left compartment of the box. After 5 sec, a tone (Sonalert, 2800 Hz) was sounded and the
guillotine door raised. If the rat moved to the right compartment within 10 sec
from the onset of the tone, the tone terminated and no shock was delivered; otherwise, the grid of the left compartment was electrified with 1 mA current. As
soon as the rat performed the avoidance or the escape response, the door was
closed, the rat left in the right compartment for 15 sec, and then carried to the
left side for the next trial. In Session 1, the rats were trained to reach the
learning criterion of 9 consecutive avoidances. In Session 2, 3 days after the
acquisition session, retention was tested by re-training the rats to the same
criterion as in acquisition. The next day, extinction training was started: the
procedure was the same as before, except that shock never followed the tone. The
rats were given daily sessions of 30 trials until they reached the extinction
criterion of 4 consecutive avoidance omissions. The original shock contingency

was then re-instituted, and the rats trained to reacquire the avoidance criterion
in a single session. The next day the shock contingency was reversed. The rat
was inserted in the left compartment, the tone was sounded and the door opened
after 5 sec. If the rat moved to the right compartment within 10 sec of tone onset, it received continuous footshock there, until it went back to the left compartment (which now was the safe compartment). If the rat remained in the left
compartment for 10 sec after the tone onset, the tone was terminated, the door
closed, and no shock delivered. The rats were trained to the criterion of 3
consecutive trials in which they passively avoided footshock, by remaining in the
left compartment during the 10-sec tone. One week after completion of avoidance
training, footshock detection thresholds were determined with the procedure
already described.

The results are shown in Figure 4. The KA-treated rats did not significantly
differ from the controls in either retention or re-acquisition performance, t = 1
or less. However, they took significantly more trials than the controls to reach
the criteria of acquisition, extinction and reversal (or passive avoidance),
t(16)=2.15, 2.16, and 2.49, respectively, p < .05, indicating an impairment of
both learning of avoidance responses and suppression of nonreinforced and punished
avoidance responses.

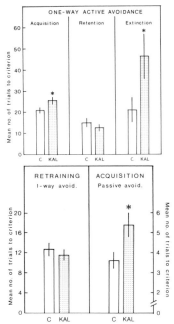

Fig. 4.   Mean ± SE trials of control (C) and KA-lesioned (KAL) rats to
          reach the criteria of acquisition, retention, extinction (upper
          panels), re-acquisition and reversal (lower panels) of active
          avoidance.

Exploration and reaction to novel stimuli. The effects of KA striatal injections
on exploratory locomotion and novelty reactions were examined in two experiments.

In the first experiment, groups (N = 10) of nine control and KA-treated rats were
tested for locomotor exploration and spontaneous alternation in the T-maze already
described. In the daily Sessions 1 to 5, the rats were placed at the choice point
and the entries into the stem and the goal arms recorded during each of 5, 1-min

periods. In the daily Sessions 6 to 10, the rats were first given a trial to
establish their initial goal arm preference, and then 2 trials of spontaneous
alternation. In each trial, the rats were placed in the start box and given the
opportunity to run to the choice point and enter a goal arm, where they were
confined for 10 sec. The rats were then moved to a waiting box, where they spent
a 20-sec ITI. Rats that failed to select a goal arm within 5 min in one or more
trials were given a make-up session on Day 11.

Locomotor performance in the T-maze is shown in Fig. 5. There was a significant
lesion x sessions interaction effect on the number of entries $F(4,72)=1.6$,
$p < .05$, with Neumann-Keuls post-hoc comparisons ($p < .05$) revealing that the
KA-treated rats made significantly less entries than the controls in Session 1,
although not in the subsequent sessions. The KA-treated also made significantly
less entries than the controls in the first 1-min period of the daily sessions
($p < .05$), although not in the subsequent periods.

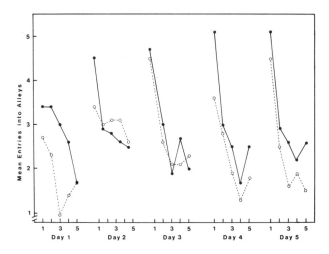

Fig. 5. Mean ± SE entries of control (filled circles) and KA-treated (open
         circles) rats into the alley of a T-maze in the 5 sessions of
         locomotor exploration. Numbers in abscissa indicate 1-min
         periods (from Pisa et al., 1980).

In the test of spontaneous alternation (Table II), the KA-treated rats failed to
leave the start box in several trials, thus making significantly less choices
than the controls. However, there was no significant difference between groups
in spontaneous alternation performance in either the first or the second alternation trial, $U = 35.0$ and 46.5, respectively, $p > .1$.

In the second experiment, groups (N=9) of naive control and KA-treated rats were
tested first in a maze with multiple alleys, and then in an open field. The maze
had wooden, gray-painted floor and walls, and a Plexiglas top. It consisted of a
central square area of 80 cm side, with a start box and a goal box (both squares
of 30 cm side) at two opposite corners. The central square was divided by
wooden partitions into 5 alleys parallel to the diagonal joining the start box
to the goal box. A cup with 8 Noyes pellets (which were a novel food for the
rats) was placed at the rear end of the goal box. The maze was illuminated by
a 100-W bulb 2 m above its center. After 24 h of food deprivation, the rats
were inserted in the start box and given the opportunity to ambulate in the
maze for 21 min after their exit from the start box.

TABLE II

Choice behavior and spontaneous alternation in a T-maze

Group	N	Number of choices		% alternation	
		Trial 1	Trial 2	Trial 1	Trial 2
Control	10	5(4-5)	5(4-5)	60(40-100)	80(60-100)
Striatal					
kainic	10	4(1-5)*	3(1-5)*	60(0-100)	87.5(20-100)

Note. Data are medians and ranges.
*significantly different from control, p < .05 (Mann-Whitney U test, two-tailed).

The KA-treated rats took significantly longer than the controls both to exit from the start box and to start eating food after entering the goal box (Table III). Analyses of the entries into the alleys showed that the KA-treated rats entered significantly less alleys than the controls in the first 3-min period (Neumann-Keuls test, p < .05), but not in the subsequent periods (Fig. 6).

Two weeks later, the rats were tested in the open field, which consisted of a white-painted wooden board illuminated by a 100-W bulb, 2 m above its center, and was divided into a grid of 16 squares of 30 cm side by black lines. The rats were placed in the center of the board and given the opportunity to ambulate for 5 min.

TABLE III

Mean ± SE start latencies and latencies to eat
novel food in the maze with multiple alleys

Group	N	Start latency (sec)	Latency to eat food (sec)
Control	9	29.2 ± 6.1	37.3 ± 7.2
Striatal kainic	9	75.0 ± 10.5*	74.5 ± 12.4**

* significantly different from control, t(16) = 3.7, p < .002.

** significantly different from control, t(16) = 2.6, p < .02.

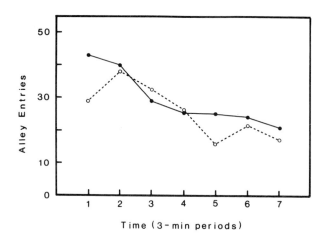

Fig. 6. Mean alley entries of control (filled circles) and KA-treated
(open circles) rats in the maze with multiple parallel alleys.

The rats of the two groups did not significantly differ in either number of
entries into the squares, number of rearings, number of fecal boli, or time spent
grooming (Student's t test, two-tailed, p < .05 for all comparisons between group
means). However, the KA-treated rats showed increased thigmotaxis, i.e., they
preferred to ambulate at the periphery of the open field more than the controls,
as indicated by the significant difference between groups in the ratio of entries
into the outer squares to entries into the inner squares (control 4.5 ± .05,
striatal kainic 10.4 ± 1.5, t(16) = 3.4, p < .005). Consistent with this result,
the KA-treated rats showed a significantly higher ratio of rearings in the peripheral squares to rearings in the inner squares than the controls, t(16) = 2.7,
p < .02.

An increase of thigmotactic behavior in open fields has been shown in rats with
electrolytic lesions of the neostriatum (Kirkby, 1973). This behavioral alteration has been interpreted to reflect increased fear (Ross et al. 1966). Consistent with the interpretation that the KA striatal lesions increased neophobia,
the KA-treated rats took longer to start exploration and to eat novel food in the
mazes, and showed less locomotor exploration in the initial period of exposure to
the mazes than the control rats.

Histology. The brains of the KA-treated rats showed markedly enlarged forebrain
ventricles and bilateral shrinkage of the striatal nuclei. The neostriatal
lesions were usually ovoidal, centered approximately at A 7.8 - 8.2 (Konig and
Klippel, 1963), and with rostrocaudal extent of 2.0 - 2.5 min. The core of the
dorsal neostriata was almost completely devoid of neurons. A rim of apparently
normal neurons remained in the dorsomedial and ventrolateral regions of the
nuclei. The fiber bundles of the internal capsule traversing the area of neuronal loss appeared to be more packed than in normal tissue, but their size and
stain density were not appreciably altered. The space around the fiber bundles
was densely infiltrated with astrocytic glia. The rostral pole of the globus
pallidus usually showed similar glial infiltration and partial neuronal loss. In
addition to the striatal damage, unilateral or bilateral degenerative changes and
partial neuronal loss were often detected in the deep layers of the frontal
cortex and, less frequently, in the CA$_1$ and CA$_3$ fields of the dorsal hippocampus,
and in the olfactory tubercle. The brains of the control rats appeared to be
intact except for a slight glial infiltration along the cannula track.

DISCUSSION

At the time when the present investigations were started, KA striatal injections
had been reported to induce selective destruction of neostrial neurons, with
sparing of the fibers of passage, and no detectable damage to neurons outside the
neostriatum (Coyle et al., 1977; Mason and Fibiger, 1978; Schwarcz and Coyle,
1977). In fact, in a discussion of their attempts to obtain a morphological model
of HD, Coyle and coworkers noted with some disappointment that, unlike in HD,
"in the striatal kainic acid lesion the pallidum and cerebral cortex are spared"
(Coyle et al., 1977). Our results confirmed that KA striatal injections cause
extensive loss of neostriatal neurons, with no apparent damage to the fiber
bundles of the internal capsule. However, in agreement with the results of more
recent investigations, (Coyle et al., 1978; Wuerthele et al., 1978; Zaczeck
et al., 1980) we also found that the KA injections frequently induced a partial
loss of neurons in the deep layers of the frontal cortex and in the rostral globus
pallidus. Also, neurodegenerative changes were detected in the hippocampus and
the olfactory tubercle, although these limbic lesions occurred less frequently,
and were usually less symmetrical than those in the neostriatum, pallidum and
frontal cortex.

The observation that the neuronal loss in the neostriatum occurred more constant-
ly and was more severe than in other brain structures might be taken to suggest
a major contribution of the neostriatal degeneration to the behavioral impairments of the KA-treated rats. It is clear, however, that the frequent multifocality of the KA-induced lesions prevented us from fulfilling the objective to
elucidate the behavioral effects of "pure" loss of neostriatal neurons. On the
other hand, the finding of a systemic frontocortical-neostriatal-pallidal degeneration after KA injections indicates an anatomical parallelism between KA
striatal preparation and HD that is even more remarkable than it was originally
thought. Do our findings also suggest a behavioral parallelism?

In recent investigations of patients with HD (Caine et al., 1978; Butters et al.,
1979; Oscar Berman et al., 1973; Weingartner et al, 1979) a behavioral syndrome
has been delineated, which includes these alterations: i) psychomotor: a failure
to initiate activities spontaneously, unless strongly motivated; ii) emotional:
disphoric reactions and, especially, hyperirritability and labile affect; iii)
associative: cognitive inflexibility and amnesia for discrete events. Our
results suggest similar disorders of locomotion, emotional reactivity, behavioral
flexibility and working memory in the rats with KA-induced brain lesions.

The finding that the KA-treated rats ran for food reward more slowly than the
controls especially at the onset of the daily sessions, and decreased their
running speed more than the controls in extinction, can be taken as evidence of
bradykinesia -- a motor alteration that has been defined as "hesitancy in initiation of a movement, slowness in its execution, and rapid fatiguing" (Duvoisin,
1978). It is also likely that the bradykinesia partly accounts for the finding
that, on exploring both the T-maze and the multiple-alley maze, the KA-treated
rats showed a longer start latency and less initial exploratory activity than the
control rats. However, not all the alterations of locomotor exploration can be
readily interpreted to reflect a bradykinetic disorder. A purely motoric impairment would be expected to reproduce the same effects on locomotor activity, independent of practice. In contrast, the KA-treated rats showed a prolonged decrease of locomotor exploration (i.e., a decrease not limited to the initial
1-min period) in the first session of T-maze exploration, but not in the subsequent sessions. Since aversive (presumably fear-inducing) stimuli, have been
shown to inhibit exploration of novel mazes in normal rats (Lippman and Thompson,
1977; Russell, 1973) the low level of locomotor exploration of the KA-treated
rats in the first test session can be interpreted to indicate an increased fear

reaction to novelty. In support of this interpretation are also the findings
that the KA-treated rats took longer to start eating novel food in the multiple-
alley maze, and showed increased thigmotaxis in the open field. Collectively
taken, these results suggest that the locomotor alterations induced by the KA
striatal injections reflected both a bradykinesia and an aversive hyperreactivity
to novel stimuli.

Coagulative lesions of the neostriatum in rats have been shown to induce resistance to extinction of CRF bar pressing without altering acquisition performance
(Schmaltz and Isaacson, 1972). The KA-induced loss of neurons produced the same
effect in the present study. However, the KA-treated rats were not impaired in
either learning or extinction of CRF running. In fact, the lesions had a slightly facilitatory effect on extinction of running. Thus, although the KA-induced
neuronal loss did not affect learning of relatively simple appetitive responses,
it altered their extinction.

The resistance to extinction of bar pressing indicates a behavioral disinhibition, i.e., a decreased sensitivity to the inhibitory effects of reinforcement
omission. Why was this impairment not manifested in extinction of running?
Length of the interresponse interval did not seem to be a relevant factor,
because the KA-treated rats failed to show resistance to extinction of running
both with relatively short (10-sec) and relatively long (10-min) ITI_s (Pisa
et al., 1981). An alternative explanation is suggested by the evidence that the
kainate lesions resulted in bradykinesia. This locomotor disorder would tend
to antagonize the manifestation of behavioral disinhibition. Thus, different
effects of the lesions on extinction performance might be expected, depending on
the balance between strength of the conditioned response and effort required for
its performance. The occurrence of both behavioral disinhibition and bradykinesia could, therefore, reasonably account for the lesion-induced resistance to
extinction of a relatively effortless response, such as bar pressing, and the
slightly facilitated extinction of a relatively effortful response, such as fast
running.

The effects of KA striatal injections on avoidance performance were consistent
with those found in rats with coagulative lesions of the neostriatum (Kirkby and
Polgar, 1974; Rothman and Glick, 1976; Thomas and Hill, 1973; Winocur and Mills,
1969). The bradykinesia may have contributed to the modest impairment of learning performance in the task of active avoidance. However, it cannot account for
the inability to suppress both the punished, step down responses and the nonreinforced or punished shuttle responses. Taken collectively, the latter alterations of avoidance performance, like the resistance to extinction of appetitive
bar pressing, indicate a behavioral disinhibition overriding the attendant brady-
kinesic disorder.

The kainate brain lesions impaired working memory performance, as indicated by
the failures of both spatial alternation and speed alternation learning. These
effects cannot be attributed to a general impairment of learning and memory. First,
the kainate brain lesions did not alter learning performance of either bar pressing or running. Second, they did not appreciably alter performance of spontaneous spatial alternation, which is thought to be sensitive to alterations of
place memory (Douglas, 1966). Third, the KA-treated rats gave evidence of
hedonic memory in the early daily trials of the speed alternation task, although
not in the late trials. An increased susceptibility of working memory to proactive interference, with resulting inability to maintain reliable levels of
alternation over a series of trials, would appear to be the more likely explanation of the impairments of alternation learning.

Thus, in addition to the anatomical similarities, there seems to be a considerable correspondence between the bradykinesia, increased neophobia, behavioral disinhibition and working-memory impairment apparently induced by kainate brain lesions, and the psychomotor apathy, disphoria, cognitive inflexibility and failure of episodic memory described in patients with HD. The proposed anatomical and behavioral parallelism between the two conditions is certainly not perfect. Thus, the hippocampal and basal forebrain neurodegeneration induced by kainic acid, probably on account of its potent epileptogenic properties (Ben Ari et al., 1980), does not appear to occur in HD. On the other hand, the choreatic dyskinesias of HD patients do not seem to be manifested in the KA striatal preparation (Pisa, 1982). Nonetheless, a detailed understanding of the behavioral effects of kainate striatal injections should prove to be relevant to the psychopharmacologic evaluation of drugs with prospective antagonistic actions on the neurobehavioral alterations induced by kainic acid. On the other hand, kainic acid does not seem to be an appropriate tool for behavioral studies of neostriatal functions. For this purpose, ibotenic acid should prove to be especially useful, because recent studies (Guldin and Markowitsch, 1981; Schwarcz et al., 1979) indicate that intracerebral injections of this neurotoxin can produce axon-sparing neuronal loss in the neostriatum, with no damage to other brain structures.

ACKNOWLEDGEMENTS

The collaborative efforts of Drs. H.C. Fibiger and P.R. Sanberg are greatly appreciated. The author is a Research Scholar of the Ontario Mental Health Foundation.

REFERENCES

Ben-Ari, Y., E. Tremblay, O.P. Ottersen and B.S. Meldrum (1980). Brain Res. 191, 79-97.
Bruyn, G.W., G.T.H.A.M. Bots and R. Dom (1979). Adv. Neurol., 23, 83-94.
Butters, N., M.S. Albert and D. Sax (1979). Adv. Neurol., 23, 203-214.
Caine, E.D., R.D. Hunt, H. Weingartner and M.H. Hebert (1978). Arch. Gen. Psychiat., 35, 377-384.
Capaldi, E.J. (1971). In Animal Memory (Honig, W.K. and P.M. James, eds.), pp. 111-154, Academic Press, New York.
Coyle, J.T., M.E. Molliver and M.J. Kuhar (1978). J. Comp. Neurol., 180, 301-324.
Coyle, J.T. and R. Schwarcz (1976). Nature (London) 263, 244-246.
Coyle, J.T., R. Schwarcz, J.P. Bennett and P. Campochiaro (1977). Prog. Neuropsychopharmac., 1, 13-30.
Divac, I., H.J. Markowitsch and M. Pritzel (1978). Brain Res., 151, 523-532.
Douglas, R. (1966). J. Comp. Physiol. Psychol. 62, 171-183.
Duvoisin, R.C. (1978). Parkinson's Disease. Raven Press, New York.
Flaherty, C.F. and J.W. Davenport (1972). J. Exp. Psychol., 96, 1-9.
Forno, L.S. and C. Jose (1973). Adv. Neurol., 1, 453-470.
Guldin, W.O. and H.J. Markowitsch (1981). Brain Res., 225, 446-451.
Honig, W.K. (1978). In Cognitive Processes in Animal Behavior (Hulse, S., H. Fowler and W.L. Honig, eds.), pp. 211-248, Lawrence Erlbaum, Hillsdale.
Kirkby, R.J. (1973). J. Comp. Physiol. Psychol., 85, 82-96.
Kirkby, R.J. and S. Polgar (1974). Physiol. Psychol., 2, 301-306.
Konig, J.F.R. and R.A. Klippel (1963). The rat brain. Williams and Wilkins, Baltimore.
Kluver, H. and E.A. Barrera (1953). J. Neuropathol. Exp. Neurol., 12, 400-403.
Lange, H., G. Thorner, A. Kopf and K.F. Schroeder (1974). J. Neurol. Sci., 28, 401-425.
Lippman, L.G. and R.W. Thompson (1977). Am. J. Psychol., 90, 363-382.
Mason, S.T. and H.C. Fibiger (1978). Brain Res. (155), 313-329.
McGeer, E.G. and P.C. McGeer (1976). Nature (London) 263, 517-519.

Oberg, R.G.E. and I. Divac (1979). In The Neostriatum (Divac, I. and R.G.E. Oberg, eds.), pp. 291-313, Pergamon Press, New York.

Oscar-Berman, M., D.S. Sax and L. Opoliner (1973). Adv. Neurol., 1, 717-728.

Pisa, M. (1982). Trends Neurosci., 5, 36-37.

Pisa, M., P.R. Sanberg and H.C. Fibiger (1980). Physiol. Behav. 24, 11-19.

Pisa, M., P.R. Sanberg and H.C. Fibiger (1981). Exp. Neurol., 74, 633-653.

Ross, S., Z.M. Nagy, C. Kessler and J.P. Scott (1966). J. Comp. Physiol. Psychol., 62, 338-340.

Rothman, A.H. and S.D. Glick (1976). Brain Res., 118, 361-369.

Russell, P.A. (1973). British J. Psychol., 64, 417-433.

Sanberg, P.R., M. Pisa and H.C. Fibiger (1979). Pharmacol. Biochem. Behav., 10, 137-144.

Schmaltz, L.W. and R.L. Isaacson (1972). Physiol. Behav., 9, 155-159.

Schwarcz, R. and J.T. Coyle (1977). Brain Res. 127, 235-249.

Schwarcz, R., T. Hokfelt, K. Fuxe, G. Johnson, M. Goldstein and L. Terenius (1979). Exp. Brain Res., 37, 199-216.

Thomas, R.K. and A.S. Hill (1973). Bull. Psychon. Soc., 1, 346-348.

Weingartner, H., E.D. Caine and M.H. Ebert (1978). Adv. Neurol., 23, 215-226.

Winocur, G. and J.A. Mills (1969). J. Comp. Physiol. Psychol., 68, 552-557.

Wuerthele, S.M., K.L. Lovell, M.Z. Jones and K.E. Moore (1978). Brain Res., 149, 489-497.

Zaczeck, R., S. Simonton and J.T. Coyle (1980). J. Neuropathol. Exp. Neurol., 39, 245-264.

EFFECTS OF NEUROTOXIC EXCITATORY AMINO ACIDS ON NEUROENDOCRINE REGULATION

CHARLES B. NEMEROFF

Biological Sciences Research Center, Department of Psychiatry, University of North Carolina, School of Medicine, Chapel Hill, North Carolina, U.S.A.

ABSTRACT

This report summarizes the available literature concerning the effects of glutamate and related excitatory amino acids on neuroendocrine function. The majority of investigators in this field have pursued two lines of inquiry: (1) evaluation of the effect of administration of monosodium glutamate (MSG) and related excitotoxic amino acids to neonatal rodents on endocrine regulation in adulthood and (2) assessment of the acute neuroendocrine effects of MSG and related compounds in adult rodents. The use of these compounds as tools in neuroendocrine research is described.

KEYWORDS

Monosodium glutamate (MSG); n-methyl aspartate (NMA); growth hormone (GH); prolactin (PRL); luteinizing hormone (LH); follicle-stimulating hormone (FSH); thyrotropin (TSH); hypothalamic releasing hormones; dopamine; acetylcholine.

INTRODUCTION

The discovery by Olney (1969) that parenteral administration of relatively high doses of monosodium l-glutamate (MSG) to neonatal mice produces a hypothalamic lesion which is associated with the development of marked obesity, skeletal stunting, anterior pituitary hypoplasia, sterility in females and pathological changes in female reproductive organs has stimulated considerable research both on the effects of these excitatory amino acids, on the one hand, and the use of these substances as tools to unravel the complex hypothalamic neural circuits which play a major role in neuroendocrine regulation. These data have previously been reviewed by our group (Nemeroff et al., 1978a; Kizer et al., 1978; Nemeroff, 1981) and by Olney and his colleagues (Olney and Price, 1978; Olney, 1980; Olney and Price, 1980).

EFFECTS OF ADMINISTRATION OF MSG IN THE NEONATAL PERIOD ON NEUROENDOCRINE REGULATION IN THE ADULT

The appearance of endocrine alterations in adult rodents treated in the neonatal period with MSG have been questioned by a few researchers, though the general consensus is indeed in favor of significant endocrinopathies. For the sake of brevity I have not discussed these few negative studies. In an early study in rats,

Redding et al. (1971) noted decreased body weights and nasoanal lengths in 40 and 110 day old rats treated neonatally with MSG. Calculation of the Lee Index ($\sqrt[3]{Body\ wt}$/nasoanal length), a measure of stuntedness and obesity, indicated a significant increase in carcass fat in the MSG-treated rats. Furthermore, the following organs showed absolute decreases in weights in the MSG-treated rats when compared to age- and sex-matched controls: thyroid, adrenal, gonads, and anterior pituitary. Finally anterior pituitary content of growth hormone (GH) and luteinizing hormone (LH), but not thyrotropin (TSH), was significantly reduced in MSG-treated rats at 40 days of age. Nagasawa et al. (1974) confirmed and extended the findings previously reported by Olney (1969) in mice. Female neonatal mice treated with a single SC injection of MSG exhibited, as adults, marked obesity, increased Lee indices, decreased pituitary content of prolactin (PRL) and GH and marked disturbances in estrous cycles and mammary development. Although pituitary weight was decreased significantly, no difference in the absolute weights of the thyroid, adrenal, ovary, spleen, kidney or liver were noted, though relative organ weights may well have been different. Holzwarth-McBride et al. (1976b) reported that administration of 2.5 g/kg MSG on days 5-10 in neonatal mice resulted in adults that were obese and stunted in growth and had ovaries and testes (but not adrenals) significantly smaller than age- and sex-matched controls.

Our research group has conducted extensive studies to characterize the nature and locus of the endocrine deficit in rats treated with MSG (4 g/kg IP on alternate days in the first ten days of life) in the neonatal period. In early studies (Nemeroff et al., 1975, 1977a) we confirmed and extended the findings of increased Lee index, stuntedness, obesity and decreased (absolute and relative) organ weights of the ovaries, uteri, and pituitary, of MSG-treated rats. The testes, adrenal and thyroid showed decreases in absolute, but not in relative, organ weights. Both serum tri-iodothyronine (T3) and the free thyroxine index were significantly reduced in the MSG-treated rats. We extended these findings in subsequent studies (Nemeroff et al., 1977b; Greeley et al., 1978) and have reviewed these data (Nemeroff et al., 1978a; Nemeroff, 1981). In our initial studies, MSG-treated rats were found to have normal basal levels of LH, FSH and TSH (despite hypothyroidism and gonadal atrophy), greatly reduced levels of GH and elevated PRL levels, the latter finding in the males only. In a more recent study (Nemeroff et al., 1981) male rats treated with MSG in the neonatal period, showed, as adults, significant reductions in serum levels of LH, FSH and testosterone whereas female MSG-treated rats showed marked reductions in serum levels of FSH and estradiol 17-β.

Terry et al. (1981) also observed diminished GH levels in MSG-treated rats and noted marked reductions in the normal pulsatile secretion of GH as well. Our group (Nemeroff et al., 1977b) also reported that MSG-treated rats show normal or enhanced LH and TSH responses to their respective releasing hormones [luteinizing hormone-releasing hormone (LHRH), and thyrotropin-releasing hormone (TRH)]. In addition, the hypothalamic content of LHRH, TRH and somatostatin was unchanged in adult rats treated neonatally with MSG. Finally, we observed the normal light-induced depression and dark-induced elevation of pineal serotonin n-acetyl-transferase in both control and MSG-treated rats, indicating that any endocrinopathies observed are not secondary effects attributable to the retinal lesion induced by the MSG treatment. It therefore appears that MSG-treated rodents, though exhibiting optic nerve atrophy, possess a functional retinal-hypothalamic projection which is responsive to changes in environmental lighting. In later work we showed that MSG-treated male rats show the expected rises in serum gonadotropin concentrations after castration; MSG-treated females exhibit a normal FSH, but somewhat subnormal LH, rise after castration. A more detailed analysis (Greeley et al., 1980) revealed that the rise in gonadotropins in adult and peripubertal MSG-treated male and female rats is significantly delayed when compared to age- and sex-matched controls; however, these animals eventually achieve the post-castration gonadotropin levels observed in control animals. In addition, MSG-treated adult female rats exhibited a delayed TSH rise after thyroidectomy when compared to controls. Clemens et al. (1978) also observed smaller gonads, uteri, anterior pituitary and seminal vesicles in adult rats treated with MSG in the neonatal period. These workers obtained similar results to those of Greeley et al. (1978, 1980) concerning the diminished post-castration rise in serum gonadotropins in MSG-treated rats. Of particular interest was their finding that neonatal MSG treatment resulted in a marked attenuation of the estradiol benzoate-induced increase in serum LH and PRL concentrations in ovariectomized rats. In contrast MSG-treated rats exhibited an enhanced PRL response to 5-hydroxytryptophan when compared to controls. It would therefore appear that the MSG-treated rat exhibits an impaired release mechanism for LH and PRL when estrogen is the inducer and an enhanced PRL response to manipulations that increase brain serotonergic tone.

Bakke et al. (1978) also studied the endocrine status of adult rats treated neonatally with MSG. They reported the MSG-treated rats to be obese and stunted (significantly increased Lee indices) and to have reduced pituitary, thyroid, adrenal, gonadal, and prostate weights and reduced serum GH concentration. In addition they observed reduced serum, pituitary and hypothalamic TSH levels in the glutamate-treated males and reduced serum thyroxine and elevated PRL levels in the MSG-treated females. Although they observed normal fertility in the MSG-treated females (when mated with normal males), the MSG-treated males (when mated to normal females) exhibited a marked reduction in fertility. Matsuzawa et al. (1979) reported that MSG-treated female rats exhibit precocious puberty, disturbed estrous cycles and small ovaries and pituitaries. They confirmed the previous findings of normal basal levels of LH and FSH in the MSG-treated rats but found lowered pituitary levels of the gonadotropins.

Rodriguez-Sierra et al. (1980) determined the effects of neonatal MSG administration on endocrine function in the female rat. They noted a delay in vaginal opening, an absence of ovulation at the time of vaginal opening and a failure to exhibit compensatory ovarian hypertrophy in MSG-treated rats. They also noted a reduction in sexual receptivity of MSG-treated female rats. In a more recent study, this same group (Sridaran et al., 1981) confirmed the previous observations of Greeley et al. (1980) that MSG-treated female rats exhibit an increase in plasma LH levels after ovariectomy that is significantly smaller than that observed in saline-treated controls.

Dyer et al. (1981) studied the secretion of LH in ovariectomized adult rats treated neonatally with MSG. The MSG-treated ovariectomized rats had significantly lower basal LH plasma levels; estradiol treatment significantly reduced plasma LH levels in the control rats to a greater extent than that observed in the MSG-treated animals.

Pizzi et al. (1977) treated neonatal mice with MSG and noted severe reproductive dysfunction in adulthood in both males and females. The females had significantly fewer pregnancies and smaller litters, and the males were significantly less fertile. In addition, the MSG-treated mice had significantly smaller pituitary, thyroid, ovary and testes weights and increased obesity.

The disruption of neuroendocrine regulation by treatment with MSG in the neonatal period is not limited to mice and rats. The effects of neonatal MSG treatment in hamsters has been examined. Lamperti and Blaha (1976) reported that MSG-treated hamsters had significantly smaller ovaries, uteri, adrenals, and anterior pituitary, and a significant reduction in the number of tubal ova. MSG-treated female hamsters were acyclic; their ovaries contained small follicles and no corpora lutea. Of paramount importance was their findings that administration of pregnant mare's serum (PMS) to these MSG-treated females induced follicular maturation and, furthermore, administration of human chorionic gonadotropin (HCG) induced ovulation. MSG-treated male hamsters exhibited atrophic seminiferous tubules and very low activity of Δ^5-3β steroid dehydrogenase in the interstitial cells. Treatment of the MSG-treated males with HCG resulted in normalization of both the histological appearance of the seminiferous tubules and the enzyme activity. Lamperti and Baldwin (1982) studied pituitary responsiveness to LHRH in adult female hamsters treated neonatally with MSG. Although LH responsiveness to LHRH was found to be similar in MSG-treated and control hamsters, FSH responses to the decapeptide were greatly attenuated. The MSG-treated hamsters also had lower basal serum FSH levels than control animals, confirming our findings in rats (Nemeroff et al., 1981).

Lastly, Olney and Price (1978) reported that MSG-treated mice and rats have very high corticosterone levels when compared to controls.

A final summary statement concerning the loci at which neonatally administered MSG produces neuroendocrine disturbances might clarify this complex problem. The endocrinopathies are almost certainly not due to a direct effect of MSG on endocrine target organs since the ovaries and testes of MSG-treated animals respond normally to HCG administration (vide supra). The primary lesion is not at the pituitary level since the gonadotropin and thyrotropin response to their respective releasing hormones, LHRH and TRH, is not subnormal. The neuroendocrine disturbance appears then to be related to the MSG-induced hypothalamic lesion. Since the hypothalamic content of at least two of the releasing hormones (TRH, LHRH) is unchanged after neonatal MSG treatment, but dopamine concentrations and choline acetyltransferase activity are severely diminished (vide infra), it would appear that the primary fault in the glutamate-treated animals is in those hypothalamic or circumventricular organ neurotransmitter systems that play a prominent role in maintenance of neuroendocrine homeostasis.

There are several naturally occurring and synthetic analogs of glutamate that share its excitatory effects on CNS neurons and these structure-activity relations have been well studied (Curtis and Watkins, 1963; Curtis et al., 1972; Kizer et al., 1978; Honoré et al., 1981). In several studies Olney and his associates (Olney et al., 1971, 1974; Olney, 1976, 1979) reported that many of these excitatory acidic amino acid analogs of glutamate share its neurotoxic properties; in fact many of these (e.g. aspartate, kainic acid, homocysteic acid, n-methyl-aspartate) are considerably more potent neurotoxic agents than MSG. In general there is close correspondence between their potencies in exciting central neurons and in inducing the characteristic retinal, hypothalamic and circumventricular organ lesions in neonatal mice (Olney et al., 1971). For example, both Schainker and Olney (1974) and Pizzi et al. (1978) treated neonatal mice with sodium-1-aspartate and noted obesity, skeletal stunting and reduced testicular, ovarian, and pituitary weights. Reproductive dysfunction was also present in aspartate-treated mice.

THE EFFECTS OF MSG ADMINISTRATION IN THE NEONATAL PERIOD ON THE CONTENT OF HYPOTHALAMIC NEUROTRANSMITTERS AND HYPOTHALAMIC RELEASING HORMONES

As noted in the introduction, Olney (1969, 1971, 1979) and Olney and his associates (Olney et al., 1971), in a series of studies have reported that MSG, administered in relatively high doses to mice, produce destruction of neurons (but not glia or ependyma) in the arcuate nucleus of the hypothalamus. Both light and electron microscopic techniques have been utilized.

In 1975 our laboratory utilized the histochemical technique of Falck and Hillarp for visualization of catecholamines in frozen tissue sections and noted loss of arcuate nucleus dopamine (DA) neurons in adult rats who were treated with MSG in the neonatal period. Since DA neurons comprising the tuberoinfundibular DA system originate in the arcuate-periventricular region and project primarily to the median eminence, it was postulated that neonatal MSG administration selectively destroys all tuberoinfundibular system neurons, by definition, since in rodents 90-95% of arcuate neurons are destroyed after high dose MSG treatment. This finding allowed correlation of MSG-induced destruction of specific neurotransmitter systems with the observed endocrine alterations present in MSG-treated animals (Nemeroff et al., 1975, 1977). Glial cell infiltration makes Nissl-stained light microscopic identification of the arcuate lesion in adult animals treated with MSG as neonates difficult. In contrast, the loss of DA neuronal histofluorescence in the arcuate nucleus of adult rats treated with MSG as neonates is readily observed. These results have been confirmed in the mouse; Holzwarth-McBride et al. (1976b) found a marked decrease in both the number and intensity of DA histofluorescence in the perikarya of arcuate neurons.

In subsequent studies we utilized both light and electron microscopic histochemistry and found a similar destruction of arcuate perikarya that exhibited specific staining for acetylcholinesterase, a putative cholinergic neural marker (Carson et al., 1977, 1978). These data implied the existence of a previously undiscovered tuberoinfundibular cholinergic system that was destroyed by neonatal MSG administration. Biochemical evidence (vide infra) supported this hypothesis.

In addition our group has reported that adult rats treated neonatally with MSG exhibit, as expected, a marked reduction in the neuronal accumulation of ^{3}H-estradiol in the arcuate nucleus, as assessed by autoradiographic methods (Grant et al., 1978).

The data obtained in the histochemical studies described above provided evidence for destruction of dopaminergic and cholinergic tuberoinfundibular systems in rats treated neonatally with MSG. Our laboratory sought to determine the extent and specificity of these effects using more sensitive and specific neurochemical assay techniques and a microdissection technique to remove individual brain nuclei (Nemeroff et al., 1977b). Although MSG-treated rats showed no alterations in the concentration of norepinephrine (NE), serotonin (5HT) or in the three hypothalamic hypophysiotropic hormones (TRH, LHRH and somatostatin), there was a substantial reduction in the concentration of DA in the arcuate nucleus and median eminence (Table 1). Consistent with these findings are the observations of Kizer and Youngblood (1978) of diminished tyrosine hydroxylase activity in the median eminence of MSG-treated rats (Table 1). Moreover the activity of choline acetyltransferase (CAT) in the arcuate nucleus and median eminence (Table 1) was markedly reduced in the MSG-treated rats. The regional specificity of these MSG effects is highlighted by the normal levels of DA in other brain nuclei including the paraventricular, dorsomedial, caudate, $A_{8,9,10}$, and normal CAT activity in the dorsomedial hypothalamus, habenula and lateral amygdaloid nuclei. Of particular interest was the finding that neonatal MSG treatment produces a greater depletion of mediobasal hypothalamic DA than does the catecholamine neurotoxin 6-hydroxydopamine (6OHDA) and does not, like 6OHDA, alter brain NE concentration (Nemeroff et al., 1977b). This led to the use of MSG as a tool to unravel hypothalamic neurocircuitry and the involvement of specific neurotransmitter systems in neuroendocrine regulation. Much of these neurochemical data have been repeatedly confirmed both in our laboratory (Greeley et al., 1978) and by others; thus, Lechen et al. (1976) found normal levels of LHRH and TRH in MSG-treated mice and Clemens et al. (1978) confirmed the 60% reduction in the concentration of DA in the mediobasal hypothalamis. Walaas and Fonnum (1978) treated neonatal rats with MSG and confirmed both the marked diminution of CAT activity in the arcuate nucleus and median eminence and the loss of AChE staining in the arcuate nucleus.

Krieger et al. (1979) measured brain levels of ACTH and β-endorphin in adult rats treated with MSG in the neonatal period and found significant reductions in the levels of both peptides in the mediobasal hypothalamus, medial preoptic area and amygdala. Hong et al. (1981) confirmed the reduction of hypothalamic β-endorphin in MSG-treated rats; no MSG-induced alteration in the hypothalamic concentration of neurotensin, substance P or met-enkephalin was observed. Eslay et al. (1979) reported that rats treated with MSG in the neonatal period exhibit marked reduction in hypothalamic MSH levels.

Table 1. Effect of MSG Treatment in the Neonatal Period on the Concentration
           of Neurotransmitters, Neurotransmitter-Related Enzymes and Releasing
           Hormones.[1]

	Control Males	MSG-treated Males
Releasing hormones in the medio-basal hypothalamus, ng/mg protein ± SEM[2]		
TRH	5.5 ± 0.5 (n=6)	5.9 ± 0.7 (n=6)
LH-RH	4.2 ± 0.7 (n=12)	4.2 ± 1.5 (n=11)
Neurotransmitters, ng/mg protein ± SEM		
Serotonin (arcuate	11.8 ± 1.1 (n=6)	12.1 ± 0.9 (n=6)
Serotonin (median eminence)	30.7 ± 3.1 (n=6)	24.0 ± 3.0 (n=6)
Norepinephrine (arcuate)	17.0 ± 0.6 (n=6)	14.0 ± 0.7 (n=6)
Norepinephrine (median eminence)	14.0 ± 1.1 (n=6)	14.0 ± 1.3 (n=6)
Dopamine (arcuate)	17.0 ± 1.4 (n=6)	8.3 ± 0.5*(n=6)
Dopamine (median eminence)	85.0 ± 3.4 (n=6)	52.0 ± 6.9*(n=6)
Neurotransmitter-related enzymes		
Glutamic acid decarboxylase (arcuate)[3]	228 ± 25 (n=6)	250 ± 40 (n=6)
Glutamic acid decarboxylase (median eminence)[3]	119 ± 10 (n=6)	114 ± 40 (n=6)
Choline acetyltransferase (arcuate)[4]	3.6 ± 0.3 (n=5)	1.3 ± 0.1*(n=5)
Choline acetyltransferase (median eminence)[4]	26.0 ± 0.5 (n=5)	5.9 ± 0.4*(n=5)
Tyrosine hydroxylase (median eminence)[5]	24.0 ± 5.5 (n=5)	15.1 ± 0.5*(n=5)

[1]Data were analyzed by one-way analysis of variance and Student's t-test (two-tailed); *$p < 0.05$.
[2]Concentrations of releasing hormones were determined by radioimmunoassay. Because of inherent problems of specificity associated with immunoassay procedures, it is best to refer to these measures as 'TRH-like,' and 'LHRH-like' immunoreactive materials.
[3]pmol/h/μg protein ± SEM.
[4]pmol[^{14}C]-acetylcholine formed/h/mg protein.
[5]nmoles L-DOPA formed/hr/mg protein.

Adapted from Nemeroff, 1981.

EFFECTS OF ACUTE ADMINISTRATION OF MSG AND RELATED EXCITATORY AMINO ACIDS TO ADULT RATS ON NEUROENDOCRINE REGULATION

Olney et al. (1976) reported that MSG administration (1 g/kg SC) induced a rapid rise (15 min) in serum LH and testosterone in adult rats. The steroid remained significantly elevated six hours after MSG treatment. Our group (Nemeroff et al., 1978b), using the exact protocol of Olney et al. (1976), did not observe an acute rise in serum LH levels after MSG. However, serum levels of GH were markedly diminished and PRL levels significantly elevated after acute MSG treatment, effects reminiscent of those observed in adult rats treated with MSG in the neonatal period (Table 2). Pretreatment with neither haloperidol (a DA antagonist), nor atropine (an anticholinergic), blocked these endocrine sequalae observed after acute MSG treatment. No MSG-induced changes in serum levels of FSH or TSH were noted.

Table 2. The Effect of Monosodium Glutamate (MSG), Haloperidol or Atropine on Serum Levels of Anterior Pituitary Hormones

	Prolactin (PRL)	Growth Hormone (GH)	Thyroid-stimulating Hormone (TSH)	Follicle-stimulating Hormone (FSH)
Non-injected control	7.2 ± 2.0	51.6 ± 16.9	290 ± 90	548 ± 45
Saline + saline	4.7 ± 1.7	53.6 ± 8.6	221 ± 49	508 ± 58
Saline + MSG	20.0 ± 7.4*	31.8 ± 3.8*	269 ± 58	435 ± 33
Atropine + saline	13.1 ± 4.6*	8.4 ± 2.6*	108 ± 24*	454 ± 17
Atropine + MSG	27.5 ± 8.1*	11.5 ± 4.4*	173 ± 33	468 ± 14
Haloperidol + saline	79.8 ± 7.2*	6.4 ± 1.0*	122 ± 19*	455 ± 28
Haloperidol + MSG	86.8 ± 4.3*	10.2 ± 2.3*	151 ± 26	454 ± 31

Data is expressed as ng/ml SEM; n=6/group. Treatment regimens: MSG, 1 g/kg SC; atropine, 700 mg/kg SC; haloperidol, 0.5 mg/kg IP. All of the serum samples were assayed for LH, but none of the samples contained more than 15-20 ng/ml, the sensitivity level of the radioimmunoassay. $p < 0.05$, one-way ANOVA, Newman-Keuls test. When compared with saline + saline. (From Nemeroff, et al., 1978b)

Terry et al. (1981) also observed a significant diminution in serum GH levels in adult rats after acute MSG treatment. They also noted a rapid, transient release of PRL after acute MSG treatment. Yonetoni and Matsuzawa (1978) reported that MSG (1 g/kg SC) produced significant reductions in serum concentrations of LH and testosterone when measured 1 hour after treatment in adult male rats.

Carillo and Alcantara (1981) have reported that in ovariectomized, estrogen-progesterone primed rats, intravenous (but not subcutaneous) administration of MSG (1 g/kg) resulted in a significant elevation of plasma LH levels. Peter et al. (1980) reported that intraperitoneal injection of MSG (2.5 g/kg) to adult male goldfish produced a significant elevation in serum gonadotropin levels, 6, 24 and 48 hrs after injection. This effect was reversible.

After infusion into the third ventricle of rats, both glutamate and aspartate produce significant elevations in serum levels of LH (Ondo, 1981).

Olney, Price and their associates have studied the acute effects of n-methyl-DL-aspartate acid (NMA), kainic acid and DL-homocysteic acid on LH secretion in the rat. These data have been comprehensively reviewed (Olney and Price, 1980). Price et al. (1978a, 1979) reported that SC administration of NMA (15-40 mg/kg) to young male rats produces a significant elevation in serum LH levels. These doses of NMA are considered to be below those required to produce hypothalamic destruction. It is of interest to note that the order of potency of the excitatory amino acids to stimulate LH release is identical to their order of potency both in exciting CNS neurons and in destroying arcuate neurons (Price et al., 1978a). Price et al. (1978b) reported that the LH releasing action of NMA is blocked by SC injection of GABA or taurine, but not by the DA antagonists, pimozide or chlorpromazine. From this concatenation of data, Price et al. (1978b) concluded that NMA produces LH release by an action "on dendritic or somal surfaces of a subpopulation" of arcuate neurons that may be cholinergic (but not dopaminergic). In a comprehensive study Schainker and Cicero (1980) confirmed and extended the original observations of Price, Olney and their associates concerning the LH releasing effects of NMA and have investigated the site of action of this substance. They reported that in 42

day old rats, SC injection of NMA (66 mg/kg) produced a marked increase in serum LH
levels by 7.5 min post-injection; serum LH levels returned to normal by 30-45 min
post-injection. They observed similar effects of NMA in rats of different ages
(25, 40 or 55 days old). However, older animals weighing more than 171 g consistently showed attenuated LH responses to NMA. Since one possible mechanism by
which NMA might produce LH release is a blockade of the negative feedback exerted
by testosterone, Schainker and Cicero (1980) evaluated the effects of NMA in castrated male rats. This excitatory amino acid produced significant elevations in
serum LH in the castrated rats. To assess whether NMA might act directly on the
pituitary to release LH, hemipituitaries were incubated in vitro with NMA (10^{-5}M).
No effect of NMA on LH release was observed in vitro; LHRH produced its characteristic effects in this system. Recently the hypothesis that the NMA-induced release
of LH is dependent on intact arcuate nucleus neurons was substantiated by the
finding that this excitatory amino acid does not produce its characteristic effect
on serum LH levels in rats that had sustained arcuate nucleus lesions by administration of MSG in the neonatal period (Olney and Price, 1980). They also
investigated the possibility that NMA acted by exciting arcuate cholinergic
neurons; this is apparently not the case since both muscarine and nicotinic cholinergic antagonists (atropine, mecamyline) did not block the LH releasing effect of
NMA.

Carillo and Alcantura (1981) reported that SC administration of NMA (25 mg/kg) produced a significant elevation of serum LH, but not FSH, in 25 day old rats; this
effect was not observed in adult female rats. Intravenous injection of the same
dose of NMA to ovariectomized, estrogen-progesterone primed rats produced a significant elevation of plasma LH levels. These workers confirmed the null effect of
NMA (5×10^{-3}M) on LH release in a hemipituitary preparation in vitro. In a subsequent study Carillo (1982) reported that pretreatment of ovariectomized, steroid-
primed female rats with pentobarbital completely suppressed the NMA-induced release
of LH in the conscious rat. In order to localize the central nervous system site
of action of NMA, rats were microinjected with NMA into the diagonal band of Broca-
medial preoptic area or into the third ventricle with NMA (0.2-35 nm). At both
sites, plasma LH elevations were observed. Infusion of NMA into more posterior
sites produced no elevation of plasma LH levels.

Our group has recently evaluated the effects of NMA on anterior pituitary hormone
secretion. Adult male Sprague Dawley rats (250-300 g) were injected SC with NMA
(10, 25 or 66 mg/kg) or 0.9% NaCl (10 ml/kg) and decapitated 7 1/2 min post-
injection, with care taken to minimize stress as previously described (Nemeroff
et al., 1978b). Trunk blood was collected and serum concentrations of LH, FSH, GH
and PRL were measured using materials produced by the NIAMDD as previously described (Nemeroff et al., 1977b, 1978b). The data were analyzed with Dunnett's test
for multiple comparisons after ANOVA. The results are illustrated in Table 3.

Table 3. The Effect of n-Methyl-DL-Aspartic Acid (NMA) on Serum Concentrations of
          Anterior Pituitary Hormones

Treatment	N	LH (ng/ml ± SEM)	FSH (ng/ml ± SEM)	GH (ng/ml ± SEM)	PRL (ng/ml ± SEM)
Vehicle	8	18.5 ± 4.9	195.6 ± 19.0	22.2 ± 6.9	8.8 ± 2.5
NMA 10 mg/kg SC	8	29.1 ± 3.5	228.9 ± 21.0	36.8 ± 11.4	11.0 ± 2.4
NMA 25 mg/kg SC	8	33.3 ± 6.0	251.8 ± 23.3	78.9 ± 20.4*	9.0 ± 1.6
NMA 66 mg/kg SC	8	49.9 ± 8.0*	251.1 ± 29.8	160.0 ± 46.5*	9.3 ± 2.0

*$p < 0.05$ when compared to vehicle-treated controls.

N-methyl-DL-aspartate produced a significant elevation of serum LH levels only at
the highest dose tested (66 mg/kg SC), a dose previously reported to be neurotoxic

(Schainker and Cicero, 1980). The failure of lower doses of NMA to significantly increase serum LH levels may be due to the older age of the rats used in this study compared to those of Price et al. (1978, 1979) as discussed by Schainker and Cicero (1980). Of interest is our findings, similar to those of Carillo and Alcantura (1981), that NMA produced no elevation in serum levels of FSH. Since there is considerable controversy over the issue of whether LHRH solely controls secretion of both gonadotropins or alternatively whether a separate FSH-releasing factor exists, these data revealing a selective effect of NMA on LH release appear to support the latter hypothesis.

The effect of NMA on serum GH and PRL levels is also of particular interest for several reasons. First the lack of effect on serum PRL levels appears to rule out non-specific stress as one mechanism of action of NMA on adenohypophysial hormone secretion. The marked dose-dependent increase in serum GH concentrations is a previously unreported finding. The high dose of NMA (66 mg/kg) produced a greater than seven-fold increase in serum GH levels. This finding is surprising in view of the fact that both our group (Nemeroff et al., 1978) and Terry et al. (1980) reported that MSG produced a significant diminution in serum GH levels (vide supra). Thus NMA and MSG may indeed act at different receptor populations—the former perhaps predominantly at aspartate receptors, the latter at glutamate receptors. This view has been promulgated by Olney and Price (1980).

CONCLUSIONS

Administration of MSG or related excitatory amino acids to neonatal rodents results in destruction of neurons in the arcuate nucleus of the hypothalamus. Mice or rats treated with MSG as neonates exhibit, as adults, a syndrome characterized by obesity, stunted growth, reproductive dysfunction and a marked reduction in the weight of the pituitary, gonads and accessory sexual organs. Although both the anterior pituitary and gonads appear atrophic, they both respond appropriately to their natural hormonal stimuli. Thus MSG treated rats exhibit normal or enhanced pituitary hormone secretion after exogenous releasing factor administration and MSG-treated hamsters respond appropriately to exogenously administered HCG. These data taken together with the observation of normal dark-induced increase and light-induced decrease in pineal serotinin n-acetyl transferase activity, strongly implicate the central nervous system as the site of the defect in neuroendocrine regulation in MSG-treated rats. Both histochemical and biochemical techniques have provided strong evidence to support this hypothesis. Thus tuberoinfundibular dopamine-, β-endorphin-, MSH- and acetylcholine-containing neurons are destroyed by neonatal MSG administration whereas noradrenergic, serotonergic and releasing hormone-containing circuits appear to be spared.

Acute administration of MSG and related excitatory amino acids to adult rats produce marked, reversible alterations in adenohypophyseal hormone secretion. Our research group and others have demonstrated a reduction in serum GH and elevation in serum PRL after acute MSG treatment in adult rats. In contrast NMA produced a significant rise in serum GH and LH levels. These data support the view that MSG and NMA may act preferentially on different receptor populations within the central nervous system.

ACKNOWLEDGEMENTS

I am grateful to Dori Yarbrough for aid in preparation of this manuscript. The research described in this report represents collaborative work with Drs. G. A. Mason, J. S. Kizer, A. J. Prange, Jr., G. Bissette, K. A. Carson and S. C. Bondy. I wish to acknowledge the advice and encouragement of Morris A. Lipton, Ph.D., M.D., Director of The Biological Sciences Research Center of the University of North Carolina. The author is supported by NICHHD HD-03110, NIMH MH-33127, MH-34121 and MH-32316.

REFERENCES

Bakke, J.L., N. Lawrence, J. Bennett, S. Robinson, and C.Y. Bowers (1978). Neuroendocrinology, 26, 220-228.

Carrillo, A.J. (1982). The effect of n-methyl aspartic acid on plasma LH levels in the conscious female rat. Proc. Intl. Conf. on Integrative Neurohumoral Mechanisms. Budapest, Hungary.

Carrillo, A.J., and O. Alcantara (1981). Soc. Neurosci. Abst., 108, 7.

Carson, K.A., C.B. Nemeroff, M.S. Rone, W.W. Youngblood, A.J. Prange, Jr., S. Hanker, and J.S. Kizer (1977). Brain Res., 129, 169-173.

Carson, K.A., C.B. Nemeroff, M.S. Rone, G.F. Nicholson, J.S. Kizer, and J.S. Hanker (1978). J. Comp. Neurol., 182, 201-220.

Clemens, J.A., M.E. Roush, R.W. Fuller, and C.J. Shaar (1978). Endocrinology, 103, 1304-1312.

Curtis, D.R., and J.C. Watkins (1963). J. Physiol. (London), 166, 1-14.

Curtis, D.R., A.W. Duggan, D. Felix, G.A.R. Johnston, A.K. Tebēcis, and J.C. Watkins (1972). Brain Res., 41, 283-301.

Dyer, R.G., R.F. Reick, S. Mansfield, and H. Corbet (1981). J. Endocr. 91, 341-346.

Eskay, R.C., M.J. Brownstein, and R.T. Long (1979). Science, 205, 827-829.

Grant, L.D., W.E. Stumpf, M. Sar, C.B. Nemeroff, and J.S. Kizer (1978). Fed. Proc., 37, 297.

Greeley, G.H., Jr., G.F. Nicholson, C.B. Nemeroff, W.W. Youngblood, and J.S. Kizer (1978). Endocrinology, 103, 170-175.

Greeley, G.H., Jr., G.F. Nicholson, and J.S. Kizer (1980). Brain Res., 195, 111-122.

Holzwarth-McBride, M.A., E.M. Hurst, and K.M. Knigge (1976a). Anat. Rec., 186, 185-196.

Holzwarth-McBride, M.A., J.R. Sladek, Jr., and K.M. Knigge (1976b). Anat. Rec., 186, 197-206.

Hong, J-S, C. Lowe, R.E. Squibb, and C.A. Lamartiniere (1981). Reg. Peptides, 2, 347-352.

Honoré, T., P. Krogsgaard-Larsen, J.J. Hansen, and J. Lauridsen (1981). Mol. Cell. Biochem., 38, 123-128.

Kizer, J.S., and W.W. Youngblood (1978). Psychopharmacology: A Generation of Progress, Raven Press, New York, 465-486.

Kizer, J.S., C.B. Nemeroff, and W.W. Youngblood (1978). Pharmacol. Rev., 29, 301-318.

Krieger, D.T., A.S. Liotta, G. Nicholson, and J.S. Kizer (1979). Nature, 278, 562-563.

Lamperti, A.A., and D.M. Baldwin (1982). Neuroendocrinology, 34, 169-174.

Lamperti, A., and G. Blaha (1976). Biol. Reprod., 14, 362-369.

Lechan, R.M., L.C. Alpert, and I.M.D. Jackson (1976). Nature, 264, 463-465.

Matsuzawa, Y., S. Yonetani, Y. Takasaki, S. Iwata, and S. Sekine (1979). Toxicol. Lett., 4, 359-371.

Nagasawa, H., R. Yanai, and S. Kikuyama (1974). Acta Endocrinol., 75, 249-259.

Nemeroff, C.B. (1981). Monosodium glutamate-induced neurotoxicity: Review of the literature and call for further research. Nutrition & Behavior, The Franklin Institute Press, Philadelphia.

Nemeroff, C.B., L.D. Grant, L.E. Harrell, G. Bissette, G.N. Ervin, and A.J. Prange, Jr. (1975). Neurosci. Abst., 1, 434.

Nemeroff, C.B., L.D. Grant, G. Bissette, G.N. Ervin, L.E. Harrell, and A.J. Prange, Jr. (1977a). Psychoneuroendocrinology, 2, 179-196.

Nemeroff, C.B., R.J. Konkol, G. Bissette, W.W. Youngblood, M.S. Rone, J.B. Martin, P. Brazeau, G.R. Breese, A.J. Prange, Jr., and J.S. Kizer (1977b). Endocrinology, 101, 613-633.

Nemeroff, C.B., G. Bissette, G.H. Greeley, R.B. Mailman, J.B. Martin, P. Brazeau, and J.S. Kizer (1978a). Brain Res., 156, 198-201.

Nemeroff, C.B., M.A. Lipton, and J.S. Kizer (1978b). Devel. Neurosci., 1, 102-109.

Nemeroff, C.B., C.A. Lamartiniere, G.A. Mason, R.E. Squibb, J-S Hong, and S.C. Bondy (1981). Neuroendocrinology, 33, 265-267.

Olney, J.W. (1969). Science, 164, 719–721.

Olney, J.W. (1971). J. Neuropathol. Exp. Neurol., 30, 75–90.

Olney, J.W. (1976). Adv. Exp. Med. Biol., 69, 496–506.

Olney, J.W. (1979). Excitotoxic amino acids: Research applications and safety implications. Glutamic Acid: Advances in Biochemistry and Physiology, Raven Press, New York.

Olney, J.W. (1980). Experimental and Clinical Neurotoxicology, 272–294.

Olney, J.W., and M.T. Price (1978). Excitotoxic amino acids as neuroendocrine probes. Kainic Acid as a Tool in Neurobiology, Raven Press, New York.

Olney, J.W., and M.T. Price (1980). Brain Res. Bull., 5, 361–368.

Olney, J.W., O-L Ho, and V. Rhee (1971). Exp. Brain Res., 14, 61–76.

Olney, J.W., V. Rhee, and O-L Ho (1974). Brain Res., 77, 507–512.

Olney, J.W., T.J. Cicero, E.R. Meyer, and T. deGubareff (1976). Brain Res., 112, 420–424.

Ondo, J.G. (1981). Brain Res. Bull., 7, 333–335.

Peter, R.E., O. Kah, C.R. Paulencu, H. Cook, and A.L. Kyle (1980). Cell Tissue Res., 212, 429–442.

Pizzi, W.J., J.E. Barnhart, and D.J. Fanslow (1977). Science, 196, 452–454.

Pizzi, W.J., J.M. Tabor, and J.E. Barnhart (1978). Pharmacol. Biochem. Behav., 9, 481–485.

Price, M.T., J.W. Olney, and T.J. Cicero (1978a). Neuroendocrinology, 26, 352–358.

Price, M.T., J.W. Olney, M.V. Mitchell, T. Fuller, and T.J. Cicero (1978b). Brain Res., 158, 461–465.

Price, M.T., J.W. Olney, M. Anglim, and S. Buchsbaum (1979). Brain Res., 176, 165–168.

Redding, T.W., A.V. Schally, A. Arimura, and I. Wakabayashi (1971). Neuroendocrinology, 8, 245–255.

Rodriguez-Sierra, J.F., R. Sridaran, and C.A. Blake (1980). Neuroendocrinology, 31, 228–235.

Schainker, B.A., and T.J. Cicero (1980). Brain Res., 184, 425–437.

Schainker, B., and J.W. Olney (1974). J. Neural. Transm., 35, 207–215.

Sridaran, R., J.F. Rodriguez-Sierra, and C.A. Blake (1981). Proc. Soc. Exper. Biol. Med., 168, 38–44.

Terry, L.C., J. Epelbaum, and J.B. Martin (1981). Brain Res., 217, 129–142.

Walaas, I., and F. Fonnum (1978). Brain Res., 153, 549–562.

Yonetani, S., and Y. Matsuzawa (1978). Toxicol. Lett., 1, 207–211.

Session IV

CLINICAL ASPECTS

Chairman: L. Wetterberg

ADVERSE REACTIONS IN HUMANS THOUGHT TO BE RELATED TO INGESTION OF ELEVATED LEVELS OF FREE MONOSODIUM GLUTAMATE (MSG)
(Chinese Restaurant Syndrome and Other Reactions)

LIANE REIF-LEHRER, PhD

*Eye Research Institute of Retina Foundation and Harvard Medical School,
Boston, Massachusetts, U.S.A.*

ABSTRACT

Monosodium glutamate is widely used as a flavor enhancer. A number of adverse effects in humans have been attributed to ingestion of this substance. The most well known of these is the so-called Chinese Restaurant Syndrome. Various studies have been done to attempt to substantiate that glutamate is indeed the etiologic factor responsible for the reported symptoms. No measurable signs appear to be associated with the syndrome. Symptoms can be quite frightening but appear to be transient and rely on subjective reports of reactors. Other adverse reactions, presumably associated with ingestion of glutamate, are also discussed.

KEYWORDS

Glutamate; monosodium glutamate; adverse reactions; Chinese restaurant syndrome; humans; ingestion; food additives.

Glutamic acid is a natural component of proteins (about 14–17% of most food is protein and approximately 20% of most protein is glutamic acid) and also exists in the free form in many natural foods. It is ingested at an estimated daily level of 38–40 gm in protein. Only somewhere between approximately 1 and 10% is in the form of free glutamate.

Foods such as mushrooms and tomatoes have a high endogenous concentration of free glutamate. For example, the total glutamate in tomatoes is 0.238 gm (including 140 mg free glutamate) per 100 gm of tomato. [Fresh foods may lose much of their natural free glutamate content (as much as 50% or more) within 24 hours.] An 8 lb baby consuming 21 oz of human milk per day has an intake of 1.5 gm (1/4 teaspoon) total glutamate, including about 150 mg free glutamate.

Virtually all glutamate sold in the United States is derived from food sources. The most common source is from fermentation of

molasses derived from sugar beets or sugar cane. Glutamate has
also been extracted directly from sugar beets, corn or wheat
gluten.

The MSG content of various food products tested by Conacher et al
(1979) ranged from 0.2% in some condensed soups to 13.1% in bouillon cubes. According to Consumer Reports (1978), common commercially available soups contain up to 1.3 gm of glutamate per 6
oz serving which, for a 10 kg child, would be a dosage of 130 mg
glutamate per kg body weight.

It is quite possible in a typical meal to consume on the order of
10 gm total glutamate, including approximately 1 gm of free glutamate. If MSG is used in such a meal as a flavor enhancer, it is
easy to increase the intake of free glutamate by an additional 4-6
gm. Twenty-thousand tons of MSG are manufactured and used in the
United States each year.

It has been known for some time that glutamate possesses a
somewhat unique flavor-enhancing property (Sjöström, 1955), probably related to its known neuroexcitatory properties (Olney, 1980;
Reif-Lehrer, 1976a).

To enhance the flavor of foods, Orientals have for many years used
a seaweed named Laminaria Japonica in their cooking. In 1908, a
Japanese chemist, Ikeda, showed that the active component in the
seaweed responsible for flavor enhancement was free MSG (Marshall,
1948). Shortly thereafter, glutamate began to be produced commercially and has been used in increasing amounts as a flavor enhancing condiment, not only in the Orient, but in cooking of many
nationalities. MSG became commercially available in the United
States in the early 1950s, and in 1955 the National Restaurant
Association "endorsed and encouraged" the use of MSG in the "public feeding industry." MSG is on the FDA so-called GRAS list
(generally recognized as safe), is sold in unlimited quantities
under a variety of trade names (In the United States a popular
form of glutamate is sold in supermarkets under the trade name of
"Accent." In some countries, the Japanese product, under the trade
name of "Ajinomoto," can be found.), and is unregulated in
restaurant food preparation. (Restaurants of many different
nationalities in the U.S. have been found to use this amino acid
salt in their cooking. Label listing is required for most
packaged foods, with some exceptions, e.g. freshly slaughtered
poultry is apparently dusted with MSG (Tracor-Jitco, 1974) and MSG
may be used without label declaration in mayonnaise, French
dressing and salad dressing (Department of Health, Education and
Welfare, 1974). The highest per capita consumption of glutamate
is in Okinawa, Japan, and the Philippines; the United States is
also high on the list. Additional glutamate is added to foods in
the form of hydrolyzed vegetable protein (HVP); this material
contains more glutamate, by far, than any other single amino acid.
According to a Food and Drug Administration report (Tracor-Jitco,
1974), the content of MSG in two brands of HVP was 11 and 20%.
(The next most abundant amino acids were alanine and proline, at
3-4% each; aspartate content was 3%.) The percent of Nestles Maggi
Hydrolyzed Plant Protein (HVP) (by weight) used in Worcestershire
sauce (Trauberman, 1960) is 20%; therefore, 1 oz (28.4 gm) of

Worcestershire sauce would contain 5.7 gm HVP. Even if this HVP only contains 10% glutamic acid, then 1 oz of Worcestershire sauce would contain about 0.57 gm glutamic acid, which is equivalent to 0.66 gm MSG. Thus, in determining the total free glutamate in foods, one must take into account 1) the endogenous free amino acids, 2) those added in the form of hydrolyzed protein, and 3) added MSG.

Several decades ago monosodium glutamate was considered to have a number of beneficial effects. It was thought to enhance I.Q. in mentally retarded children (Albert et al, 1946) and was used to treat psychiatric disorders (Himwich et al, 1955), epilepsy (Goodman, 1946; Tursky et al, 1976; Nitsch, 1976), hypoglycemic coma (Mayer-Gross, 1949; Weil-Malherbe, 1949), and more recently, Lesch-Nyhan syndrome (Ghadimi et al, 1970).

As early as 1949, however, some adverse effects of glutamate were reported: Levey et al (1949) suggested a correlation between glutamate and aspartate in intravenously administered amino acid solutions and the incidence of nausea and vomiting in individuals fed with such solutions. (See also M.E. Rubini, 1971.)

Chinese restaurant syndrome (CRS) was first described in April 1968 by a Chinese physician, Robert Ho Man Kwok, in the New England Journal of Medicine (Kwok, 1968). In the ensuing months, numerous letters to the editor of the New England Journal (1968, pp. 1123, 1124) appeared indicating that others also experienced similar symptoms. In the same year, two small experiments were reported that strongly implicated free monosodium glutamate (MSG) as the etiologic factor in this syndrome (Ambos et al, 1968; Schaumburg et al, 1968). (It should be noted that other components of Chinese food have recently aroused interest: Hammerschmidt, 1980.)

In 1969 the first serious study of the effects of MSG in humans was a reported by Schaumburg et al (1969). This study reported on the acute reaction to MSG in 56 normal subjects (30 males and 26 females, ranging in age from 21 to 67 years) and also presented evidence that glutamate causes headaches. While many symptoms were noted as components of CRS, Schaumburg et al suggested that three categories of symptoms were elicited by MSG: burning, facial pressure, and chest pain. Headache was considered to be a consistent complaint in a minority of individuals. Symptoms appeared only if the meal containing free MSG was taken on an empty stomach by a susceptible individual. Such individuals responded to 3 gm of free glutamate or less. (This amount was found to be present in a 200 ml serving of wonton soup in one New York restaurant.) Schaumburg et al determined that the attacks in their subjects were caused by L-glutamate; the D-form appeared to be inactive at 7 gm, as were L-aspartate (5 gm), sodium chloride (10 gm) and glycine (5 gm). Intensity and duration of the symptoms were related to the dosage of MSG. In 36 subjects used to determine a dose response curve, all but one individual reported symptoms. The one individual who had no symptoms, even at 21 gm by oral ingestion, showed definite symptoms following an intravenous dose of 50 mg. While symptoms to oral MSG usually had an onset 15 to 25 minutes after ingestion, the first symptom after intravenous

administration (13 subjects) generally appeared in 17 to 20 seconds, with a threshhold of minimum symptoms ranging from 25 to 125
mg. The first symptom to appear after intravenous injection was
the burning sensation. The second was the chest pressure (an extremely alarming sensation causing some people to think they are
having a heart attack; subjects who received 500 mg infusion
showed no EKG changes despite presence of severe chest pain). The
last symptom to appear was the sensation of tightness and pressure
over the cheek areas, occasionally extending into the temple. This
symptom had the longest duration, lasting about 2 to 3 minutes
after intravenous injection, but as long as 30 minutes after oral
administration. Oral threshhold appeared to bear no relationship
to the intravenous threshhold in the same person. The oral threshhold in the 36 subjects tested for dose response ranged from 1.5 to
12 gm. In two subjects intravenous injection of MSG in the forearm, while the arterial circulation was occluded by an axillary
cuff, produced burning of the subject's entire arm. Seventeen
seconds after the cuff was removed, the subject felt the burning
sensation over the chest and neck. Schaumburg et al concluded that
the burning sensation was a peripheral phenomenon and not due to
central nervous system stimulation. Six subjects who complained
about headache after oral administration of MSG came from a group
of nine individuals who had a history of either common migraine or
vascular-muscle tension headaches. A double-blind experiment on
eight individuals with headache history, including five of the six
reactors, revealed that two consistently suffered headaches after
MSG ingestion. The pain was described as pressure throbbing over
the temples and a "band-like" sensation around the forehead,
starting 20 to 25 minutes after ingestion of MSG and lasting for
one hour. No nausea or warning preceded the headaches. Prior
ingestion of food, which delays absorption of MSG, protected even
the most susceptible individuals from this syndrome. Reaction to
MSG was not affected by pretreatment with diphenhydramine (an
antihistamine), making it unlikely to be an allergic reaction.

In 1971 Ghadimi et al published a study entitled "Studies on Monosodium Glutamate Ingestion: I. Biochemical Explanation of Chinese
Restaurant Syndrome." This paper reported an expanded list of
symptoms following ingestion of MSG, including headache, sweating,
nausea, weakness, thirst, flushing of the face, a sensation of
burning or tightness, abdominal pain and lacrimation. (In subsequent studies by others, additional symptoms have been noted;
these included numbness of the neck, "heaviness" of the eyelids,
drowsiness, numbness of the legs, substernal pressure, urgency of
urination, palpitation, urgency of bowel evacuation, retro-orbital
pain, vomiting, and prolonged headache.) Ghadimi et al tested 14
healthy adults (10 males and 4 females). The initial challenge
was with 150 mg MSG/kg body weight (8.2 gm for a 120 lb person)
dissolved in 150 ml of water and administered orally after an
overnight fast. Volunteers were informed that the study concerned
CRS, but were supposedly not aware of the identity of sequence of
the test substances used. (However, it is difficult to imagine
that anyone would not be able to guess immediately the presence of
this concentration of MSG in water administered orally!) Ghadimi
et al concluded that their study, like that of Schaumburg, showed
that appearance and severity of symptoms were dose related. All
subjects in this study, with one possible exception, developed

definite signs and symptoms. Certain complaints were not mentioned by the volunteers but were obvious to observers. For example, one individual had a striking mood change from lively and talkative to quiet and subdued, although he himself was apparently not aware of this change. EKG, blood pressure and pulse rate were normal in all subjects during a 3-hour post ingestion test period. The highest test dosage used in this study was 250 mg MSG/kg body weight (13.7 gm/120 lb individual). Two subjects primed with atropine, an anticholinergic drug, exhibited only mild reactions even though a larger dose of MSG was administered. On the other hand, volunteers who received prostigmine, a cholinergic drug, in addition to MSG, exhibited marked to severe reactions. Control subjects tested with 150 mg histidine/kg body weight, did not have any observable clinical response. However, while no changes in plasma levels of cholinesterase activity were observed in control subjects treated with histidine, a 30% decrease in this enzyme occurred 1 hour after MSG ingestion, but the effect was reversible after 3 hours.

(Ghadimi et al (1971) injected a healthy 44 lb dog with 7.5 mg acetylcholine in 10 ml of saline intravenously over a period of 4 minutes. The dog showed a rapid drop in cholinesterase activity (by about 3 minutes) and the animal's heart rate was simultaneously reduced from 104 to 60 with the rhythm becoming irregular and respiration deepening. Both heart rate and respiratory rate came back to normal within 40 minutes. Unna and Howe (1945) reported that a dog injected with 1 gm of glutamic acid (2.5-5 mg/kg/body weight/min) exhibited salivation, vomiting, and bradycardia.) While no changes in heart rate were observed in the human volunteers tested with MSG in this study, changes in heart rate in individual human subjects have been reported by several other investigators (Gann, 1977; Neumann, 1976; Alston, 1976). In our hands, a single test on a 15-month-old child (with, however, definite developmental problems) who was challenged with MSG, also resulted in a profound decrease in heart rate within minutes. The same child showed no response to a similar challenge of sodium chloride on the following day. (Liane Reif-Lehrer and Ira Lott, unpublished observations; see below.)

In the Ghadimi study, even 25 mg MSG/kg body weight (approximately 1.4 gm in a 120 lb individual) produced mild but definite symptoms in four instances. Ghadimi et al pointed out that the mode of appearance, duration and recovery as well as the diverse nature of the symptoms following MSG ingestion, were remarkably similar to the action of acetylcholine in humans and suggested that CRS syndrome be renamed "transient acetylcholinosis." (See also Ghadimi and Kumar, 1972.) He did not comment on the difference in cardiac effects reported with acetylcholine compared to those found with MSG in his study.

In a study by Rosenblum et al (1971), 99 male volunteers aged 21 to 59 were given 5 gm of MSG in 100 ml of water (5% solution), or the same concentration in chicken stock, on an empty stomach. Controls received an osmotically equivalent amount of sodium chloride (1.7 gm) in 100 ml of chicken stock or just 100 ml of chicken stock alone. Subjects received a questionnaire to fill out one hour after ingestion of the test fluid. Eleven subjects were re-tested with 8 gm of MSG or 2.8 gm of sodium chloride in chicken stock.

Ten of these individuals were subsequently tested with 12 gm of MSG
in 200 ml of diluted chicken stock (8% solution, or 4.2 gm sodium
chloride in the same amount of chicken stock). While some complaints were reported by both the control and MSG groups, a significantly greater (p < 0.01) incidence of complaints were reported
in subjects receiving MSG than in control subjects. Complaints
reported were headache, itching, light headedness, drowsiness, dry
mouth, and tightness in the face. However, only the light headedness and tightness in the face appeared with a significantly
greater (p < 0.05) frequency in the MSG compared to the control
subjects. In no case in this study were all three symptoms of CRS
(burning, chest pain, and facial pressure) reported by a given
subject. These authors reported that nausea became more common
with the higher doses (8-12 gm) but was not followed by vomiting.

This study as well as one by Morselli et al (1970) concluded that
there were no differences in parameters such as arterial blood
pressure, heart rate, and respiratory frequency, following ingestion of broth containing MSG, compared to broth which did not contain MSG. Morselli and co-workers also reported no difference in
symptoms.

Kenney and Tidball (1972) reported on a placebo control study conducted on 77 normal volunteers. The subjects in this study included both males and females, blacks as well as whites. Subjects
were tested with either 5 gm of MSG or 0.8 gm of sodium chloride in
150 ml tomato juice in such a way that each person got MSG on one
day and sodium chloride on two other days. Subjects were questioned 2 hours later about their reactions. A total of 40 symptoms
were reported following ingestion of MSG while only 17 symptoms
were reported after placebo. Of the whole sample, 32% were found
to be reactors (25% of the 44 males and 42% of the 33 females).
(In a questionnaire study done by me [discussed later], 22% of the
males reported reactions compared to 34% of the females.) Subjects
were over 20 years old, with the predominant sample (38 out of 77)
being between 20 and 25 years. Of the nine blacks in the study
(two females and seven males) none reported a reaction after either
MSG or placebo. Type of breakfast eaten 2 hours prior to testing
appeared to have no effects on the outcome. A significant
difference in plasma level of MSG after glutamate compared to
placebo ingestion (p < 0.01) was observed in this study, but the
increase in plasma level of glutamate was not significantly different between reactors and non-reactors. Stegink (1979) recently
confirmed that 20-fold elevation of plasma glutamate in adult
humans can result after glutamate ingestion in tomato juice.
However, when glutamate was ingested with large amounts of carbo-
hydrates, absorption of glutamate decreased. Of the various species that have been tested, man appears to have a much greater
increase of blood glutamate levels after oral loading than other
species, including even monkey.

While Kenney and Tidball found that the symptoms described by their
subjects matched those previously reported, only in a few cases
did they find the combination of symptoms described by Schaumburg
et al in the range of doses used in their experiments. A dose-
response relationship was particularly marked with the stiffness/

tightness symptoms and less marked for the pressure/tingling sensation, which exhibited a clear threshold of appearance at the 2-3 gm level. If the skin was mildly abraded, the site of the abrasion became the site for the first appearance of sensation during the development of the response. Kenney and Tidball suggested that the symptoms were largely peripheral and might involve the subcutaneous free-nerve endings of primitive chemical sense. The headaches were frequently described as migraine-like with similar prodromata.

Kenney and Tidball suggested that MSG taken as the free salt is probably not physiologically equivalent to glutamate ingested as a component of protein. (Glutamic acid released during hydrolysis of protein is readily transaminated to α-ketoglutaric acid, a reaction in which pyruvate is converted to alanine. A bolus of free glutamate, however, may overload the capability of the gut to convert the total amino acid.) Kenney and Tidball also suggested that the lack of correlation of symptoms with blood glutamate level might suggest that MSG per se is not the effective agent.

In 1979 Kenney reported additional placebo-controlled studies of human reaction to oral MSG which confirmed the previous observations of Kenney and Tidball (1972) in that 33% of men and 50% of women reported symptoms following MSG (5 gm) administration (reaction to placebo juice occurred in 1 out of 6 trials). Kenney (1979) also confirmed that in reactor subjects, symptoms are related to MSG dose. No tremor or visual change and no significant difference in blood chemistry was seen in reactors. Kenney reported on an additional series of experiments in which individuals were tested with MSG (upper dose = 6 gm) in a formulated soft drink given after fasting. Fifty-seven individuals began in this second study (9 blacks, 4 Orientals, 44 whites; 22 males, 35 females; 20 to 56 years of age). Symptoms of headache, thirst, light headedness or gastric discomfort, appeared approximately equal in groups given MSG and placebo. However, reactions that could be described as sensations of warmth or burning, stiffness or tightness, weakness in the limbs, or tingling, were seen only in individuals tested with MSG and were found in 16 of the 57 subjects (28%) (15 females, 1 male; 1 black, 1 Oriental). In no cases were sensations accompanied by objective signs; blood pressure remained stable. Kenney concluded that the failure to demonstrate objective correlated symptoms could be interpreted as being indicative of sensations that are transferred to the body surface from a visceral rather than a peripheral area and suggested that symptoms to MSG are similar to those to which esophageal pain is often referred. He points out that heartburn, for example, believed to arise from spastic irritation of the gastro-esophageal junction, is felt at the lower end of the sternum while upper esophageal pain is experienced in the midline at the upper sternal border, from where the sensation spreads to involve the face, head, neck, upper chest and back, shoulders and upper arms. Such esophageal pain generally comes in two varieties, burning and pressure, and results from spasms of the muscle coats and chemical stimulation of free nerve endings of the mucous surface by 1. direct exposure to an irritant after swallowing, 2. reflux of gastric juices from the stomach, and 3. from the circulation. He suggested that MSG reaction may be "Transient Esophagalgia".

Kenney retested four individuals who had experienced reaction at
the 6 gm (3%) level, but had not responded at the 3 gm (1.5%) level; three out of the four subjects experienced symptoms at the
lower dose, i.e., 3 gm, when given at equal concentration, i.e., 3
gm in 100 ml as opposed to 3 gm in 200 ml.

Kenney also reported that of three individuals who had reacted at a
level of 3 gm in 200 ml and were subsequently tested with 3 gm MSG
in gelatin capsules in order to avoid contact with nerve endings of
the oropharynx and esophagus (placebo controls contained lactose),
one experienced the typical reaction of burning in the upper chest
and shoulders. The woman who showed reaction to the latter treatment had a history of heartburn while the two individuals who
showed no reactions denied a history of heartburn.

The 20 minute usual latency of symptoms following MSG ingestion has
frequently been considered time needed for absorption; such latency would also be compatible with gastroesophageal reflux. A lack
of good saliva flow to dilute away the MSG, and a tendency toward
gastroesophagael reflux, would be expected to predispose
individuals toward reactions to MSG. Kenney concluded that at a
0.75% level of MSG, even sensitive individuals are unlikely to
react; at 1.5% only a few individuals would be affected; but that
at the 3% level (6 gm in 200 ml) about 30% of individuals respond
to MSG.

Rippere (1981) criticized certain aspects of Kenney's use of place-
bos on the grounds that some of them may themselves be food allergens, the effects of which are not necessarily dose-related, i.e.,
minute traces of allergens may trigger severe symptoms in sensi-
tized individuals. She points out that the symptoms designated by
Kenney and Tidball as non-specific reaction (headache, light-head-
edness, gastric discomfort, nausea, heartburn) are amongst those
commonly found in food allergy reactions.

In a study by Marrs et al (1978), six subjects (healthy adults, age
20-35) were given 60 mg MSG/kg body weight, dissolved in 200 ml of
water, while six others were given an amount of casein hydrolysate
containing an equivalent amount of glutamic acid (=440 mg casein
hydrolysate/kg body weight). Blood samples taken from a peripheral
vein at zero time and subsequent time points up to 2 hr showed a
rapid increase in blood glutamate from the normal of approximately
43 micromoles per liter up to 155 micromoles per liter at 30 minutes post-ingestion. Levels of both glutamate and aspartate were
back to pretreatment levels by 2 hours. Blood aspartate also rose
from 5 to 15 micromoles per liter in the same time period, while
blood alanine did not change. After pancreatic hydrolysate ingestion, there were no dramatic increases in any of the free amino
acids.

Marrs et al pointed out that absorption of glutamic acid into plasma was quite different after ingestion of free MSG compared to
comparable doses when accompanied by other amino acids. Their
argument was that MSG is normally consumed as a food additive and
this is accompanied by other material including protein, thus
giving rise to much lower concentrations of blood glutamate than
after doses of the pure compound when ingested on an empty

stomach.

Ghezzi et al (1980) reported that in 109 healthy adult volunteers, the average basal plasma glutamic acid level was 0.06 = 0.003 S.E. micromol/ml (they measured 10 mg glutamate/100 ml in bouillon and 200 mg MSG/100 ml in tomato juice). After the volunteers fasted overnight, MSG was given as a 2% solution in bouillon or tomato juice to be consumed within 3 minutes. After 60 mg MSG/kg, the plasma area under the curve was 5.6 $\pm$ 0.34 (S.E.) micromol/ml/min. In most volunteers the peak was reached between 15 and 30 minutes. The highest value obtained was 0.24 micromol/ml after 15 min. Levels of blood glutamate in subjects who developed symptoms were not statistically different from those in subjects who did not develop symptoms. These authors also reported that MSG taken along with other nutrients leads to considerably lower plasma glutamic acid levels than when free MSG is consumed alone on an empty stomach.

Ghezzi et al point out that an oral dose of 30 mg MSG/kg represents 15 times the average daily intake of a person in the United States. Infants' plasma glutamic acid levels are higher than those of adults. Aspartate acts in a manner similar to that of glutamate when given parenterally, but apparently is benign when fed. Glutamic and aspartic acid in quantities usually ingested are transaminated in intestinal mucosa to alanine (Ghadimi, 1973).

When large quantities of MSG are ingested, especially in the absence of other foods, rapid absorption may surpass the transamination capability of intestinal mucosa and an excessive amount of MSG appear in the circulation, just as it does if MSG is injected.

A study by Gore and Salmon (1980) of 30 men and 25 women again indicated that while symptoms were not exactly as described by Schaumburg, reactions to MSG were significant when 1.5, 3, or 6 gm of MSG in 150 ml of cold water were ingested after an overnight fast: 16 subjects reported reactions to MSG out of the total of 55; 11 responded only at the highest level; three responded at 6 and 3 gm; and two responded at 6, 3 and 1.5 gm.

A number of other studies corroborated adverse reactions to glutamate, while several studies reported no reaction even at quite high levels of free MSG. In none of the studies from the early 1970s were changes noted in parameters such as arterial blood pressure, heart rate, and respiratory frequency.

Unfortunately, a definitive study on CRS has yet to be done. This would involve a double-blind study using free MSG after an overnight fast on a group of subjects known to be susceptible to MSG. This may be difficult to accomplish. According to one anecdotal report (Himms-Hagen, 1970) susceptible individuals tend to some extent to estimate the amount of MSG ingested as judged from the severity of symptoms. Other sensitive individuals maintain that they can recognize the "feel" of MSG in their mouth regardless of the type of vehicle used to disguise the taste. We have some evidence in our laboratory (unpublished results) that individuals who react to glutamate may also have the ability to taste, i.e.

detect the taste of, MSG. Thus, it is difficult to do a double-
blind study using simple ingestion. A study on a sizable population of susceptible individuals using free MSG in capsule form (to
avoid contact with taste receptors) would probably be optimal. To
date, capsules have only been used in two studies on a very small
number of individuals (Kenney, 1979; Allen and Baker, 1981).

In 1974, in the course of some studies of the effects of MSG on the
isolated embryonic retina, I became interested in CRS. In an attempt to determine how common CRS is in the general population I
devised a questionnaire study (Reif-Lehrer, 1977b). Of 2091
individuals who received questionnaires, 1491 (71%) responded. In
addition, 38 individuals voluntarily contacted me directly to report adverse reactions of CRS. This gave a total of 1529 respondents. Twenty-five percent of the adult population sampled (excluding the 38 who had contacted me), had some adverse symptoms,
presumably (but not necessarily) caused by the MSG contained in
food; 30% of those who specified eating Chinese restaurant food, or
other food containing exogenously added free MSG, reported adverse
reactions.

The age group of seemingly highest overall sensitivity was 26 to 30
(41 people belonged to this age group, and 66% reported symptoms). The lowest frequency of symptoms was in the over-60 age
group.

Of the 280 individuals who reported experiencing CRS, 35 (12%)
stipulated that they experienced it every time they ate in a
Chinese restaurant, 128 (45%) only sometimes, and 103 (36%) only in
certain restaurants.

Seventy-three percent of those reporting symptoms experienced them
within 30 minutes after the meal. Twenty percent said symptoms
last less than 30 minutes, 28% said they last 3-4 hours, and only
10% reported symptoms lasting more than 3-4 hours.

Forty-three percent of the sample were females (not including the
38 individuals who contacted me, of whom 29 were women). Thirty-
four percent of women and 22% of men reported symptoms.

Of 317 grade school children I interviewed, 267 had eaten Chinese
restaurant food and 51 (19%) reported some adverse reaction. (In
1980 Asnes reported a presumed case of CRS in an 18-month-old boy.
Ten minutes after having been fed noodles and broth from wonton
soup in a Chinese restaurant known to use MSG in the preparation of
this food, the child began to cry and scream, assume a crouching
position and hold his hands tightly against the side of his head
with his knees drawn up to his abdomen, obviously in distress. The
child's face was slightly flushed and his conjunctivae were injected; the child was extremely irritable. The physical and neurological exam were normal. The child (who had not previously eaten
Chinese food nor previously experienced a similar illness) became
asymptomatic two hours after the onset of symptoms.)

In our study we found that Orientals also experienced CRS. In
addition, I sent questionnaires to the various associations for
twins; 200 usable questionnaries were returned, and a rough

hand-tabulation of these indicates that adverse reactions to MSG probably are hereditary.

In a questionnaire study by Kerr et al (1979), which attempted to define the prevalence of symptoms characteristic of CRS in the general adult population, 43% of more than 3000 respondents associated unpleasant symptoms with certain types of foods, but only 1 to 2% reported symptoms characteristic of CRS, and only 0.2% associated these characteristic symptoms with consumption of Chinese food. Since the results of my study were in good agreement (30% reactors) with the results of the laboratory study of Kenney and Tidball (32% when subjects were challenged with 5 gm of glutamate) and since one can easily consume 4 to 6 gm of glutamate in a single meal if one follows the instructions on the "Accent" package, my estimate of the number of responders in the population may be closer to the correct number than the values reported by Kerr et al.

A variety of other reactions presumed to result from MSG ingestion have been reported in recent years; e.g. MSG has been reported to decrease serum cholesterol and associated beta-lipoproteins in man (Bazzano et al, 1970).

Neumann (1976) pointed out that MSG experiments had only been done on healthy adults and not on individuals with cardiovascular disorders. He reported having seen reactions involving frequent ventricular premature beats and considerable discomfort in such individuals shortly after eating in Chinese restaurants, with arrhythmia continuing for hours and triggering a long period of reduced functional capacity of the heart.

Alston (1976) reported that a 52-year-old man arriving in Tokyo for a vacation with a well-documented idiopathic subaortic stenosis (which had responded well to propranolol) and who was maintained on a low salt diet, responded to a Japanese meal within 20 minutes with a flushed sensation, general uneasiness, tightness about the face, and palpitations, progressing to severe pressure-like pain. He continued to have palpitations, dyspnea and dull chest pain. On hospitalization, his blood pressure was normal, pulse 90; a systolic murmur that increased with hand grip was noted. EKG showed changes characteristic of ischemia or left ventricular hypertrophy (or both). Serum enzymes showed no changes. A repeat EKG showed no changes. Symptoms abated after rest, oxygen and increased propranolol dosage. Alston suggested (personal communication) that tachycardia may be a frequent concomitant of CRS and may precipitate additional problems in patients with underlying heart disease.

Gann (1977) reported on a patient who developed CRS and on admission to the emergency room was found to have a ventricular tachycardia. A 36-year-old white male, previously in good health with no history of significant medical problems, had eaten in a Chinese restaurant 4 hours prior to admission; the meal began with wonton soup. Symptoms included burning feeling in chest, face and neck, diaphoresis and extreme weakness. At the time of admission only severe weakness and diaphoresis remained. No peripheral pulse or blood pressure could be recorded. EKG showed regular rhythm of

210, which was compatible with ventricular tachycardia. Lidocaine
(100 mg) converted the rhythm back to normal within 3 minutes.
The patient had no further problems during a 6-month follow-up.
(Severe palpitations had also been reported earlier by Rath (1968),
Kandall (1968), Schaumburg (1968), and Ghadimi and Kumar (1972),
and might have resulted from ventricular tachycardia.) Gann suggested that MSG might produce potential arrhythmia in susceptible
individuals.

The possibility that the effects noted in the three preceding reports may be due to excess sodium should be considered.

In 1978, a California physician (Colman, 1978a) reported on two
individuals with possible psychiatric reactions to MSG ingestion
which, in one of them (a 38-year-old woman), followed the usual CRS
symptoms by about 48 hours. The symptoms lasted about 2 weeks and
apparently were "reminiscent of the occasional psychopathology seen
after large doses of corticosteroids." In the second individual (a
nine-year-old boy), the typical acute CRS reaction was reported to
be accompanied by bladder and bowel incontinence and intermittent
hyperactivity.   Both individuals apparently responded to dietary
regulation of MSG intake. (See also Kenney, 1978; and Colman,
1978b).

A case report from Poland describes a severe case of glutamic acid
poisoning of a 17-year-old girl who apparently attempted to commit
suicide by ingestion of 17.5 gm of glutamic acid. She was hospitalized with "transient excitation of the central nervous system and
atrioventricular block" (Sworczak et al, 1980).

Most recently Allen (Allen and Baker, 1981), an allergist from
Australia, has reported a possible correlation between MSG ingestion and asthma attacks in certain individuals. A delay time of
about 12 hours to onset of asthma (as measured by decrease in air
flow rates) was reported in two female patients, following ingestion of capsules containing 2.5 gm MSG in single-blind oral challenge studies. The long delay time is puzzling, and the possibility of stress-induced asthma should be considered.

A recent report of a degenerative neurological disorder has been
associated with elevated plasma glutamate (Plaitakis et al, 1982).

I have collected information about some 8 children who, according
to anecdotal information from either the parents or the physician,
appeared to react adversely to ingestion of food known to contain
MSG, either with shudder attacks (in the younger children) or with
migraine headaches (in the older children).   In each of these
cases, eliminating foods known to contain exogenously added free
MSG or hydrolized vegetable protein from the diet eliminated many,
and in some cases all of the symptoms as reported to me by either
the parents or the physician (Reif-Lehrer and Stemmermann, 1975;
Reif-Lehrer, 1976b; Andermann et al, 1976; Reif-Lehrer, 1977a).

In December, 1977, an 8-month-old child who had been brought to a
Boston hospital for further evaluation of atypical seizures was
challenged with 1 gm of glutamate in a small amount of commercially prepared broth. The child vomited after 20 minutes and

experienced one of her characteristic episodes at 45 minutes.

In July of 1978, we arranged to have this child, then about 15 months old, (date of birth: April, 1977) brought back to Boston for testing. The history was as follows: The child's maternal grandfather had late onset diabetes. A second cousin had early onset diabetes. The father's grandfather on his mother's side was diabetic (probably late onset). All four of the child's mother's grandparents had late onset diabetes. Thus, there was a strong history of diabetes in the family.

The child's paternal grandfather died of a heart problem in his late 40s. The paternal grandmother had a radical mastectomy in 1976.

The mother also reported having a second cousin who at age 12 developed epilepsy, which was apparently completely controlled by diet.

Both parents reported having unpleasant reactions after eating Chinese food. The mother reported diarrhea and excessive thirst; the father reported being "Thirsty after Chinese food in a way which is quite different from what happens after I eat in any other kind of restaurant," and feeling as though he has a "film" on his tongue.

The parents had a completely normal 4-year-old daughter. During that first pregnancy the mother reported that she was unable to "hold things down".

In contrast, during the second pregnancy, she had no problems with nausea and, therefore, was able to eat as usual.

The family apparently consumes many of the commercially prepared foods that tend to contain exogenously added glutamate. The mother recalled, in particular, the ample use of Hickory salt, (which apparently contains MSG) during the pregnancy.

The only untoward happening during this second pregnancy was bronchitis during the third month, for which the mother was given ampicillin and terpin hydrate.

The child's birthweight was 7 lbs 4 oz, and delivery was apparently normal.

The mother reported that in addition to eating much prepared food, she also ate a lot of chocolate and pizza during the breast feeding. Although she got headaches from the chocolate, she continued to eat it.

The shudder attack episodes had begun in the second child at the age of 1 month, seemed to increase dramatically after each breast feeding, and seemed to be especially bad if the mother had consumed, e.g., pizza, prior to breast feeding. The child was taken to a hospital in upstate New York for a seizure work-up, and the parents were told that there was no evidence of real seizures. The child was put on phenobarbital, as a precaution, but the attacks continued. (The child is on poly-vi-fluor, a multivitamin preparation.) During an episode of meningitis for which the child was hospitalized some months prior to our seeing her, she was fed intravenously and apparently had only one shudder attack during the time she was off oral feeding.

The mother perceived that shudder attacks were most common 2 hours after meals, but in some cases seemed to occur 20 minutes after the end of a meal. As a result, the mother had further and further restricted the child's diet to goat's milk, apple juice, oatmeal, meat and potatoes, and yogurt. (The mother also reported that about once a week blood was visible in the child's stool.)

When the child was brought to Boston, it was immediately evident that she had multiple problems, was appreciably mentally retarded and had sporadic shudder attacks.

In fact, prior to the beginning of our test the child had a brief seizure during which Dr. Ira Lott, a pediatric neurologist, assessed that there was a momentary loss of consciousness. The child was tested by Dr. Lott and myself in a hospital setting after overnight fasting.

The child's temperature, blood pressure, heart rate and EEG were monitored during the experiment. Temperature before the experiment was normal, pulse rate was 150 and blood pressure was 130/86.

At 12:10 the child was fed 0.75 gm MSG in 15 ml of chicken broth prepared in my laboratory, followed by 15 ml of broth free of MSG. The 30 ml was consumed in approximately 3 minutes.

At 12:20, the temperature remained normal, pulse rate dropped down to about 90, then 80, and the mother reported that the child's hand was twitching.

At 12:23, there was a noticeable jerk.

At 12:25, there were one or two more big jerks.

By 12:29, the heart rate was down to 40, and by 12:30, down to 20; then it suddenly began to beat very fast.

There were several more definite jerks between 12:36 and 12:38.

At 12:48, the heart rate had leveled off, and by 1:15, it was very steady at about 154.

At 1:20, the mother fed the child her normal feed, which consisted of apple sauce, beef and broth (Gerber).

At 1:40, the child had just started drinking goat's milk and there was another big jerk; yet another at 1:55, at 2:00 and at 2:19.

In the evening, the child had a last feeding at 8 pm followed by phenobarbitol at 10 pm, accompanied by a teaspoon of applesauce; a single shudder episode occurred about 1/2 hr after this medication was given.

At 10:22 the next morning, the child was given 0.26 gm of sodium chloride in 15 ml of chicken broth followed by 15 ml of chicken broth without added sodium chloride or MSG. It took 3 minutes for the child to ingest the 30 ml of fluid.

Prior to the test the blood pressure was 104/72. Immediately after the child consumed the broth, the pulse was 132.

At 10:29, the mother reported the child was having small twitches over her whole body; I was unable to detect these when I put my hand on the child's leg.

At 10:50, the heart rate was still very stable and there were no signs of any kind of discomfort.

By 11:10, the heart beat was very slightly irregular, varying from 108 to 132. (The previous day, at peak time, the heart rate had been vacillating from almost 0 to 204.)

By 11:30, the heart rate was at 132, the same as the start of the experiment; blood pressure was 104/54-56.

The EEG was continuously recorded throughout both test sessions and showed no paroxysmal discharges and was remarkable only for a movement artifact.

In summary then, following MSG consumption, the child had extreme and abrupt changes in cardiac rate, going from 200/minute with drops close to asystole. There was no compromise in blood pressure or any other disturbance in EKG other than the changing rate. One hour after MSG consumption, the child was back to normal and resumed her baseline status. No such changes were observed following the test with NaCl-broth (cf dog experiment in Ghadimi et al, 1971).

A further test of the child at her home by a pediatric gastro-enterologist using a commercially prepared soup apparently produced no reaction, but was difficult to interpret in the absence of details.

Folkers et al (1981) reported that supplemental Vitamin B$_6$ effectively prevents CRS in those who respond to MSG. In this study, pyridoxine hydrochloride as a tablet and a matching placebo were used. (The MSG dosage and that of the matching placebo were formulated and provided by Nestle Products, but no mention is made of what the vehicle for the MSG was.) An oral dose of MSG was administered double-blind to fasted subjects (approximately 7 gm MSG per 120 lb individual). A group of 158 students, who did not take any vitamin supplements, were tested for glutamic oxaloacetic transaminase (EGOT) in their erythrocytes. The mean basal specific activity was 0.32 ± 0.08. Twenty-seven of the students with basal activity of the enzyme equal to 0.26 or below were used in the double-blind study and were challenged either with MSG or with placebo; 12 of these 27 showed symptoms in response to MSG. Of these 27, those showing and not showing symptoms had similar enzyme specific activities. Of the 12 students who had symptoms to MSG, 12-week treatment (double-blind) with either pyridoxine (50 mg daily) or a matching placebo showed, upon decoding, that nine out of 12 had received pyridoxine and the other three had received placebo. At the end of 12 weeks they were rechallenged with MSG. Eight of nine treated with pyridoxine showed no symptoms after MSG and one continued to show symptoms. All three students exposed to placebo showed symptoms to MSG. The one student who continued to show symptoms to MSG after Vitamin B_6 treatment had a very severe erythrocyte deficiency of Vitamin B_6. After further treatment with Vitamin B_6 at 100 mg pyridoxine daily for 4 weeks, she still continued to show symptoms. The authors warned that it was difficult to monitor compliance with the daily Vitamin B_6 regimen. The authors also cautioned that a blood deficiency of Vitamin B_6 may not necessarily have a quantitative correlation with deficiencies of tissues in the brain, face, and chest, which may account for CRS. However, the individuals treated with pyridoxine for 12 weeks did show an increase in the specific activity of EGOT of 0.23 ± 0.12, while the three individuals receiving placebo showed an increase in the enzyme specific activity of only 0.03 ± 0.03 (difference is significant at the $p < 0.001$ level).

Folkers' explanation of why only 12 of the 27 students with low EGOT activities reacted to MSG was based on the fact that the tissues of the brain, face, and chest might have greater deficiencies of Vitamin B_6 in those who reacted than in those who did not react.

It is interesting that Vitamin B_6 supplementation has also been reported to reduce epileptic seizures in children (Reinken, 1975) as well as the more specific so-called Vitamin B_6-dependent seizures (Scriver and Whelan, 1969; Lott et al, 1978). Glutamate was found to be elevated (and GABA reduced) in the brain of one child who died during a Vitamin B_6-dependent seizure (Lott et al, 1978).

In 1981 the US Food and Drug Administration approved the use of an artificial sweetening agent, Aspartame, (G.B. Searle, Co.) in certain foods (breakfast cereals, chewing gum, powdered beverages, whipped toppings, puddings, gelatins, and table-top sweeteners. It will not be used in liquid soft drinks because it is unstable in that vehicle) (Smith, 1981). This ester of a dipeptide of aspartic acid and phenylalanine is expected to occupy about 25% of the market presently held by saccharin.

From studies by Olney and by Reynolds et al (1976), as well as some very preliminary studies in my own laboratory, it would appear that Aspartame affects both retinal (Table I) and hypothalamic tissue (Moneysworth, 1975; Olney 1975, 1976, 1980) in a manner similar to that seen subsequent to treatment with glutamate. Whether or not Aspartame will cause symptomatology in humans similar to that seen with glutamate is as yet unknown.

TABLE I

Effect of Aspartame (ATM) on GS Induction in Retinas from 12-Day
Chick Embryo

Additions	S.A. (GS)[a] after 24-hour in-cubation	% inhibition of induction due to MSG or Aspartame
none	0.12 + 0.01	———
0.01 g/ml cortisol	0.83 + 0.05	(fold of induction = 6.9)
cortisol + 2.4 mM MSG	0.28 + 0.06	67
cortisol + 0.1 mM ATM	0.86 + 0.04	-3
cortisol + 0.3 mM ATM	0.63 + 0.09	24
cortisol + 1.2 mM ATM	0.21 + 0.03	75
cortisol + 2.4 mM ATM	0.16 + 0.02	81

Aspartame is L-aspartyl-L-phenylalanine methyl ester
              (1-methyl N-L-α-aspartyl-L-phenylalanine)

a.) The values in the table are specific activity (S.A.) of glutamine synthetase (GS) (as measured by its γ-glutamyltransferase
activity) + the average deviation from the mean.
     S.A. is defined as μg γ-glutamylhydroxamate formed per hour
per μg protein in the retinal lysate.

An interesting question — but one which would be difficult to
pursue for ethical reasons — is the following: diabetics are
known (from fluorescein angiography studies) to have a leaky blood
retinal barrier. This might allow molecules which normally do not
get to the retina to reach this tissue; e.g., glutamate and aspartate. Do elevated levels of glutamate in the diet of such individuals perhaps "spill" into the retina and cause further damage to
the already damaged retina? If this were the case, it would be
important to consider that it would be precisely these diabetic
individuals who would be most inclined to use the new artificial
sweetener, Aspartame.

Glutamate and some of its structural analogues have long been known
to stimulate firing of neurons in many regions of the central
nervous system. In the 1970s, it was demonstrated that such neuroexcitatory amino acids, systemically administered to immature
rodents, act as convulsants, and appear to vary in potency in proportion to their known neuroexcitatory activities. Many of these
findings have recently been concisely reviewed by Olney (1980). In

general, the literature on effects of MSG in animals has been adequately reviewed in recent years (Tracor-Jitco, 1974; Reif-Lehrer,
1976a; Reif-Lehrer, 1977c; Reif-Lehrer, 1982, in press; Olney,
1980). Animal effects include convulsions (Johnston, 1973), behavioral changes (Berry et al, 1974; Carter and Levesque, 1979),
retinal and hypothalamic damage, specifically neurotoxicity (Olney,
1980), retardation of retinal blood vessel development (Bellhorn et
al, 1981), effects on high affinity neurotransmitter uptake (Dawson
et al, 1982), possible blood-brain barrier effects (Nemeroff and
Crisley, 1975; McCall et al, 1980; Bellhorn et al, 1981), inhibition of glucose uptake into brain (Creasey and Malawista,
1971), and a variety of endocrine disorders, (e.g. Nemeroff and
Crisley, 1975; Cooper, 1977; Krieger et al, 1979; Bodnar et al,
1980; Komeda et al, 1980; Olney, 1980; Peter et al, 1980;
Rodriguez-Sierra et al, 1980; Schubert et al, 1980; Utsumi et al,
1980; Saphier and Dyer, 1981; Terry et al, 1981; Dhindsa, 1981).
Only minimal cardiovascular effects have been reported (Kirkendol
et al, 1980).

Berry et al (1974) suggested that although many of the abnormalities reported to be due to MSG occur only in neonates, they may
well have the possibility of altering the structural development of
the central nervous system and thus induce a long-lasting impairment of brain function at the time in the animals' development when
enzyme and transport systems are still immature. Olney (1980) has
also argued that while no overt signs of damage are seen at the
time when circumventricular organs (i.e. those not protected by a
blood-brain barrier) are damaged due to glutamate, such damage may
well be manifest at a later stage, e.g., in adulthood. Examples of
this are the obesity and disturbances in the neuroendocrine system
that have been reported. In humans, it would be extremely difficult to establish at some adult age that such effects might have
been related to ingestion of neurotoxic amino acids in infancy or
early childhood.

Recent evidence that glutamate may be a neurotransmitter substance
in certain types of neuronal cells (Roberts et al, 1981) is also of
interest. It is now thought that neurotoxicity is an excitatory
receptor-mediated phenomenon and the flavor-enhancing properties
that have been attributed to glutamate, in all likelihood, stem
from its excitatory (depolarizing) action on sensory taste receptors.

Olney (1980) has suggested that the artificial sweetner, Aspartame
(1-methyl-N-L-α-aspartyl-L-phenylalanine), probably also interacts
with taste receptors in such a way that a sweet flavor is perceived. He has suggested the possibility of a significant hazard
in combining ingestion of glutamate, aspartate (which largely
mimics the action of glutamate), and Aspartame, especially for
young children. A detailed analysis of the possibilities may be
found in Olney (1980). (See also Stegink et al, 1981.)

An increasing body of information from laboratory studies as well
as from anecdotal reports seems to indicate that ingested free
glutamate (and possibly related compounds) may have adverse effects
on an appreciable number of individuals. Unfortunately, the only
question that has usually been asked in relation to this is whether

glutamate is, or is not, safe for human consumption in general. (It seems unlikely, for example, that MSG even in large doses is overtly harmful to normal adult individuals.) The more interesting question: Are there subgroups of individuals for whom glutamate ingestion is not safe, or at least not advisable?, has not, as yet, been adequately explored. In general, one can conjecture that individuals with certain minor inborn "errors" of metabolism that may go unnoticed under normal circumstances, might be subject to symptoms under increased MSG load. For example, individuals with marginal levels, or frank deficiences of Vitamin B_6, might not metabolize glutamate at an adequate rate. Another possibility relates to transient or permanent impairment of the blood-brain and blood-retinal barriers (Bakay, 1972), which may allow glutamate, normally excluded by these barriers, to enter the CNS, especially when the plasma levels of the amino acid are appreciably increased. A particular example of this might be early breakdown of the blood-retinal barrier known to occur in diabetes (Cunha-Vaz et al, 1975). Numerous other factors are now thought to impair these CNS barriers (Pardridge et al, 1975; Albert, 1979). These include certain drugs, diseases (including viral infections) and environmental factors (e.g. possibly microwave radiation; Albert, 1979; Justesen, 1980; Merritt et al, 1978). The recent report of elevated plasma glutamate in olivopontocerebellar degeneration associated with a partial glutamate dehydrogenase deficiency is also of interest in this regard (Plaitakis et al, 1982).

An important current practical consideration is to increase public awareness of the fact that although there are common overall metabolic mechanisms, each of us may also have unique metabolic properties that may respond differentially to various elements of our environment. The anxiety that has been caused to some individuals with CRS (due to lack of proper diagnosis) before they knew of such a syndrome may well be one of the worst known documentable effects of glutamate. Possible additive effects of glutamate, hydrolyzed vegetable protein and Aspartame should be brought to the attention of individuals who may be especially sensitive to glutamate.

Additional studies on glutamate metabolism in humans and, in particular, possible adverse reactions, are certainly needed. However, conceivable long-range effects of this amino acid on subtle developmental phenomena in humans such as endocrine disturbances, learning disabilities and hyperactivity may be important but are likely to be difficult to establish.

REFERENCES

Albert, E.N. (1979). J. Microwave Power, 14, 281-285.
Albert, K., P. Hoch and H. Waelsch (1946). J. Nerv. Ment. Dis., 104, 263-274.
Allen, D.H., and G.J. Baker (1981). N. Engl. J. Med., 305, 1154-1155.
Alston, R.M. (1976). N. Engl. J. Med., 294, 225.
Ambos, M., N.R. Leavitt, L. Marmorek and S.B. Wolschina (1968). N. Engl. J. Med., 279, 105.
Andermann, F., M. Vanosse and L.S. Wolfe (1976). N. Engl. J. Med., 295, 174.
Asnes, R.S. (1980). Clin. Pediatr. (Philadelphia), 19, 705-706.
Bakay, L. (1972). In: Handbook of Neurochemistry, Laitha, A., ed. Plenum Press, New York, 417-427.

Bazzano, G., J.A. D'Elia and R.E. Olson (1970). Science, 18, 1208-1209.

Bellhorn, R.W., D.A. Lipman, J. Confino and M.S. Burns (1981). Invest. Ophthalmol. Vis. Sci., 21, 237-247.

Berry, H.K., R.E. Butcher, L.A. Elliot and R.L. Brunner (1974). Dev. Psychobiol., 7, 165-173.

Bodnar, R.J., G.M. Abrams, E.A. Zimmerman, D.T. Krieger, G. Nicholson and J.S. Kizer (1980). Neuroendocrinology, 30, 280-284.

Carter, L.T., and L. Levesque (1979). Neurobehav. Toxicol., 1, 247-251.

Colman, A.D. (1978a). N. Engl. J. Med., 299, 902.

Colman, A.D. (1978b). N. Engl. J. Med., 300, 503.

Conacher, H.B., J.R. Iyengar, W.F. Miles and H.G. Botting (1979). J. Assoc. Off. Anal. Chem., 62, 604-609.

Consumer Reports (1978). 615-619.

Cooper, P. (1977). Fd. Cosmet. Toxicol., 15, 347-356.

Creasey, W.A., and S.E. Malawista (1971). Biochem. Pharmacol. 20, 2917-2920.

Cunha-Vaz, J., F. De Abreu, A.J. Campos and G.M. Figo (1975). Br. J. Ophthalmol. 59, 649-656.

Dawson, R., Jr., J.J. Valdes and Z. Annau (1982). Neuroendocrinology, 34, 292-296.

Department of Health, Education and Welfare (1974). FDA publication #74-2043. Washington, D.C.

Dhindsa, K.S., R.G. Omran and R. Bhup (1981). Acta Anat., 109, 97-102.

Folkers, K., S. Shizukuishi, S.L. Scudder, R. Willis, K. Takemura and J.B. Longenecker (1981). Biochem. Biophys. Res. Comm., 100, 972-977.

Gann, D. (1977). South. Med. J., 70, 879-881.

Ghadimi, H. (1973). Am. J. Clin. Nutr., 26, 686-687.

Ghadimi, H., C.L. Bhalla and D.M. Kirchenbaum (1970). Acta Paediatr. Scand. 59, 233-240.

Ghadimi, H., and S. Kumar (1972). Am. J. Clin. Nutr., 25, 643-646.

Ghadimi, H., S. Kumar and F. Abaci (1971). Biochem. Med., 5, 447-456.

Ghezzi, P., M. Salmone, M. Recchia, G. Dagnino and S. Garattini (1980). Toxicol. Lett., 5, 417-421.

Goodman, L.S., E.A. Swinyard and J.E.P. Toman (1946). Arch. Neurol. Psychiat., 56, 20.

Gore, M.E., and P.R. Salmon (1980). Lancet, 1, 251-252.

Hammerschmidt, D.E. (1980). N. Engl. J. Med., 302, 1191-1193.

Himms-Hagen, J. (1970). Nature, 228, 97.

Himwich, H.E., K. Wolff, A.L. Hunsicker and W.A. Himwich (1955). J. Nerv. Ment. Dis., 121, 40.

Johnston, G.A.R. (1973). Biochem. Pharm. 22:137-140.

Justesen, D.R. (1980). Proc. IEEE, 68, 60-67.

Kandall, S.R. (1968). N. Engl. J. Med., 278, 1123.

Kenney, R.A. (1978). N. Engl. J. Med., 300, 503.

Kenney, R.A. (1979). In: Glutamic Acid: Advances in Biochemistry and Physiology. Filer, L.J. Jr. et al, eds. Raven Press, New York, 363-373.

Kenney, R.A., and C.S. Tidball (1972). Am. J. Clin. Nutr., 25, 140-146.

Kerr, G.R., M. Wu-Lee, M. El-lozy, R. McGandy and F.J. Stare
    (1979). J. Am. Diet Assoc., 75, 29-33.
Kirkendol, P.L., J.E. Pearson and N.W. Robie (1980). Clin. Exp.
    Pharmacol. Physiol., 7, 617-625.
Komeda, K., M. Yokote and Y. Oki (1980). Experientia, 36, 232-
    234.
Krieger, D.T., A.S. Liotta, G. Nicholsen and J.S. Kizer (1979).
    Nature, 278, 562-563.
Kwok, R.H.M. (1968). N. Engl. J. Med., 278, 796.
Levey, S., J.E. Harroun and S.J. Smyth (1949). J. Lab. Clin.
    Med., 34, 1238-1248.
Lott, I.T., T. Coulombe, R.V. DiPaolo, E.P. Richardson Jr. and
    H.L. Levy (1978). Neurology, 28, 47-54.
McCall, A., B.S. Glaeser, W. Millington and R.J. Wurtman (1980).
    Neurobehav. Toxicol., 1, 279-283.
Marrs, T.C., M. Salmone, S. Garattini, D. Burston and D.M.
    Mathews (1978). Toxicology, 11, 101-107.
Marshall, A.E. (1948). Monosodium Glutamate, A Symposium.
    Quartermaster Food and Container Institute for the Armed
    Forces, and Associates. Chicago, Ill. 4.
Mayer-Gross, W., and J.W. Walker (1949). Biochem. J., 44, 92-97.
Merritt, J.H., A.F. Chamness and S.J. Allen (1978). Radiat.
    Environ. Biophys., 15, 367-377.
Moneysworth (Feb. 1975), 23.
Morselli, P.L., and S. Gara Hini (1970). Nature, 227, 611.
Nemeroff C.B., and F.D. Crisley (1975). Environ. Physiol.
    Biochem., 5, 389-395.
Neumann, H.H. (1976). Am. Heart J., 92, 266.
New York International Glutamate Technical Committee (1974). The
    Remarkable Story of Monosodium Glutamate, Food and Drug Ad-
    ministration, Washington, D.C.
Nitch, C. (1976). Acta Neurochir. (Wien) 23:Suppl, 101.
Olney, J.W. (1975). In: Sweetners: Issues and Uncertainties.
    National Academy of Science Forum, G.P.O., Washington, D.C.
Olney, J.W. (1976). In: Transport Phenomena in the Nervous
    System: Physiological and Pathological Aspects (Advances in
    Experimental Medicine and Biology 69) Levi G. et al, eds.
    Plenum Press, New York, 497-506.
Olney, J.W. (1980). Neurotoxicology, 2, 163-192.
Pardridge, W.M., J.D. Connor and I.L. Crawford (1975). CRC Crit.
    Rev. Toxicol., 3, 159-199.
Peter, R.E., O. Kah, C.R. Paulencu, H. Cook and A.L. Kyle (1980).
    Cell Tissue Res., 212, 429-442.
Plaitakis, A., S. Berl, and M.D. Yahr (1982). Science, 216, 193-
    196.
Rath, J. (1968). N. Engl. J. Med., 278, 1123.
Reif-Lehrer, L. (1976a). Fed. Proc. 35, 2205-2212.
Reif-Lehrer, L. (1976b). Pediatrics, 58, 771.
Reif-Lehrer, L. (1977a). Yearbook of Pediatrics, 309-310.
Reif-Lehrer, L. (1977b). Fed. Proc., 36, 1617-1623.
Reif-Lehrer, L. (1977c). Testimony, Federation of American
    Societies for Experimental Biology, Bethesda, Md.
Reif-Lehrer, L. (1982, in press). Chapter in: Current Topics in
    Eye Research. Academic Press, New York.
Reif-Lehrer, L., and M.G. Stemmermann (1975). N. Engl. J. Med.,
    293, 1204-1205.
Reinken, L. (1975). Acta Vitaminol. Enzymol. (Milano), 29, 252-

254.
Reynolds, W.A., V. Butler and N. Lemkey-Johnston (1976). J. Toxicol. Environ. Health, 2, 471-480.
Rippere, V. (1981). Med. Hypotheses, 7, 819-823.
Roberts, P.J., J. Storm-Mathisen and G.A.R. Johnston, eds. (1981). Glutamate: Transmitter in the Central Nervous System. John Wiley & Sons, New York.
Rodriguez-Sierra, J.F., R. Sridaran and C.A. Blake (1980). Neuroendocrinology, 31, 228-235.
Rosenblum, I., J.D. Bradley and F. Coulston (1971). Toxicol. Appl. Pharmacol., 18, 367-373.
Rubini, M.E. (1971). Am. J. Clin. Nutr. 24, 169-171.
Saphier, D.J., and R.G. Dyer (1981). J. Endocrinol., 89, 379-387.
Schaumburg, H.H. (1968). N. Engl. J. Med., 278, 1122.
Schaumburg, H.H., and R. Byck (1968). N. Engl. J. Med., 279, 105.
Schaumburg, H.H., R. Byck, R. Gerstl and J.H. Mashman (1969). Science, 163, 826.
Schubert, F., J.M. George and M. Bhaskar Rao (1980). Life Sciences, 26, 651-656.
Scriver, C.R., and D.T. Whelan (1969). Ann. N.Y. Acad. Sci., 166, 83-86.
Sjöström, L.B. (1955). Monosodium Glutamate: A Second Symposium. Research and Development Associates, Food and Container Inst., Inc. 31.
Smith, R.J. (1981). Science, 213, 986-987.
Stegink, L.D., L.J. Filer, Jr., G.L. Baker, S.M. Mueller and MY-C Wu-Ridout (1979). In: Glutamic Acid: Advances in Biochemistry and Physiology, Filer L.J., Jr. et al, eds. Raven Press, New York, 333-351.
Stegink, L.D., L.J. Filer, Jr. and G.L. Baker (1981). Am. J. Clin. Nutr., 34, 1899-1905.
Sworczak, K., M. Siekjerska and R. Komarnicka (1980). Pol. Tyg. Lek., 35, 991-992.
Terry, L.C., J. Epelbaum and J.B. Martin (1981). Brain Res., 217, 129-142.
Tracor-Jitco, Inc. (1974). Scientific literature reviews on generally recognized as safe (GRAS) food ingredients — glutamates. Food and Drug Administration, Washington, D.C.
Trauberman, L. (1960). Food Engineering.
Tursky, T., M. Lassanova, M. Sramka and P. Nadvorink (1976). Acta Neurochir. (Wien) 23:Suppl., 111.
Unna, D., and E.E. Howe (1945). Fed. Proc., 4, 138.
Utsumi, M., Y. Hirose, K. Ishihara, H. Makimura and S. Baba (1980) Biomed. Res. 1, Suppl., 154-158.
Weil-Malherbe, H. (1949). J. Ment. Sc., 95, 930-944.

TEMPORAL LOBE EPILEPSY, EXCITOTOXINS AND THE MECHANISM OF SELECTIVE NEURONAL LOSS

T. GRIFFITHS, M. C. EVANS and B. S. MELDRUM

Departments of Neurology and Neuropathology, Institute of Psychiatry, De Crespigny Park, London SE5 8AF, and Rayne Institute, King's College Hospital Medical School, 123 Coldharbour Lane, London, SE5 9NU (U.K.)

ABSTRACT

The pattern of selective neuronal loss associated with temporal lobe epilepsy is reproduced in the rat by administration of kainic acid or of drugs acting on GABA-mediated inhibition (L-allylglycine, bicuculline). The sequence of cytological change in astrocytes and neurons is the same after kainic acid and after the GABA antagonists. A common pathophysiological mechanism is proposed, involving burst firing, excessive Ca^{2+} entry, and the cytotoxic action of raised cytosolic Ca^{2+}. Calcium accumulation within vulnerable neurons can be demonstrated electron microscopically. It predominates in swollen mitochondria in cell bodies, and focally in zones of the dendritic tree.

KEY WORDS

Epilepsy; hippocampal damage; kainic acid; allylglycine; calcium toxicity; mitochondria; dendrotoxicity.

INTRODUCTION

The histological appearances known as "Ammon's horn sclerosis" or "hippocampal sclerosis" have been recognised as a common pathological finding in patients with chronic epilepsy for more than 100 years (Sommer, 1880; Corsellis & Meldrum, 1976).

Their significance has however been a matter of continuing controversy (Meldrum, 1975, 1982). Children dying acutely after prolonged status epilepticus show "ischaemic cell change" or neuronal loss in the hippocampus with the same selective pattern as in patients with chronic epilepsy (i.e. involving pyramidal neurons of H_1 and H_{3-5}, with relative sparing of dentate granule cells) (Fowler, 1957; Zimmerman, 1938; Norman, 1964). Additionally such children show similar pathological changes involving small pyramidal neurons in the neocortex (principally in the IIIrd lamina) and Purkinje cells in the cerebellum.

Ten years ago we showed that a similar pattern of pathological change occurs in experimental primates following prolonged seizures (duration $>$ 90 min) induced by the GABA antagonist, bicuculline, or closely recurrent seizures induced by allylglycine (which inhibits GABA synthesis) (Meldrum & Brierley, 1973; Meldrum et al., 1973; Meldrum et al., 1974). Interestingly, as in man, the H_1 (C_{A1} or 'Sommer sector') lesions in the hippocampus were usually asymmetrical.

Subsequently we observed similar unilateral hippocampal lesions after limbic
seizures induced by the intra-amygdaloid injection of kainic acid in baboons,
marmosets or rats (Menini et al., 1980; Meldrum, and Pedley, 1981; Ben-Ari et
al., 1980).

Systemic or intracerebroventricular administration of kainic acid also leads to
selective neuronal loss in the hippocampus with the same pattern as in patients
with chronic epilepsy or status epilepticus (Olney et al., 1974; Nadler et al.,
1978). Ultrastructural studies of the early cytological changes have emphasised
"dendrotoxic" changes, particularly involving the basal dendrites of pyramidal
neurons (Olney et al., 1979). This is consistent with a primary toxic mechanism
involving excitatory receptors, and suggests that the sequence of cytological
change may be different in the syndromes involving failure of GABA-mediated
inhibition (bicuculline and allylglycine). In order to study the mechanism by
which different primary mechanisms lead to a common pattern of selective
neuronal loss we have begun a comparison in the rat of the different stages of
cytological change in the hippocampus during prolonged seizures induced by
systemic administration of bicuculline, L-allylglycine or kainic acid. We have
used paralysed mechanically-ventilated animals, with monitoring and control of
arterial pressure and blood gases to eliminate any contribution of systemic
factors to differences between the convulsant agents. Perfusion fixation after
specific periods of seizure activity permits an electron microscopic comparison
of the sequence of cellular changes.

A raised cytosolic $[Ca^{2+}]$ is thought to be the critical step in determining
pathological change in various myopathies and in hypoxic-ischaemic damage in
cardiac or vascular smooth muscle. (Wrogemann and Pena, 1976; Emery and Burt,
1980; Flameng et al., 1980). In the neocortex and hippocampus during burst
firing of neurones there is a marked fall in extracellular $[Ca^{2+}]$ (Heinemann et
al., 1978). These and other observations led to the formulation of the
hypothesis (put forward at various Meetings in 1980, - Meldrum, 1981, 1982) that
"ischaemic cell change" and neuronal loss in status epilepticus were the
consequence of the cytotoxic action of a raised intracellular $[Ca^{2+}]$, and that
selective vulnerability was primarily determined by the occurrence of burst
firing and the excessive entry of Ca^{2+} into the neurons.

The recent development of an electron microscopic technique for the visualisation
of Ca^{2+} in muscle (Borgers et al., 1977, 1981) has allowed us to make a direct
test of this hypothesis. Preliminary results in allylglycine-induced seizures
have already been reported (Griffiths et al., 1982). We now describe the
application of this technique to the experimental material obtained in the
comparative study of seizures induced by bicuculline, allylglycine and kainic
acid.

METHODS

Adult male Wistar rats (200-300 g) were anaesthetised with 2% halothane, while
breathing a mixture of 70% N_2O and 30% O_2. Right and left femoral arteries were
cannulated to allow continuous pressure monitoring, and sampling for arterial
blood gas determinations. A femoral vein was cannulated for infusion of drugs
or of donor blood (to maintain mean arterial pressure above 100 mm Hg). Animals
were given atropine (240 µg/kg, i.m.) tracheotomised, paralysed with tubocurarine
(2 mg/kg, i.v.) and mechanically ventilated with N_2O 70%, O_2 30%. Body temperature was recorded by a rectal probe and maintained by a heating blanket. The
EEG and ECG were continuously recorded via subcutaneous platinum electrodes.
Animals were maintained in a steady state for 30 min following completion of the
operative procedures. Arterial P_{CO_2} was adjusted to 35-45 mm Hg.

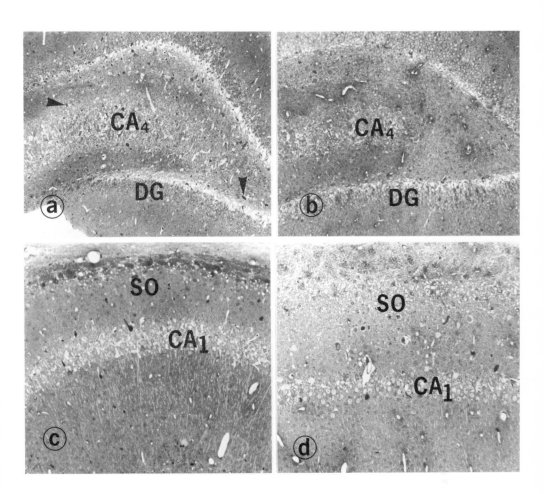

Figure (1a) Light micrograph of CA4 pyramidal neurons and dentate granule cells
(DG) from a rat hippocampus following 2 h of LAG-induced seizures. Astrocytic
swelling can be seen in and around the pyramidal neurons and at the inner
layer of the granule cells. Some ischaemic cell change is also visible
(arrowheads). Mag x 76.5 (1b) Similar changes to those shown in (1a),
following 2 h of KA-induced seizures. Mag x 98. (1c) LAG-induced changes in
the CA1 region. Astrocytic swelling and ischaemic cell change can be seen,
together with swelling of basal dendrites in the stratum oriens (SO). Mag 380.
(1d) Very similar pathological changes in the CA1 region following KA-induced
seizures. Mag x 120.

Bicuculline (1.2 mg/kg, i.v.) or L-allylglycine (276 mg/kg, i.v.) or kainic acid
10 mg/kg, i.v.) were infused, and blood withdrawn or infused to minimise the early
ictal rise in arterial pressure and to prevent late hypotension. Blood gases were
determined at intervals, and ventilation rate or the gas mixture was adjusted as
appropriate.

After 0.5 - 3.5 hours of EEG seizure activity animals were given pentobarbitone
(45 mg/kg) and perfused with ice-cold 2% glutaraldehyde/3% paraformaldehyde
solution (250 ml, via an aortic cannula preceded by a brief saline wash). For the
calcium studies the glutaraldehyde perfusion fixative contained potassium oxalate
(Borgers et al., 1977). Bilateral hippocampal blocks were removed from each brain
and embedded in araldite for light and electron microscopy. Blocks for the
calcium study were post-fixed in osmic acid/potassium pyroantimonate. Control
material was prepared from sham-operated rats, mechanically ventilated for 2 hours.
Control blocks for calcium localisation were washed in oxalate solution
containing 5 mM EGTA.

Light microscopy sections (0.75 μm) were stained with toluidine blue; EM
sections (50-80 nm) with uranylacetate and lead citrate.

              RESULTS

Light Microscopy

The earliest and most widespread pathological change was vacuolation around
pyramidal cell bodies (at 0.5-1 h with all 3 convulsants). After 2 hours of
seizures this change is seen more or less uniformly throughout the pyramidal cell
regions (i.e. C_{A1-4}), and also on the inner aspect of the dentate granule cell
layer (see Fig 1).

Vacuolation was also evident after 1-2 h seizure activity in the basal dendritic
system (stratum oriens), being most evident in the outer third of the stratum in
the Ca_3 region, but also occurring in the inner third (CA_3) and the outer third
in CA_1 (Fig 1).

Scattered dark neurons ('ischaemic cell change') occurred, most frequently in CA_3
and CA_4 but also in CA_1 after 2 hours of seizure activity.

Electron Microscopy

Control material conformed to well fixed ultrastructural appearances. In the
experimental material distended electron-lucent processes of atrocytic
processes surrounded pyramidal cell bodies.

Dentate granule cells were structurally unaltered, as were the majority of
pyramidal neurons. Within the CA_3 and CA_4 regions after 1-2 hours of seizure
activity changes of varying severity were apparent in some pyramidal neurons.
The minimal change was a slight increase in electron density associated either
with normal mitochondria and slight distension of the endoplasmic reticulum and
Golgi apparatus, or with swollen disrupted mitochondria. Occasional neurons
showed severe changes with dense shrunken cyto- and karyo-plasma with loss of
ultrastructural detail, and multiple vacuoles.

Within the stratum oriens there was focal swelling of some dendritic processes.
These swellings contained grossly distended mitochondria (Fig 2C), and were
contacted by synaptic terminals, which contained mitochondria and vesicles of
normal morphology (although a slight clumping of vesicles was sometimes apparent).

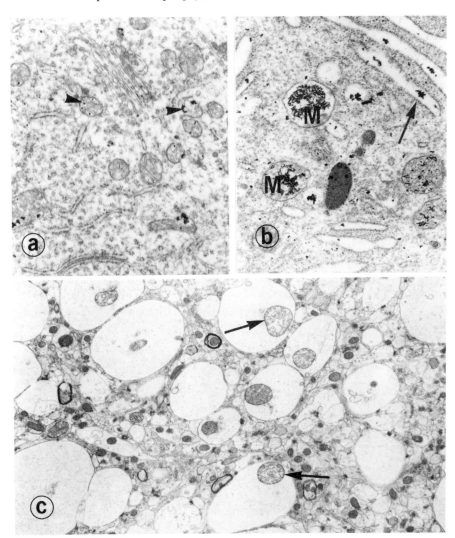

Figure (2a) Electron micrograph of part of a pyramidal neuron cell body, from a control hippocampus treated with potassium pyroantimonate. Small amounts of electron dense calcium pyroantimonate precipitates are visible in the mitochondria (arrows). Mag x 27,500. (2b) Following 2 h of LAG-induced seizures a pyramidal neuron shows swelling of mitochondria (M) and endoplasmic reticulum (arrow), both containing dense calcium pyroantimonate deposits. Mag x 27,500. (2c) Swollen dendrites in the stratum oriens containing disrupted and enlarged mitochondria (arrows) after LAG-induced seizures. Mag x 7,000.

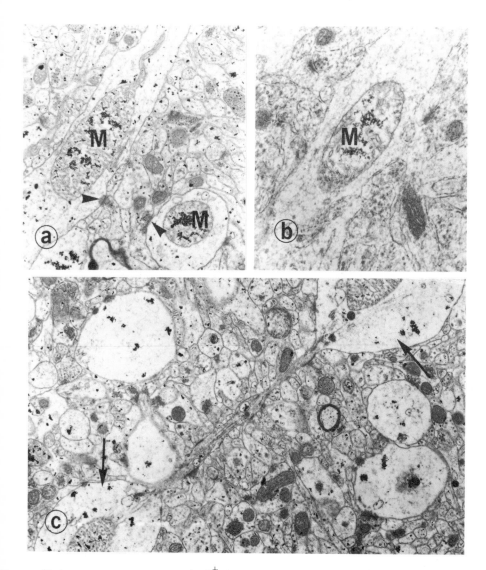

Figure (3a) Same region as Fig (2c)[+] after treatment with potassium pyroantimonate. The mitochondria (M) contain dense calcium pyroantimonate deposits. Arrowheads point to nerve terminals. Mag x 16,500. (3b) KA-induced seizures also produced occasional swollen mitochondria with calcium pyroantimonate deposits in the stratum oriens. Mag x 31,000. (3c) Stratum oriens after 2 h of LAG-induced seizures, showing a dendrite with 2 zones of distention containing swollen mitochondria and dense calcium pyroantimonate deposits. Mag x 12,800.

[+]2 h of LAG induced seizures.

Calcium pyroantimonate deposits

In control material calcium pyroantimonate deposits are most prominent in synaptic vesicles in the neuropil (see Griffiths et al., 1982). In neuronal somata occasional fine deposits are seen in mitochondria and other organelles (Fig 2a).

Following seizure activity (0.5-2 hours) enhanced calcium pyroantimonate deposits occur selectively in vulnerable pyramidal neurons. In the soma, dense deposits occur in all swollen mitochondria and sometimes in the endoplasmic reticulum (Fig 2b). Similar dense deposits are seen within the swollen motochondria, and in the cytosol, in the zones of distension in basal dendritic processes of the pyramidal neurons (Fig 3).

DISCUSSION

Comparison of early cytological changes after kainic acid and after GABA related convulsants

The changes we observe in hippocampal morphology after systemic kainic acid administration are closely similar to those previously reported in light and electron microscopic studies (Olney et al., 1974, 1979; Schwob et al., 1980). They do not differ significantly from the changes induced by bicuculline or L-allylglycine (reported here and by Evans et al., 1983). Specifically, the three types of change (astrocytic, dendritic and somatic in pyramidal neurons) are indistinguishable in distribution, morphology and severity after 2 hours of seizures induced by kainic acid or by L-allylglycine. The mechanism and significance of these three types of cytopathology will be discussed separately.

Swelling of astrocytic processes

This is the earliest change associated with seizure activity, and is presumably closely related to the movement of K+ out of neurons during the abnormal burst firing of seizure activity.

The rise in extracellular $[K^+]$ associated with burst discharges activates the astrocytic uptake of K+, so that the early rise in extracellular $[K^+]$ stabilises at 9-10 mM. The extracellular fluid volume decreases, (by about 30%), extracellular fluid osmolarity increases, and there is a net movement of K+, Cl- and water into astrocytes (Heinemann et al., 1978; Dietzel et al., 1982). The initial slight increase in electron density of pyramidal neurons is presumably the neuronal counterpart of these ion and fluid movements.

Perineuronal astrocytic swelling is sometimes selective within the pyramidal cell zones of the hippocampus and sometimes occurs diffusely throughout CA_1 - CA_4. A similar pattern of swelling can be produced by sustained electrical stimulation of the perforant pathway (Sloviter and Damiano, 1981). As severe degrees of astrocytic swelling can occur in the absence of neuronal pathological change, the contribution of such changes to neuronal alterations remains uncertain.

Dendritic swelling

The similar distribution and nature of the dendritic swelling seen after seizures induced by agents interfering with GABA-mediated inhibition suggests that the "dendrotoxic" lesions associated with kainic acid are not the local consequence of kainic acid acting on specific receptors in the dendritic membrane. They are more probably the result of local excitatory transmitter action (possibly glutamate or aspartate, released from commisural pathway). The focal swelling observed at the EM level (Fig 3c) is equivalent to the globular distension observed in light microscope Golgi preparations by Sloviter. The sharply focal changes suggest that the neurotransmitter involved could be identified by EM autoradiography using either labelled receptor antagonists to identify post-synaptic sites on swollen zones of dendrites, or a labelled transmitter (or analogue) to identify the presynaptic terminals.

There is no evidence so far to link dendritic swelling to 'ischaemic cell change' or 'dark cell degeneration' at the level of the soma. Golgi studies of hippocampi in surgical material from patients with temporal lobe epilepsy (Scheibel et al., 1974) have suggested that there is a continuous process of dendritic degeneration (loss of spines, simplification of branching pattern) occurring in patients with intractable seizures. Acute focal distension of dendrites as a result of sustained excitatory activation may be the immediate cause of such changes.

Neuronal degeneration

The light and electron microscope appearances of dense, pyknotic neurons described here conform to those described by Brown & Brierley (1973) as 'ischaemic cell change'. However as it is now clear that there is no cerebral ischaemia or hypoxia during seizures induced in paralysed ventilated animals with full physiological control (Meldrum, 1981, 1982) it is more appropriate to use the descriptive term 'dark cell degeneration'. This appearance involves, selectively, those neurons that suffer loss in chronic studies using similar seizure models (Meldrum et al., 1974). Study of our material does not allow conclusions about which intermediate neuronal changes (i.e. condensed cytoplasm and swollen mitochondria) indicate irreversibility of the pathological process.

Excitation versus failure of inhibition

These results (and those reported by Olney, 1982 this volume) indicate that the pattern of damage in the hippocampus induced by kainic acid is typical of epileptic activity of any origin. It is by no means certain that kainic acid is acting as an 'excitotoxin'. The possibility that it impairs inhibitory transmission is suggested by the studies of Sloviter and Damiano (1981) and of McLennan (this volume). It is probably more useful to think in terms of the effects of burst discharges (on metabolism and ionic movements) rather than in terms of 'excitoxins'.

Calcium movements in seizures

A decrease in extracellular Ca^+ activity (as measured by ion-selective micro-electrodes) occurs during seizure activity in the neocortex or the hippocampus (Heinemann et al., 1978; Benninger et al., 1980). Quantitatively greater decreases in extracellular$[Ca^{2+}]$can be induced by iontophoretic application of excitatory amino acids at the dendritic level in the neocortex (Heinemann & Pumain, 1980) or at the somatic and basal dendritic level in the hippocampus (Marciani et al., 1982).

The use of the calcium oxalate/pyroantimonate method in this experimental situation allows visualisation of the intracellular localisation of free Ca^{2+}. This shows that Ca^{2+} accumulates post-synaptically during seizure activity, and is powerfully accumulated by mitochondria in both pyramidal cell somata and dendrites. Calcium uptake or efflux in mitochondria is largely dependent on extramitochondrial $[Ca^{2+}]$ so that mitochondria provide a Ca^{2+} buffer system (Nicholls and Crompton, 1980). Ca^{2+} can be exchanged for H^+, or accumulated with Po_4^{2-}. In the latter case accumulation is osmotically active and may lead to mitochondrial swelling. Normal recovery following mitochondrial calcium accumulation depends on the cytosolic$[Ca^{2+}]$being reduced to normal (i.e. 50-150 nMol) by active transport across the somatic membrane, permitting Ca^{2+} efflux from mitochondria. The maximal rate of outward transport of Ca^{2+} (either by a Ca^{2+}/Na^+ antiport or by Ca^{2+} ATPase) is substantially less than the maximal rate of Ca^{2+} entry during burst firing in pyramidal neurons. As the capacity of intracellular proteins (calmodulins), the endoplasmic reticulum and the mitochondria to sequester calcium is limited, burst firing sustained beyond a certain time will cause intracellular $[Ca^{2+}]$ to rise beyond physiological limits. Grossly distended mitochondria massively loaded with Ca^{2+} probably indicate that this point has been reached. Deficiency of ATP will limit both extrusion and sequestration of Ca^{2+}.

Cytotoxicity of Calcium

Evidence relating to the pathological role of raised $[Ca^{2+}]$ in skeletal, cardiac and vascular smooth muscle, and hepatocytes has been summarised in previous reviews (Meldrum, 1981; 1982).

A recent in vitro study of locust muscle attributes the cytotoxic effect of excitatory amino acids (Duce et al., 1982) to entry of Ca^{2+} secondary to the action of glutamate on membrane potential. Mitochondrial swelling is not a significant feature of myopathic change in this system, although it is observed in mouse diaphragm during degeneration induced by calcium ionophore treatment (Publicover et al., 1978). An increased cytosolic $[Ca^{2+}]$ leads to activation of various phospholipases and proteinases, with consequent loss of ultrastructural features, and the development of the histological appearances of myopathic degeneration or of "dark cell degeneration" in neurons.

A unified hypothesis for excitotoxic action and epileptic brain damage

The neurons that are selectively vulnerable in human epilepsy and all types of chemically induced seizures, including those due to kainic acid, very readily show burst firing and a "paroxysmal depolarising shift". Such activity often occurs spontaneously in CA_3 pyramidal neurons in vivo and in vitro hippocampal slices, and is readily provoked in CA_1 neurons. (Kandel & Spencer, 1961; Wong & Prince, 1978). It is not easily induced in dentate granule cells. Furthermore it can be induced by various patterns of stimulation in the other classes of cells specifically vulnerable in epilepsy (Cerebellar Purkinje cells and small pyramidal neurons in the neocortex) (Rushmer et al., 1976; Traub, 1979). An excessive entry of Ca^{2+} is a direct consequence of the sustained burst firing. This Ca^{2+} entry eventually overwhelms the capacity of mitochondria and other organelles to buffer or sequester Ca^{2+} and the cytotoxic effect of raised cytosolic $[Ca^{2+}]$ becomes evident.

The initiation of burst firing is controlled by the balance between excitatory inputs and inhibitory inputs, thus explaining the pathological equivalence of impaired GABAergic inhibition and enhanced excitatory inputs.

Clearly the cytotoxicity produced by ibotenic acid and related excitotoxins must be determined by a factor other than the innate capacity of the neuron to display burst firing, as the pattern of selective vulnerability with ibotenic acid is not that found in epilepsy (Köhler et al., 1979; Nadler et al., 1981). For such "non-selective" toxic action determining factors will include the presence of membrane receptors responsive to the excitotoxin (in a "non-desensitising" fashion). The direct effect of the excitotoxin appears to be depolarisation due to enhanced Na^+ conductance, but there is a secondary, voltage dependent increase in Ca^{2+} conductance. As for pathology secondary to burst firing, the Ca^{2+} entry has to be of sufficient magnitude and duration to overcome the capacity of the neuron to extrude, or sequester the Ca^{2+}. The hyperpolarising action of GABA is apparently capable of opposing this excitotoxic effect. Simultaneous iontophoresis of GABA and aspartate in the pyramidal cell layer, prevents the decrease in extracellular Ca^{2+} that normally follows the iontophoresis of aspartate alone (Marciani et al., 1982).

It is proposed that the non-selective excitotoxins such as ibotenic acid either cause those neurons that are not normally liable to display burst firing (because of the balance of their excitatory and inhibitory inputs or because of particular membrane properties) to display burst firing or induce membrane conductance changes that are equivalent to the effects of burst firing. That low concentrations of kainic acid do not do this (i.e. they induce burst firing only in cells already prone to such activity), is suggested by the persistence of selective vulnerability even when kainic acid is injected focally into the various regions of the hippocampus (Nadler et al., 1981).

Significance of hippocampal sclerosis in temporal lobe epilepsy

Sommer (1980) considered that the hippocampal lesions he described were the cause of generalised seizures. Subsequent German neuropathologists (Spielmeyer, 1927; Scholz, 1959; Peiffer, 1963) adopted the view that the lesions are the result of cerebral hypoxia or ischaemia occurring during the course of generalised seizures. The suggestion that there is a specific association between temporal lobe epilepsy ('complex partial seizures') and hippocampal sclerosis (Stauder, 1935) appeared to be confirmed when neurosurgeons adopted unilateral anterior temporal lobectomy as a treatment for intractable temporal lobe epilepsy (Bailey & Gibbs, 1951; Falconer et al., 1964; Falconer, 1974). Hippocampal sclerosis has proved to be the commonest lesion in the neurosurgical specimen and its removal is associated with a favourable prognosis. Thus neurosurgeons have stated that this lesion acts as the focal cause of complex partial seizures. This possibility is not necessarily in conflict with the interpretation that the lesions are the result of generalised seizures. Indeed prolonged febrile convulsions in infancy or early childhood (which are a known cause of hippo-campal sclerosis) are a common antecedent of complex partial seizures in adolescence (Falconer, 1974; Meldrum, 1975, 1976). However the experimental results outlined above strengthen the possibility that in many cases the hippo-campal sclerosis is a consequence of the intractable limbic seizures. The favourable outcome of resection associated with hippocampal sclerosis can be interpreted as a consequence of correct identification of the hemispheric origin of the seizures. That prolonged limbic seizures can lead to chronic neuro-logical disability has only recently achieved wide recognition (Engel, et al., 1978; Wieser, 1980; Treiman & Delgado-Escueta, 1982). On the other hand direct evidence that hippocampal sclerosis is the focal cause of complex partial seizures in man is lacking. In particular focal electroencephalographic records, either made acutely during surgical intervention, or chronically prior to anterior temporal lobectomy (Engel et al., 1975) show that the sclerotic hippocampus is relatively silent, and does not originate repetitive spike discharges.

Several authors have reported the occurrence of spontaneous or stimulus-induced limbic or generalised seizures in rats or cats 1-11 weeks after having received focal cerebral injections of kainic acid, either in the striatum (Pisa et al., 1980) or in the limbic system (Tanaka et al., 1981; Cavalheiro et al., 1982). These authors have drawn attention to the association of neuronal loss in the hippocampus and pyriform cortex with limbic seizures and proposed that limbic lesions induced by kainic acid provide an animal model of temporal lobe epilepsy. However the time course described by Cavalheiro et al. (1982) in the rat does not suggest a close parallel with the human syndrome. Thus there is a silent phase of 5-10 days after the convulsions directly induced by the kainic acid; then limbic seizures occur (spontaneously or in response to handling) during 5-50 days; finally the only epileptiform feature is focal spiking in the amygdala. This time course suggests a phenomenon linked to the supersensitivity and new synaptic formation described by Nadler (this volume), as a consequence of selective hippocampal neuronal loss. It appears less permanent than kindled amygdaloid seizures in rats, or temporal lobe epilepsy in man.

ACKNOWLEDGEMENT

We thank the Wellcome Trust and the Medical Research Council for financial support.

REFERENCES

Bailey, P. and F.A. Gibbs (1951). J. Amer. Med. Assoc., 145, 365-370.
Ben-Ari, Y., E. Tremblay, O.P. Ottersen and B.S. Meldrum (1980). Brain Research, 191, 79-97.
Benninger, C., J. Kadis and D.A. Prince (1980). Brain Research, 187, 165-182.
Borgers, M., M. De Brabander, J. Van Reempts, F. Awouters and W.A. Jacob (1977). Lab Invest., 37, 1-8.
Borgers, M., Thone, F. and Van Neuten, J.M. (1981). Acta Histochem. Suppl., 24, 327-332.
Brown, A.W. and J.B. Brierley (1973). Acta Neuropath., 23, 9-22.
Cavalheiro, E.A., D.A. Riche and G. Le Gal La Salle (1982). Electroenceph., clin. Neurophysiol., 53, 581-589.
Corsellis, J.A.N. and B.S. Meldrum (1976). In Greenfield's Neuropathology 3rd Edition, W. Blackwood and J.A.N. Corsellis (eds) Edward Arnold, London. pp. 771-795.
Dietzel, I., U. Heinemann, G. Hofmeier and H.D. Lux (1982). Exp. Brain Res., 46, 73-84.
Duce, I.R., P.L. Donaldson, and P.N.R. Usherwood (1982). Brain Research (in press)
Emery, A.E.H. and D. Burt (1980). Brit. Med. J., 280, 355-357.
Engel, J., M.V. Driver and M.A. Falconer (1975). Brain, 98, 129-156.
Engel, J., B.I. Ludwig and M. Fetell (1978). Neurology, 28, 863-869.
Evans, M., T. Griffiths and B. Meldrum (1983). Neuropath. exp. Neurobiol. (in press).
Falconer, M.A., E.A. Serafetinides and J.A.N. Corsellis (1964). Arch. Neurol. (Chic.) 10, 233-248.
Falconer, M.A. (1974). Lancet 2, 767-770.
Flameng, W., W. Daenen, R. Xhonneux, A., Van de Water, F. Thone and M. Borgers (1980). Proc. Roy. Soc. Med., 29, 89-95.
Fowler, M. (1957). Arch. Dis. Childh., 32, 67-76.
Griffiths, T., Evans, M.C. and Meldrum, B.S. (1982). Neuroscience Lett., 30, 329-334.
Heinemann, U., H.D. Lux and M.J. Gutnick (1978). In Abnormal Neuronal Discharges N. Chalazonitis and M. Boisson (eds) Raven Press, New York, pp. 329-345.
Heinemann, U. and R. Pumain (1980). Exp. Brain Res., 40, 247-250.
Kandel, E.R. and W.A. Spencer (1961). J. Neurophysiol., 24, 243-259.
Köhler, C., R. Schwarz and K. Fuxe (1979). Neuroscience Lett., 15, 223-228.
Marciani, M.G., J. Louvel, and U. Heinemann. (1982). Brain Research, 238, 272-277.
Meldrum, B.S. (1975). In Modern Trends in Neurology 6, 223-239.
Meldrum, B.S. (1976). In Brain Dysfunction in Infantile febrile convulsions, ed. M.A. Brazier, Raven Press, New York, pp. 213-222.
Meldrum, B.S. (1981). In Metabolic Disorders of the Nervous System, F.C. Rose ed. Pitman Medical, London. pp. 175-187.
Meldrum, B.S. (1982). In Advances in Neurology Vol. 34, Status Epilepticus, A.V. Delgado-Escueta, C.G. Wasterlain, D.M. Treiman and R.J. Porter, eds. Raven Press, New York, pp. 263-277.
Meldrum, B.S. and T. Pedley (1981). Neuropathol. Appl. Neurobiol., 7, 185.
Meldrum, B.S. and J.B. Brierley (1973). Arch. Neurol., 28, 10-17.
Meldrum, B.S., R.A. Vigouroux, and J.B. Brierley (1973). Arch. Neurol., 29, 82-87.

342   T. Griffiths, M. C. Evans and B. S. Meldrum

Meldrum, B.S., R.W. Horton and J.B. Brierley (1974). Brain, 97, 417-428.
Menini, C., B.S. Meldrum, D. Riche, C. Silva-Comte and J.M. Stutzmann (1980).
    Ann. Neurol., 8, 501-509.
Nadler, J.V., B.W. Perry and C.W. Cotman (1978). Nature, 271, 676-677.
Nadler, J.V., D.A. Evenson and G.J. Cuthbertson (1981). Neuroscience 6, 2505-
    2517.
Nicholls, D.G. and M. Crompton (1980). FEBS Letters, III, 261-268.
Norman, R.M. (1964). Medicine, Science and the Law, 4, 46-51.
Olney, J.W., T. Fuller and T. De Gubareff (1979). Brain Research, 176, 91-100.
Olney, J.W., V. Rhee and O.L. Ho (1974). Brain Research, 77, 507-512.
Peiffer, J. (1963). Monograph. Gesamtgeb. Neurol. Psychiat. (Berl.), 100, 1-185.
Pisa, M., P.R. Sandberg, M.E. Corcoran and H.C. Fibiger (1980). Brain Research
    200, 481-487.
Publicover, S.J., C.J. Duncan, and J.L. Smith (1978). J. Neuropathol. Exp.
    Neurol., 37, 554-557.
Rushmer, D.S., Roberts, W.J. and G.K. Augter (1976). Brain Research 106, 1-20.
Scheibel, M.E., P.H. Crandall and A.B. Scheibel (1974). Epilepsia, 15, 55-80.
Scholz, W. (1959). Epilepsia 1, 36-55.
Schwob, J.E., T. Fuller, J.L. Price and J.W. Olney (1980). Neuroscience, 5,
    991-1014.
Sloviter, R.S. and B.P. Damiano (1981). Neuropharmacol., 20, 1003-1011.
Sommer, W. (1880). Arch. Psychiatr. Nervenkr., 10, 631-675.
Spielmeyer, W. (1927). Z. Neurol. Psychiatr., 109, 501-520.
Stauder, K.H. (1935). Arch. Psychiatr. Nervenkr., 104, 181-211.

Tanaka, T., M. Kaijima, G. Daita, S. Ohgami, Y. Yonemasu and D. Riche (1982).
    Electroenceph. clin. Neurophysiol., 54, 288-300.
Traub, R.D. (1979). Brain Research, 173, 243-257.
Treiman, D.M., and A.V. Delgado-Escueta (1982). In Advances in Neurology Vol. 34,
    Status Epilepticus, A.V. Delgado-Escueta, C.G. Wasterlain, D.M. Treiman,
    and R.J. Porter (eds) Raven Press, New York.
Wieser, H.G. (1980). Electroenceph. clin. Neurophysiol., 45, 558-572.
Wong, R.K.S. and D.A. Prince (1978). Brain Research, 159, 385-390.
Wrogemann, K. and S.D.J. Pena (1976). Lancet, 1, 672-674.
Zimmerman, H.M. (1938). J. Pediatr., 13, 859-890.

HUNTINGTON'S DISEASE: ANTI-NEUROTOXIC THERAPEUTIC STRATEGIES

IRA SHOULSON

Department of Neurology, University of Rochester Medical Center,
Rochester, New York 14642, U.S.A.

ABSTRACT

The dual roles of glutamate as excitatory neurotransmitter and potential neurotoxin have prompted anti-neurotoxic therapeutic strategies aimed at slowing the neuronal degeneration and clinical decline of Huntington's disease. It is proposed that long-term pharmacologic attenuation of glutamatergic corticostriatal function in patients with Huntington's disease will prevent or postpone the clinical and radiographic correlates of neuronal death. Baclofen, a drug which preferentially blocks the neuronal release of excitatory amino acids, is undergoing systematic evaluation in an effort to test this supposition.

KEY WORDS

Huntington's disease; glutamic acid, kainic acid, baclofen.

INTRODUCTION

In the past decade, rational therapeutic strategies for Huntington's disease (HD) have been based on the assertion that restoring neurochemical balance will lead to an amelioration of signs and symptoms (Shoulson, 1979a). This approach to symptomatic therapy in HD, prompted largely by the success of dopamine replacement therapy in Parkinson's disease, has led to uniformly disappointing results. The failures of replacement therapies for HD partly reflect the complexity and extent of diverse neurochemical disturbances, which are now recognized to represent the consequences of an underlying neurodegenerative process. Our increasing awareness of the putative role of excitatory neurotoxins in disease has properly focused attention on the process of pathologic change rather than on the chemical sequelae of neuronal death. The emerging roles of glutamate as both excitatory neurotransmitter and potential neurotoxin have now prompted therapeutic strategies aimed at halting or retarding the neuronal degeneration and clinical decline of HD.

343

BIOLOGIC BASIS OF ANTI-NEUROTOXIC STRATEGIES

HD is an autosomal dominant hereditary illness expressed pathologically by
neuronal degeneration and clinically by the eventual appearance of disordered
movement, intellectual decline and a variety of psychiatric disturbances
(Shoulson, 1975). The complete penetrance and exceedingly low mutation rate
of the HD gene afford an unusually high degree of diagnostic precision.
Although neuronal degeneration is relatively widespread within the postmortem
HD brain, the striatum bears the major brunt of pathologic disruption. Recent
investigations using positron emission tomography have demonstrated metabolic
perturbations within the HD striatum which antedate the appearance of caudate
atrophy and the onset of clinical features (Kuhl, 1981). The pathogenesis of
HD is accordingly viewed as a gradually evolving process which begins when the
HD gene is passed from parent to child. The HD gene and its immediate
translation products have yet to be identified. However, excitatory
neurotoxins have provided important clues toward unraveling the pathology of
HD and for understanding the basis of developmental and regional
vulnerabilities.

Glutamic acid was demonstrated to exert neurotoxic effects before it was
established as an excitatory neurotransmitter in the mammalian brain. Olney
(1969,1971) demonstrated that systemic administration of glutamate to infant
rats produced selective neuronal degeneration particularly in those regions
which were poorly protected by the blood-brain barrier. Under certain
experimental conditions, neuronal damage can result when glutamate is injected
directly into local brain regions (Olney 1978a; Schwarcz, 1981). The
occurrence and extent of glutamate-induced neurotoxicity also depend
critically on species and maturational features. The selective nature of
these effects suggests that genetic factors play a pivotal role in influencing
neurotoxic vulnerability.

Kainic acid (KA), a rigid analogue of glutamate, is a potent neurotoxin which
induces degeneration of intrinsic neurons. When injected into the striata of
experimental animals, KA produces morphologic, chemical, pharmacologic and
behavioral disturbances closely resembling those observed in HD (Coyle, 1976;
McGeer, 1976; Sanberg, 1978; Krammer, 1980). Removal of glutamate containing
corticostriatal afferents can prevent KA neurotoxicity, while intrastriatal
application of glutamate restores the neurotoxic effects of KA (McGeer 1978a;
Biziere, 1979; Coyle, 1979; Retz, 1982). Similarly, KA-induced morphologic
disturbances are observed in tissue culture of striatal cells only in the
presence of glutamate containing cortical neurons (Whetsell, 1979). It is of
particular relevance to HD that neonatal animals are relatively resistant to
the neurotoxic effects of KA. There appears to be a maturational change in
the striatal sensitivity to KA which parallels the development of striatal
glutamatergic innervation (Campochiaro, 1978). Because the animal paradigm of
KA neurotoxicity is not based primarily on genetic predisposition, it is an
imperfect model for HD. However, the KA-induced striatal preparation has
generated the reasonable supposition that the pathogenesis of HD is related to
a glutamate dependent neurotoxic process (Divac, 1977; Coyle, 1978; Olney
1978a; Sanberg, 1981).

Schwarcz and his coworkers have recently demonstrated that quinolinic acid, an
endogenous tryptophan metabolite, produces morphologic, chemical and
behavioral alterations similar to those induced by exogenous toxins such as KA
and ibotenic acid (Schwarcz, 1982 and this symposium). Moreover, the striatal
toxicity of quinolinic acid is glutamate dependent (Whetsell, this symposium).

These studies will undoubtedly prompt an active search in HD patients for endogenous substances which exert glutamate-dependent excitotoxic effects.

There is sparse information regarding glutamatergic functions in HD patients. In the HD postmortem brain, Perry found glutamate concentrations to be reduced in the striatum but normal in frontal cortex (Perry, 1982a). Several investigators have found variably normal, increased or diminished concentrations of glutamate in the cerebrospinal fluid (CSF) of HD patients (Kim, 1981; Oepen 1982, Perry, 1982b). A preliminary screening effort has failed to detect substances in HD serum, urine and CSF which displace KA from rat brain receptors (Beutler, 1981). In platelet preparations, glutamate uptake is not significantly different in HD patients from that observed in control subjects (Mangano, 1981). However, Gray and his colleagues have reported a series of experiments demonstrating that cultured HD fibroblasts show a dose-dependent loss of viability in the presence of physiological concentrations of glutamate (Gray, 1980a, 1980b). This impressive finding suggests heightened glutamate sensitivity in extra-neural HD tissue. These controversial observations have recently been corroborated by independent investigators who found a similar vulnerability of HD fibroblasts to glutamate in association with reduced numbers of glutamate receptors and a tendency for increased glutamate binding afinity (Wong, 1982a). Although considerably more information is needed regarding glutamate functions in HD, these preliminary clinical findings suggest a pivotal role for glutamate in the pathogenesis of HD.

The so-called "glutamate hypothesis of HD" has been gradually formulated on the basis of the foregoing animal and human studies. Our lack of knowledge regarding the molecular basis of excitotoxicity and its bearing on HD limits a detailed description of the tenets of the glutamate hypothesis. In brief summary, it is assumed that a single gene, as yet unidentified, codes for a biochemical or structural defect which predisposes the HD carrier to the neurotoxic influences of glutamate. It is presumed that all cells harbor the HD gene but that neural tissue, and specifically striatal cells, posess a regional vulnerability to the effects of glutamate. It is further assumed that this neurotoxic influence is present at birth, but that certain maturational correlates account for the gradually developing neuropathologic changes, the eventual onset of illness and the inevitable clinical decline of HD patients.

At the level of the striatum, it is not known what mediates the susceptibility to glutamate or whether the degenerative process involves neurotransmitter functions, metabolic alterations or their combined influences. Based on the integral role of the corticostriatal glutamatergic pathway in the genesis of KA-induced striatal toxicity, a hypothetical model has been proposed (Figure 1).

In this perspective, glutamate-mediated toxicity in HD may arise from increased synthesis and release of glutamate, heightened sensitivity of glutamate or KA-like receptors, failure of normal glutamate uptake or a combination of these effects (Schwarcz, 1979). It is unclear whether these presumptions involve pre- or postsynaptic mechanisms or are possibly linked to neuronal-glial interactions. This latter possibility is intriguing because of the prominent gliosis attending the neuronal loss in HD and the important role of glia in the uptake of synaptically released glutamate (Nicklas, 1979; Krespan, 1982). Perhaps, the most attractive feature of the glutamate hypothesis is that its suppositions can be tested in the clinical setting as well as in the experimental animal.

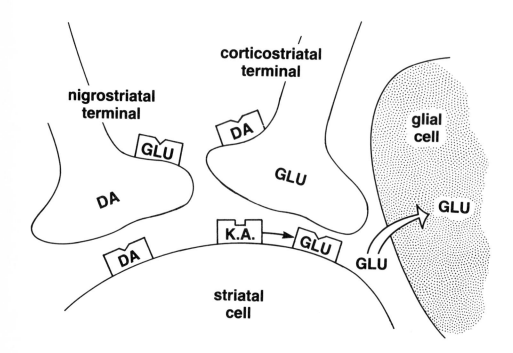

Fig. 1.   SCHEMATIC REPRESENTATION OF STRIATUM INCLUDING NIGROSTRIATAL
          AND CORTICOSTRIATAL SYNAPSES
          Glutamate uptake occurs at the corticostriatal terminal as
          well as that illustrated for the glial cell.   Kainate-like
          receptors are probably present on presynaptic
          corticostriatal terminals as well as those illustrated on
          the postsynaptic striatal cell.
          Key: DA = dopamine, GLU = glutamate, K.A. = kainate-like.
          Diagram modified after Schwarcz et al (1979).

FEASIBILITY OF ANTI-NEUROTOXIC DRUG TRIALS

The formulation and refinement of a standardized scoring system (Shoulson,
1979b, 1981, 1982a) to evaluate the functional capacities of patients has
provided an opportunity to analyze longitudinally the clinical and
radiographic correlates of HD.   Several relevant profiles have emerged from
cross-sectional and prospective analyses which are applicable to long-term
pharmacologic trials.   Our therapeutic objectives are aimed at a chronic
reduction of striatal glutamate availability in an effort to halt or lessen
the pathologic and clinical progression of HD.   The clinical data from our
preliminary studies have formed the basis for our therapeutic design.
In HD, the decline in functional capacity is relatively steady and unremitting
without remissions or exacerbations.   Although the rate of decline varies and
cannot be accurately predicted in a given patient, some general conclusions
have been made from our observations of large patient cohort   (Table 1).

TABLE 1

STAGES OF FUNCTIONAL DECLINE IN HD

Stage	Total Functional Capacity Score (units)	Characteristic Disability	Range of Duration (years)
Presymptomatic	13	none	3-70
I	11-13	gainful skills	2-4
II	7-10	domestic skills	2-4
III	3-6	self-care skills	2-4
IV	1-2	invalid	3-7
V	0	terminal	3-7

HD patients lose functional capacity at an average rate of 1.5-2.0 units per year, and spend an average of 3 years in each of the first three stages of illness (I, II, III) and 4.5 years in each of the last two stages (IV, V). Owing largely to earlier diagnosis and improved terminal care, the average length of illness for our HD patients has increased from 15 to 18 years. But, the rate of decline has remained constant and seems unaffected by the administration of antichoreic or antidepressant therapies (Shoulson, 1981). Although patients with clinical onset before the age of 35 seem to decline at a slightly faster rate than those with later onset (Shoulson, 1982a), this difference is minor in the context of the generally unyielding biologic progression of HD. The inevitable and unremitting progression of HD lends itself paradoxically to therapeutic strategies aimed at preventing or slowing clinical decline.

Although chorea is the predominant movement disorder observed in adult-onset HD patients, a changing motoric pattern is observed during the course of illness. As disease advances, the predominance of chorea lessens while dystonic and parkinsonian features intensify (Shoulson, 1982a). Progressive impairment in ocular motility also parallels the evolving motoric profile. Examination of drug-free HD populations suggests that these patterns reflect underlying neuropathologic changes and are not appreciably influenced by neuroleptic drugs. These motoric findings provide additional correlates of clinical decline. In general, drug therapies which effectively lessen clinical decline should also slow the appearance of parkinsonism, dystonia and ocular abnormalities.

Comparison of HD patients in stages I and II to those in stage III also points to an evolving pattern of intellectual decline which parallels advancing illness (Fisher, 1982). Memory impairment, as measured by the Selective Reminding Test (Buschke, 1973), is detectable in the early stages of HD (I and II) and worsens progressively (stage III). The capacity to change cognitive sets, an elaborative operation measured most sensitively by the Stroop Test (Stroop, 1935), likewise becomes progressively impaired with advancing disability. On the other hand, factual and verbal operations are relatively resistant to progressing disease. This profile of cognitive decline provides additional clinical landmarks by which the effects of protective therapies can be more meaningfully gauged.

We have also examined radiographic correlates of clinical decline. We systematically measured the extent of caudate atrophy on the computed tomography (CT) scans of 42 HD patients who were in various stages of illness (Shoulson, 1982b). The total functional capacity of our HD patients correlated significantly with the CT indices of caudate atrophy. That is, the clinical progression of HD is attended by progressive caudate atrophy. In 8 patients followed prospectively with serial CT scans, measurable increases in caudate atrophy could be detected within intervals ranging from 7 to 24 months. Although CT measurements of caudate atrophy in HD are neither sufficiently sensitive for presymptomatic detection nor sufficiently specific for distinguishing HD from allied disorders, these longitudinal indices provide an independent morphologic measure of progressing disease. Therapies which are genuinely protective in slowing clinical decline should also halt or retard progession of caudate atrophy.

We presently lack reliable neurochemical correlates of clinical decline in HD. Studies analyzing CSF samples from HD patients have generally not devoted adequate attention to stage of illness, clinical/radiographic correlates or concurrent drug therapies. Notwithstanding these concerns, neurochemical studies in HD patients are seriously hampered by the lack of reliable in vivo measures of glutamatergic function. Such measurements would certainly provide more meaningful and objective indices for use in anti-neurotoxic protective strategies. However, this obstacle should not unduly prevent the undertaking of sensible clinical trials directed towards the presumed pathogenesis of HD.

BACLOFEN AS PROTECTIVE THERAPY

The basic asumption of the "glutamate hypothesis of HD" is that glutamate vulnerability is an integral factor leading to progressive neuronal degeneration. It is unclear to what extent the neurotransmitter and metabolic functions of glutamate may contribute to this susceptibility and whether the presumed neurotoxic effects of glutamate are mediated directly or via an endogenous glutamate-dependent toxin. Regardless, pharmacologic attenuation of glutamatergic neurotransmitter function may be reasonably assumed to lead to a slowing of neuronal degeneration and clinical decline.

Glutamate availability at the postsynaptic striatal receptor (Figure 1) can be lessened by: (1) reducing brain synthesis of glutamate, (2) enhancing glutamate uptake, (3) antagonizing the postsynaptic receptor effects of glutamate or (4) retarding presynaptic release of glutamate. As indicated, these sites of neurotransmitter activity have not been examined directly in HD patients. However, there are several theoretical and practical problems in considering these alternatives for clinical study. Inhibiting synthesis of glutamate would not be feasible because of the key role of glutamate in metabolic processes and because of the multiple enzyme systems (glutaminase, aspartate aminotransferase, glutamate dehydrogenase, glutamate decarboxylase and glutamine synthetase) capable of synthesizing glutamate (Fonnum, 1981). To date, there are no drugs which specifically enhance glutamate uptake into neurons or glia. Although a variety of agents have been proposed as specific antagonists of glutamate receptors (McGeer, 1978b; Liebman, 1980; McLennan 1981; Croucher, 1982), the available drugs seem too toxic or expensive for human administration. The final alternative of reducing presynaptic glutamate release seems to be the most plausible approach for lessening the availability of striatal glutamate. This tactic is supported by the evidence that presynaptic glutamate release mechanisms are preserved after KA-induced degeneration of the postsynaptic striatum (Roberts, 1975, Olney, 1978b). By analogy, presynaptic glutamate release from corticostriatal terminals in HD patients is presumably intact. Recent findings in the postmortem HD brain suggest that corticostriatal glutamatergic neurons have partly deteriorated (Wong, 1982b), but this observation may reflect end-stage disease rather than active neuronal degeneration.

Using slices of guinea pig cerebral cortex, Potashner (1978, 1979, 1980) demonstrated that baclofen (beta-(p-chlorophenyl)-gamma aminobutyric acid) selectively inhibited endogenous glutamate and aspartate release. The preferential blocking effect of baclofen on excitatory amino acids occurred with relatively low doses of baclofen, 4 micromoles (0.85 mg/L). This dosage is pharmacologically relevant, approximating the average peak plasma concentration attained by orally administered, subsedative doses of baclofen (60-90 mg/day) in clinical trials (Knutsson, 1974). This preferential action of baclofen in blocking release of excitatory amino acids has been confirmed under a variety of experimental conditions using dosages of baclofen as low as 1 micromole (Mitchell, 1980; Johnston, 1980; Olpe, 1982; Cordingley 1982). Provided this pharmacologic action occurs in the human striatum, baclofen acting as a retardant of presynaptic glutamate release might slow striatal degeneration and thereby serve as a protective agent in HD.

Baclofen produces a variety of effects in the KA-lesioned animal. Acute pretreatment with baclofen retards KA-induced stereotypy, hypersalivation and chronic seizures (Borison, 1979; Bernard, 1980). But, this protective effect may be of a generalized nature because McGeer et al (1980) have found that acute pretreatment with baclofen results in relatively weak attenuation of KA-induced reductions in striatal choline acetyltransferase and glutamic acid decarboxylase. It is possible that chronic baclofen pretreatment of the KA-lesioned animal might produce more potent striatal protection. The relatively weak protective effects of baclofen in the KA preparation do not mitigate the rationale for baclofen therapy in HD where neuropathological changes develop more insidiously than in the KA-lesioned animal.

From a practical standpoint, the proven safety of baclofen for treatment of spasticity is a compelling reason for its selection as a protective therapy in HD. Since baclofen administration is associated with few if any adverse effects, it is a drug which lends itself to double-blind analysis. Because of the strong anticipatory influence in drug trials of HD patients, a double-blind design is required to detect genuine therapeutic effects. A systematic evaluation is also necessary because the protective influence of baclofen, if any, might be modest and otherwise escape clinical detection.

We have already embarked on a double-blind, placebo controlled study of long-term baclofen therapy in patients who are in stages I and II of HD. We plan to enter a total of 60 HD patients who will be ramdomly allocated to either chronic baclofen (60-90 mg/day) or placebo treatments. The ramdomization is blocked according to stage of illness (I or II) and age at onset of symptoms (less than or greater than 35 years old) in an effort to minimize the influence of these factors on the course of disease. Patients

are not permitted symptomatic drug therapies during this long-term study so as
to eliminate extraneous drug effects. This restriction is further justified
because current symptomatic therapies do not favorably influence the course of
HD and because neuroleptic dopamine blocking agents may theoretically increase
presynaptic glutamate release by blocking presynaptic dopamine receptors on
the corticostriatal terminal (Figure 1).

As indices of clinical decline, we are employing clinical measures of motoric
and cognitive performance and radiographic measures of caudate atrophy as well
as the evaluation of functional capacity. Assuming an average functional
decline of 1.5 - 2.0 units per year, we have calculated the anticipated power
of our analysis. A total sample of 60 patients, followed prospectively for
two years, will provide 85% probability of detecting a major therapeutic
effect from baclofen and a 68% liklihood of detecting a minor benefit.

Even if baclofen merely slows the rate of clinical decline by 10%, this would
have major practical importance for HD patients and their families. Baclofen
might then be used for comparison with other experimental drugs which are
found to exert more powerful and selective effects in reducing glutamatergic
neurotransmission. The impact of a major protective effect from baclofen
would have broader implications. A reliable test for the pre-symptomatic
detection of HD gene carriers, which is not presently available, would take on
added importance if therapy were available to prevent or postpone the
development of symptoms in presymptomatic heterozygotes.

To date, we have entered 10 HD patients into a pilot study and 7 additional
patients into a more formal evaluation of the protective effects of baclofen.
Although the double-blind design of our trial precludes premature analysis of
therapeutic results, we have not encountered major problems in the conduct of
our study. We expect to examine our preliminary findings within two years.
We are also analyzing the CSF of our HD patients at regular intervals in order
to determine concentrations of baclofen, neurotransmitters and amino acids.
These analyses will help monitor dosage and compliance and might demonstrate
neurochemical correlates of clinical decline.

It can be argued that this clinical undertaking is premature in view of the
lingering uncertainties regarding glutamate neurotransmission, excitotoxic
influences and selectivity of pharmacologic agents. Certainly, these issues
require our investigative attention. Other neurotoxic hypotheses (Brennan,
1981) also warrant exploration. At the very least, baclofen as protective
therapy in HD will provide an opportunity to explore a new strategy in
experimental therapeutics and to extend the limits of replacement therapy. In
the final analysis, the value of anti-neurotoxic strategies in HD will depend
on therapeutic outcomes and the investigative leads generated for treatment of
similar neurodegenerative diseases.

ACKNOWLEDGEMENT

These studies are supported by grants from the U.S. Public Health Service
(RO1-NS17978), the University of Rochester Clinical Research Center (RR-00044,
Division of Research Facilities and Resources, NIH) and the Hereditary Disease
Foundation (Beverly Hills, California). Dr. Shoulson is supported by NINCDS
Teacher-Investigator Development Award (KO7-NS00397). Recognition is due to
Mrs. Ruth Nobel who assisted in the preparation of this manuscript.

REFERENCES

Bernard, P.S., R. Sobiski and K. Dawson (1980). Brain Res. Bull., 5, 519-523.

Beutler, B.A., A. Noronha, M. Poon and B. Arnason (1981). J. Neurol. Sci., 51, 355-360.

Biziere, K. and J.T. Coyle (1979). J. Neurosci. Res., 4, 383-398.

Borison, R.L. and B. J. Diamond (1979). Ann. Neurol., 6, 149.

Brennan, M.J., J. van der Westhuyzen, S. Kramer and J. Metz (1981). Med. Hypotheses, 7, 919-929.

Buschke, H. (1973). J. Verbal Learning & Verbal Behavior, 12, 543-550.

Campochiaro, R. and J.T. Coyle (1978). Proc. Natl. Acad. Sci. (USA), 75, 2025-2029.

Cordingley, G. and F. Weight (1982). Soc. for Neurosci. Abstr., 8, in press.

Coyle, J.T. and R. Schwarcz (1976). Nature, 263, 244-246.

Coyle, J.T., E.G. McGeer, P.L. McGeer and R. Schwarcz (1978). Kainic Acid as a Tool in Neurobiology, Raven Press, NY, 139-159.

Coyle, J.T., E.D. London, K. Biziere and R. Zaczek (1979). Adv. Neurol., 23, Raven Press, NY, 593-608.

Croucher, M.J., J.F. Collins and B.S. Meldrum (1982). Science, 216, 899-901.

Divac, I. (1977). Acta. Neurol. Scand., 56, 357-360.

Fisher, J.M., J.L. Kennedy, E.D. Caine and I. Shoulson (1982). Recent Advances in Dementia, Raven Press, NY, in press.

Fonnum, F. and D. Malthe-Sorenssen (1981). Glutamate: Transmitter in the Central Nervous System, John Wiley and Sons Ltd., Chichester, 205-222.

Gray, P.N., P.C. May, L. Mundy, J. Elkins (1980a). Biochem. Biophys. Res. Commun., 95, 707-714.

Gray, P.N. and P.C. May (1980b). Soc. for Neurosci. Abstr. 6, 405.

Johnston, G.A.R., M.H. Hailstone and C.G. Freeman (1980). J. Pharm. Pharmacol., 32, 230-231.

Kim, J.S., H.H. Kornhuber, B. Holzmuller, W. Schmidt-Burgk, T. Mergner, G. Krzepinski (1981). Arch. Psychiat. Nervenkr., 228, 7-10.

Knutsson, E., U. Lindblom and A. Martensson (1974). J. Neurol. Sci., 23 473-484.

Krammer, E.B. (1980). Brain Res., 196, 209-221.

Krespan, B., S. Berl and W.J. Nicklas (1982). J. Neurochem., 38, 509-518.

Kuhl, D., M. Phelps, C. Markham, J. Winter, J. Metter and W. Riege (1981).
J. Cerebral Blood Flow & Metab., 1, S459-S460.

Liebman, J.M., G. Pastor, P.S. Bernard and J.K. Saelens (1980). Life Sci.,
27, 1991-1998.

Mangano, R.M. and R. Schwarcz (1981). J. Neurochem., 37, 1072-1074.

McGeer, E.G. and P.L. McGeer (1976). Nature, 263, 517-519.

McGeer, E.G., P.L. McGeer and K. Singh (1978a). Brain Res., 139, 381-383.

McGeer, E.G. and P.L. McGeer (1978b). Neurochem. Res., 3, 501-517.

McGeer, E.G., A. Jakubovic and E.A. Singh (1980). Exp. Neurol., 69, 359-364.

McLennan, H. (1981). Glutamate as a Neurotransmitter, Raven Press, NY,
253-262.

Mitchell, R. (1980). Eur. J. Pharmacol., 67, 119-122.

Nicklas, W.J., R. Nunez, S. Berl and R. Duvoisin (1979). J. Neurochem., 33,
839-844.

Oepen, G., H. Cramer, R. Bernasconi and P. Martin (1982). Arch. Psychiatr.
Nervenkr., 231, 131-140.

Olney, J.W. and L.G. Sharpe (1969). Science, 166, 386-388.

Olney, J.W., O.L. Ho and V. Rhee (1971). Exp. Brain Res., 14, 61-76.

Olney, J.W. and T. de Gubareff (1978a). Nature, 271, 557-559.

Olney, J.W. (1978b). Kainic Acid As A Tool in Neurobiology, Raven Press, NY,
95-121.

Olpe, H.R., M. Baudry, L. Fagni and G. Lynch (1982). J. Neurosci., 2, 698-703.

Perry, T.L. (1982a). Neurosci. Lett., 28, 81-85.

Perry, T.L., S. Hansen, R.A. Wall and S.G. Gauthier (1982b). J. Neurochem., 38,
766-773.

Potashner, S.J. (1978). Can. J. Physiol. Pharmacol., 56, 150-154.

Potashner, S.J. (1979). J. Neurochem., 32, 103-109.

Potashner, S. J. (1980). Brain Res. Bull., 5, 513-518.

Retz, K.C. and J.T. Coyle (1982). J. Neurochem., 38, 196-203.

Roberts, P.J. and J.C. Watkins (1975). Brain Res., 85, 120-125.

Sanberg, P.R., J. Lehmann and H.C. Fibiger (1978). Brain Res., 149, 546-551.

Sanberg, P.R. and G.A. Johnston (1981). Med. J. of Australia, 2, 460-465.

Schwarcz, R., K. Fuxe, T. Hokfelt, K. Andersson and J.T. Coyle (1979). Dopaminergic Ergot Derivatives and Motor Function, Pergamon Press, Oxford, 115-126.

Schwarcz, R., C. Kohler, R.M. Mangano and A.N. Neophytides (1981). Glutamate as a Neurotransmitter, Raven Press, NY, 403-412.

Schwarcz, R., W. O. Whetsell and R.M. Mangano (1982). Science, in press.

Shoulson, I. and T. Chase (1975). Ann. Rev. Med., 26, 419-426.

Shoulson, I. (1979a). Advances in Neurology, 23, Raven Press, NY, 751-757.

Shoulson, I. and S. Fahn (1979b). Neurology, 29, 1-3.

Shoulson, I. (1981). Neurology 31, 1333-1335.

Shoulson, I. (1982a). Movement Disorders, Butterworth Scientific, London, 277-290.

Shoulson, I., W. Plassche, and C. Odoroff (1982b). Neurology, 32, A143.

Stroop, J. (1935). J. Exp. Psychol., 18, 87-95.

Whetsell, W.O., M. Ecob-Johnston and W.J. Nicklas (1979). Adv. Neurol., 23, Raven Press, NY, 645-654.

Wong, P.T., V.K. Singh and E.G. McGeer (1982a). Soc. for Neurosci. Abstr., 8, in press.

Wong, P.T., P.L. McGeer, M. Rossor and E.G. McGeer (1982b). Brain Res., 231, 466-471.

EXCITOTOXICITY IN AGING AND DEMENTIA

D. M. BOWEN, C. C. T. SMITH and A. N. DAVISON

*Department of Neurochemistry, Institute of Neurology, The National Hospital,
Queen Square, London, WC1N 3BG*

ABSTRACT

The extracellular concentration of glutamate in the neocortex of human brain may increase progressively with ageing. Glutamergic nerve terminals seem to be a major source of the amino acid. There is no evidence that the concentration of extracellular glutamate is increased in the neocortex in Alzheimer's disease. The few remaining neocortical cholinergic terminals in Alzheimer's disease may be more metabolically active than those from normal brain. This is likely to be an adaptive change, unrelated to glutamate toxicity. Increased acetylcholine may itself be neurotoxic.

KEYWORDS

Ageing; Alzheimer's disease; acetylcholine; glutamate; excitotoxicity.

INTRODUCTION

Central to the idea of the neurotoxic effects of glutamate and aspartate is that excessively high extracellular concentrations of the amino acids cause tissue damage by excessive excitation. It has been speculated (Olney, 1978; McGeer, *et al*, 1978) that such a phenomenon may trigger the neuronal degeneration seen in normal old age and in the frequently-occurring dementing disorder of Alzheimer's disease, as well as in rarer conditions (Huntington's chorea and some of the cerebellar degenerative disorders). The widespread distribution and high concentration of glutamate and aspartate in the brain masks assessment of the amino acid transmitter pool. Total tissue content, therefore, is a very poor index of extra-cellular concentration. Thus, the purposes of the present study were:

1. To attempt to obtain information on the extracellular concentrations of glutamate and aspartate in human brain under conditions simulating high and low neuronal activity.
2. To establish whether or not the measurements are altered with ageing or in patients with Alzheimer's disease.

This has been studied by determining the concentration of amino acids in incubation media from incubations of tissue prisms (a preparation of nerve endings in the presence of disintegrated cells; Sims, *et al*, 1981), in media containing either high or low K⁺-concentrations (Sims, *et al*, 1980). The tissue prisms have been prepared from the neocortex, which in Alzheimer's disease - and to a much lesser extent in the brains of normal aged individuals - characteristically shows intense senile plaque and neurofibrillary tangle formation. This brain region in Alzheimer's disease also has evidence of loss of neurones (Colon, 1973; Bowen, *et al*, 1979; Terry, *et al*, 1981), and of a prominent cholinergic deficit (Bartus, *et al*, 1982; Marchbanks, 1982) due to probable loss of cholinergic nerve terminals (Bowen, *et al*, 1982a; Sims, *et al*, 1980, 1981, 1982).

OUTLINE OF TECHNIQUES USED

Samples of normal-appearing human neocortex removed to gain access to diseased tissue, were obtained from 21 patients undergoing surgery for either deep-seated tumours or aneurysms (table 1).

Table 1. Normal-appearing samples of human neocortex
obtained at surgery

	Number of specimens
Brain lobe	
temporal	12
frontal	6[*]
occipital	2
parietal	1
Surgery for:[**]	
glioma	9
craniopharyngioma	4
meningioma	3
aneurysm	2
suprasella tumour	1
pituitary tumour	1
dyserginoma	1

* values for amino acid release were not significantly different from data for the temporal lobe.
** comparison of release for samples separated into 3 major groups according to associated tumour type (glioma, craniopharyngioma and the other tumours) did not reveal significant differences (one-way analysis of variance), except for aspartate in 55 mM K^+ medium.

Neocortex was also obtained at diagnostic craniotomy from seven patients with presenile dementia and a clinical diagnosis of Alzheimer's disease. Histology revealed the pathological hallmarks of the disease (senile plaques and neurofibrillary tangles). Biochemistry showed that the synthesis of acetylcholine was markedly reduced (table 5).

Immediately on removal the tissue was placed in an oxygenated physiological Krebs medium containing 2.5 mM glucose and 5 mM K^+ (Sims, *et al*, 1981), and transferred to the cold-room. Grey matter was mechanically chopped and pre-incubated for 45 min. to yield tissue prism suspensions (Sims, *et al*, 1981). Rat neocortex from the entire cerebrum was from 9-month-old Porton-Wistar rats, and processed as for human tissue. Human brains excised 30-45 min. after death, were obtained from two patients (67 and 68 years old), and processed to yield tissue prism suspensions as previously described (Bowen, *et al*, 1982b).

Tissue prism suspensions were oxygenated and incubated at 37^0C. After 20 min., Krebs medium (unstimulated prisms) or Krebs medium containing KCl sufficient to raise the K^+-concentration from 5 mM to 55 mM (K^+-stimulated prisms) was added. Incubation was continued for a further 10 min., whereupon the prisms were sedimented; the resulting medium fractions were stored at -70^0C. Tissue pellets were extracted with 10% trichloroacetic acid and protein was determined. An internal standard of nor-leucine was added to thawed medium fractions and they were desalted using a methanolic extraction procedure (Dodd, *et al*, 1981a). Thirteen amino acids were determined fluorometrically as the ortho-phthalaldehyde derivatives, using a Rank-Hilger Chromaspek auto-analyzer (Norris, *et al*, 1980). The recovery of the amino acids was found to be essentially independent of the types of tissue or medium used, but varied according to the amino acid. All results are expressed as data adjusted for recovery. Data were analysed, except where stated otherwise, by Students t-test for unpaired observations. All values are expressed as mean ± S.D.

RELEASE OF ENDOGENOUS AMINO ACIDS FROM HUMAN CONTROL SAMPLES

Fig. 1 shows that on K^+-stimulation, tissue prisms prepared from human temporal neocortex respond with an enhanced and preferential efflux of only three amino acids: GABA, aspartate and glutamate.

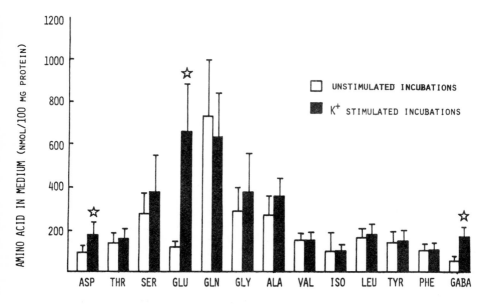

Fig. 1.   Amino acid efflux from tissue prisms of human neocortex. Incubation was carried out in Krebs medium and stimulation achieved by raising K^+-concentration from 5 mM (control incubations) to 55 mM (K^+-stimulated incubations). Values for 12 samples from temporal lobes (table 1). * significantly different from the value for control incubations, with p < 0.001.

The latter are thought to function as neurotransmitters in animal brain, and may be neurotoxic in high concentrations. Release of glutamate was found to be greatly elevated (approximately 400% over the unstimulated value), whereas the release of aspartate was increased only some 100%. A similar pattern of release was found to occur with prisms prepared from each of the other lobes (table 1) of the brain.

Raising the ionic strength of the medium by increasing the Na^+-concentration (from 141 mM to 191 mM) had no effect on the release of any amino acid, indicating that the changes observed on K^+-stimulation were not due to an alteration in osmotic pressure. The only effect on amino acid release of omitting Ca^{2+} from incubation medium containing high K^+ and human samples, was an 84% decrease in released glutamate (table 2).

Table 2. Ca^{2+}-dependance of amino acid release from human neocortical tissue prisms prepared from control neurosurgical samples

| | Amino acid content of medium (nmol/100mg protein) | | | |
| | Krebs medium | | Ca^{2+}-free medium | |
	unstimulated prisms	K^+-stimulated prisms	unstimulated prisms	K^+-stimulated prisms
Glutamate	123 ± 33	616 ± 112	146 ± 45	224 ± 27*
Aspartate	68 ± 19	180 ± 45	105 ± 17	190 ± 10
Phenylalanine	95 ± 11	104 ± 14	98 ± 16	112 ± 12
Threonine	164 ± 31	220 ± 41	198 ± 66	242 ± 56

Tissue prisms for the medium without Ca^{2+} were prepared and preincubated as described in the text, except following preincubation, they were washed three times in Ca^{2+}-free Krebs medium containing 0.5 mM ethyleneglycol-bis-(β-aminoethyl ether) N,N'-tetra-acetic acid (EGTA). Prisms for medium containing Ca^{2+} were treated similarly, substituting Krebs medium for Ca^{2+}-free-EGTA medium. Incubations were then performed in the standard way. Results expressed as mean $\pm$ S.D. for three preparations.
* identifies the only significant difference (p < 0.01) from K^+-stimulated prisms incubated in Krebs medium. The other nine amino acids (fig. 1) were also determined. The release of none of these was Ca^{2+}-dependant.

This suggests that under conditions simulating high neuronal activity, glutamate is released from nerve terminals of human brain. By contrast, release of both aspartate and glutamate from rat samples were reduced by some 70% in the Ca^{2+}-free medium. Since the same conditions were unsuccessful in demonstrating the Ca^{2+}-dependance of aspartate release from human samples, it is possible that this amino acid is not derived from nerve terminals of human brain. However, veratrine-induced efflux of aspartate from human samples was inhibited (Dodd, et al, 1981b) by an agent (tetrodotoxin), known to block sodium channels in neuronal membranes, which provides some evidence that aspartate is released from terminals of human brain.

A comparison of results for control neurosurgical samples separated into three major groups according to associated tumour type, did not reveal significant differences for the measurements made on the release of glutamate (table 1). Moreover, prisms prepared from the exceptionally fresh autopsy material of frontal and temporal neocortex, also responded to K^+-stimulation with a greatly enhanced efflux of glutamate (table 3).

Table 3.   Release (nmol/100mg protein) from tissue prisms
prepared from rapid human autopsy samples of neocortex

	unstimulated prisms	K$^+$-stimulated prisms
Glutamate	160 $\pm$ 43	493 $\pm$ 84*
Aspartate	223 $\pm$ 109	330 $\pm$ 155
Phenylalanine	143 $\pm$ 13	149 $\pm$ 17
Threonine	215 $\pm$ 47	248 $\pm$ 10

Samples (2 from frontal lobe and 1 from temporal lobe) were
obtained within 45 min. of death.
* $p < 0.01$ from unstimulated value.

These observations are consistent with the overall results for glutamate release
from neurosurgical samples. However, the release of aspartate from K$^+$-stimulated
prisms depended upon the associated tumour type (table 1), suggesting that the release of aspartate from control neurosurgical samples may not be a good indicator
of the value for normal tissue.

COMPARISON OF AMINO ACID RELEASE FROM RAT AND HUMAN SAMPLES

The amino acid concentrations for incubations with rat and human prisms (table 4)
showed greater K$^+$-stimulated release of aspartate from rodent brain.

Table 4. Release (nmol/100mg protein) from tissue prisms
prepared from neocortex of human control neurosurgical samples and rat brain

	unstimulated prisms		K$^+$-stimulated prisms	
	rat	human	rat	human
Glutamate	128 $\pm$ 42	125 $\pm$ 40	960 $\pm$ 375	718 $\pm$ 269*
Aspartate	82 $\pm$ 40	98 $\pm$ 54	337 $\pm$ 161	191 $\pm$ 67*
Glutamine	242 $\pm$ 102	665 $\pm$ 255*	258 $\pm$ 101	616 $\pm$ 197*
Phenylalanine	88 $\pm$ 21	102 $\pm$ 26	82 $\pm$ 20	105 $\pm$ 28
Threonine	160 $\pm$ 40	130 $\pm$ 43	165 $\pm$ 32	151 $\pm$ 48

$n = 21$-22.
* p at least < 0.01 from corresponding value for rat.

However, the release of glutamate from the rat samples was only slightly higher.
Hence, in view of this and the much lower packing densities of neurones in human
neocortex (Tower and Elliott, 1952), it is suggested that the amount of extracellular glutamate per nerve cell is particularly high in human brain. It is also
of interest that the concentration in the medium of glutamine, the precursor of
glutamate, was significantly higher in the incubations with human samples (table 4).

EFFECT OF AGE ON AMINO ACID RELEASE FROM HUMAN SAMPLES

A significant and positive linear correlation with ageing occurred for the release of glutamate from K⁺-stimulated prisms prepared from human samples (fig. 2).

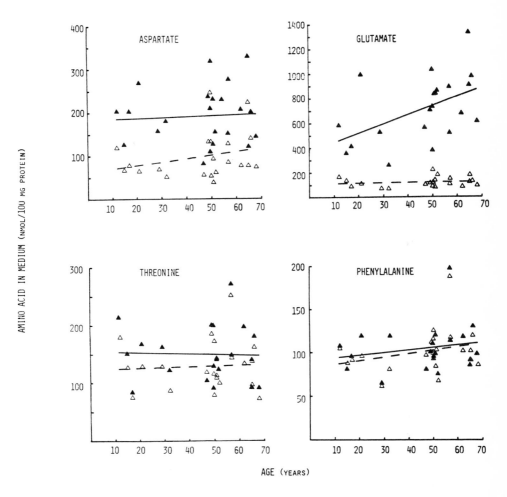

Fig. 2. Relationship between age and amino acid release. The data is for 21 neurosurgical samples (table 1). Continuous and broken lines identify plots of best fit (linear regression analysis) for incubations with 5 mM K⁺ and 55 mM K⁺ respectively. Values for individual preparations of prisms are identified by Δ (5 mM K⁺) and ▲ (55 mM K⁺). The correlation with ageing for the K⁺-stimulated release of glutamate was significant ($r = 0.49$, $p < 0.05$).

The increase was 91% for the age-range studied. No age-change was detected for unstimulated prisms. The release of no other amino acid, from either K⁺-stimulated or unstimulated prisms, significantly increased with age.

Although the atrophy of normal human brain which occurs with ageing, has been attributed to neuronal fall-out (Hanley, 1974), there was no evidence from our study that the evoked release from human samples of either glutamate or aspartate declined with ageing. On the contrary, the release of glutamate progressively increased, which may be explained by several mechanisms. Increased conversion of glutamine to glutamate could result in an increase in the releasable pool of the transmitter. As ^{3}H-GABA uptake by synaptosomes from human neocortex decreases with ageing (Goodhardt, 1980), glutamate re-uptake may be similarly affected, causing an apparent increase in the release of this amino acid. Alternatively, the density of glutamergic nerve endings may be increased due to age-related loss of other structures from the neocortex, or to neuronal plasticity (Buell and Coleman, 1979). Since releasable glutamate seems to be in excess in the ageing human brain (fig.2) the substance may have an "excitotoxic" action, as suggested by Olney (1978).

AMINO ACID RELEASE FROM ALZHEIMER SAMPLES

On K^+-stimulation, tissue prisms of temporal neocortex obtained at diagnostic craniotomy from Alzheimer patients, responded in a similar way to controls, with an enhanced and preferential efflux of only three of the 13 amino acids measured. These were the putative transmitters – aspartate, glutamate and GABA. The release of glutamate by controls (unlike aspartate) appears to be a good indicator of the normal value. The absolute amount of glutamate released by Alzheimer samples was not significantly altered from the age-matched control value, for either unstimulated or K^+-stimulated prisms, although acetylcholine synthesis was greatly reduced (table 5).

Table 5. Amino acid release (nmol/100mg protein) and acetylcholine synthesis (D.P.M./mg protein/min) by Alzheimer and control neocortical tissue prisms from age-matched patients sampled at surgery

	Alzheimer samples (n = 7)	Control samples (n = 5-6)
Acetylcholine synthesis stimulated prisms	3.21 ± 0.66*	6.33 ± 1.23
Glutamate release unstimulated prisms	152 ± 32	129 ± 36
stimulated prisms	987 ± 255	702 ± 233
Aspartate release unstimulated prisms	126 ± 35	95 ± 43
stimulated prisms	216 ± 55	185 ± 55
Phenylalanine release unstimulated prisms	116 ± 32	113 ± 44
stimulated prisms	111 ± 29	119 ± 46
Threonine release unstimulated prisms	173 ± 26	131 ± 68
stimulated prisms	187 ± 41	150 ± 68

All samples obtained from temporal lobe at neurosurgery. Mean ($\pm$ S.D.) age of the Alzheimer group was 60 ± 5 years.
* identifies the only significant difference (p < 0.01) between values for Alzheimer and control samples. Synthesis by unstimulated prisms is also reduced (Sims, *et al*, 1982).

Thus, this data fails to support the hypothesis that glutamate toxicity is involved in the pathogenesis of Alzheimer's disease. It may be possible to use

rapid autopsy brain samples (Bowen, *et al*, 1982b) to investigate the extracellular
concentrations of neurotoxic amino acids in the nucleus basalis of Meynert - a region showing cell loss and believed to be responsible for a major diffuse cholinergic projection to the neocortex (Rossor, 1981; Whitehouse, *et al*, 1982).

EXCITOTOXICITY DUE TO EXCESSIVE ACETYLCHOLINE?

Recent results obtained with Alzheimer samples indicate that the loss from the
neocortex of choline acetyltransferase activity is greater than that of choline
uptake and acetylcholine synthesis (table 6). These phenomena may conceivably reflect an enhanced metabolism and firing rate by the few remaining cholinergic
terminals. The effect may not be confined to cholinergic terminals, because the
increment in overall glucose oxidation is large (table 6). Similar phenomena
have been reported in rats lesioned electrolytically in the basal forebrain
(table 6), and a compensatory increase of activity probably also occurs in surviving dopamine neurones in Parkinson's disease (Curzon, 1976).

Table 6. Increased metabolic and cholinergic firing by nerve terminals
in neocortex of Alzheimer patients and lesioned rats?

	% change from control neocortex			
	choline acetyltransferase activity	choline uptake	acetyl-choline synthesis	overall glucose oxidation
Alzheimer's disease	- 57 *	- 43 *	- 41 *	+ 39 **
Electrolytic lesion in basal forebrain of rat †				
frontal	- 41	- 35	n.d.	n.d.
parietal	- 38	- 8	n.d.	n.d.

```
*    Sims, et al, 1982
**   Sims, et al, 1981
†    Pedata, et al, 1982 (rats 20 days after surgery)
```

Thus, it is likely that the increased cholinergic activity is an adaptive change,
unrelated to glutamate toxicity. Acetylcholine esterase activity is reduced in
Alzheimer brain (Davies and Maloney, 1976). Hence, acetylcholine may accumulate at
the remaining intact cholinergic junctions, possibly causing harmful (Harris, *et
al*, 1982) over-stimulation of receptors.

ACKNOWLEDGEMENTS

We thank Dr. R. Balázs for providing the amino acid analyzer, and Mr. D. J. Atkinson and Mr. A. Hunt for assistance in its use. The help and co-operation is gratefully acknowledged of the large number of people involved in the collection and
classification of human samples. The work was supported by the Medical Research
Council, Brain Research Trust and the Miriam Marks Trust.

REFERENCES

Bartus, R.T., R.L. Dean, B. Beer and A.S. Lippa (1982). *Science, 217*, 408-417.
Bowen, D.M., P. White, J.A. Spillane, M.J. Goodhardt, G. Curzon, P. Iwangoff,
   W. Meier-Ruge and A.N. Davison (1979). *Lancet, i*, 11-14.
Bowen, D.M., J.S. Benton, J.A. Spillane, C.C.T. Smith and S.J. Allen (1982).
   J. Neurol. Sci. (in press).

Bowen, D.M., N.R. Sims, K.A.P. Lee and K.L. Marek (1982b). *Neurosci. Lett.* (in press).

Buell, S.J., and P.D. Coleman (1979). *Science 206*, 854-855.

Colon, E.J. (1973). *Acta Neuropath. (Berl.) 23*, 281-290.

Curzon, G. (1976). *Biochemistry and Neurological Disease*, ed. A.N. Davison, Blackwell Scientific Publications, Oxford; p.186.

Davies, P., and A.J.F. Maloney (1976). *Lancet ii*, 1403.

Dodd, P., J.A. Hardy, A.E. Oakley and A.J. Strong (1981a). *Brain Res. 224*, 419-425.

Dodd, P.R., J.A. Hardy, A.E. Oakley, J.A. Edwardson, E.K. Perry and J.P. Delaunoy (1981b). *Brain Res. 226*, 107-118.

Goodhardt, M.J. (1980). *Ph.D. Thesis – University of London*.

Hanley, T. (1974). *Age and Ageing, 3*, 133-151.

Harris, L.W., D.L. Stitcher and W.C. Hey (1982). *Life Sci., 30*, 1867-1873.

Marchbanks, R.M. (1982). *J. Neurochem., 39*, 9-15.

McGeer, P.L., E.G. McGeer and T. Hattori (1978). *Kainic Acid as a Tool in Neurobiology*, ed. E.G. McGeer, J.N. Olney and P.L. McGeer, Raven Press, New York; pp. 123-139.

Norris, P.J., C.C.T. Smith, J. DeBelleroche, H.F. Bradford, P.G. Mantle, A.J. Thomas and R.H.C. Penny (1980). *J. Neurochem., 34*, 33-42.

Olney, J.N. (1978). *Kainic Acid as a Tool in Neurobiology*, ed. E.G. McGeer, J.N. Olney and P.L. McGeer, Raven Press, New York; pp. 95-121.

Pedata, F., G. Lo Conte, S. Sorbi, I. Marconcini-Pepeu and G. Pepeu (1982). *Brain Res., 233*, 359-367.

Rossor, M.N. (1981). *Brit. Med. J., 283*, 1588-1590.

Sims, N.R., D.M. Bowen, C.C.T. Smith, R.H.A. Flack, A.N. Davison, J.S. Snowden, D. Neary and A.N. Davison (1980). *Lancet i*, 333-335.

Sims, N.R., D.M. Bowen and A.N. Davison (1981). *Biochem. J., 196*, 867-876.

Sims, N.R., D.M. Bowen, S.J. Allen, C.C.T. Smith, D. Neary, D.J. Thomas and A.N. Davison (1982). *J. Neurochem.* (in press).

Terry, R.D., A. Peck, R. DeTeresa, R. Schechter and D.S. Horoupion (1981). *Ann. Neurol., 10*, 184-192.

Tower, D.B., and K.A.C. Elliott (1952). *Am. J. Physiol., 168*, 747-759.

Whitehouse, P.J., D.L. Price, R.G. Struble, A.W. Clarke, J.T. Coyle and M.R. De-Long (1982). *Science, 215*, 1237-1239.

INDEX